MANUAL OF AMBULATORY PEDIATRICS

THIRD EDITION

Rose W. Boynton, RN, CPNP

Pediatric Nurse Practitioner
Dartmouth–Hitchcock Medical Center
Nashua Division
Nashua, New Hampshire

Elizabeth S. Dunn, BSN, RNC, PNP

Pediatric Nurse Practitioner

with Charles S. Gleason, MD, FAAP

Wareham, Massachusetts

Director of Health Services
Massachusetts Maritime Academy
Buzzards Bay, Massachusetts

Consultant
Wareham School System
Wareham, Massachusetts

Geraldine R. Stephens, BS, RN, MEd, PNP

Volunteer Child Advocate
Massachusetts Society for the Prevention of Cruelty to Children
Boston, Massachusetts

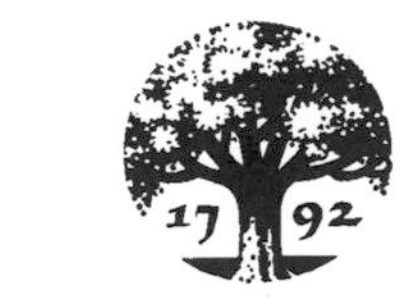

J. B. Lippincott Company
Philadelphia

Sponsoring Editor: Jennifer E. Brogan
Indexer: Maria Coughlin
Cover Designer: Tom Jackson
Production Manager: Janet Greenwood
Production Editor: Mary Kinsella
Production: Berliner, Inc.
Printer/Binder: R. R. Donnelley & Sons, Crawfordsville
Cover Printer: New England Book Components

"Children Learn What They Live," reprinted courtesy of the author.

3rd Edition

Library of Congress Cataloging-in-Publication Data

Boyton, Rose W.
Manual of ambulatory pediatrics / Rose W. Boyton, Elizabeth S. Dunn, Geraldine R. Stephens.—3rd ed.
p. cm.
Includes bibliographical references and index.
ISBN 0-397-55062-6
1. Pediatrics—Handbooks, manuals, etc. 2. Ambulatory medical care for children—Handbooks, manuals, etc. 3. Pediatric nursing—Handbooks, manuals, etc. I. Dunn, Elizabeth S. II. Stephens, Geraldine R. III. Title.
[DNLM: 1. Pediatric Nursing—handbooks. 2. Pediatrics—handbooks. WS 39 B792m 1994]
RJ48.B69 1994
618.92—dc20
DNLM/DLC
for Library of Congress 93-39333
CIP

6 5

ISBN 0-397-55062-6

Any procedure or practice described in this book should be applied by the health care practitioner under appropriate supervision in accordance with professional standards of care used with regard to the unique circumstances that apply in each practice situation. Care has been taken to confirm the accuracy of information presented and to describe generally accepted practices. However, the authors, editors, and publisher cannot accept any responsibility for errors or omissions or for any consequences from application of the information in this book and make no warranty, express or implied, with respect to the contents of the book.

Every effort has been made to ensure drug selections and dosages are in accordance with current recommendations and practice. Because of ongoing research, changes in government regulations, and the constant flow of information on drug therapy, reactions, and interactions, the reader is cautioned to check the package insert for each drug for the indications, dosages, warnings, and precautions, particularly if the drug is new or infrequently used.

MANUAL OF AMBULATORY PEDIATRICS

For Glenn W., John, Cathy, Peter, Maya, and Nathan
R.W.B.

To my grandchildren with love—
Christopher and Caroline Dunn and Brendan and Elizabeth Arkins
E.S.D.

Dedicated to my family for their understanding and loving support.
Special thanks to Susan L. McCarthy for helping to prepare the manuscript.
G.R.S.

Children Learn What They Live

If a child lives with criticism
He learns to condemn.

If a child lives with hostility,
He learns to fight.

If a child lives with ridicule,
He learns to be shy.

If a child lives with shame,
He learns to feel guilty.

If a child lives with tolerance,
He learns to be patient.

If a child lives with encouragement,
He learns confidence.

If a child lives with praise,
He learns to appreciate.

If a child lives with fairness,
He learns justice.

If a child lives with security,
He learns to have faith.

If a child lives with approval,
He learns to like himself.

If a child lives with acceptance and friendship,
He learns to find love in the world.

Dorothy Law Nolte

PREFACE

The original intent of the *Manual of Ambulatory Pediatrics* was to provide a concise reference book, in outline style, for the health care providers in ambulatory pediatric settings. The first edition was written when we were faculty members at the Northeastern University Nurse Practitioner in Boston and identified a need for a book of this type—not an in-depth reference book, but rather a handbook for pediatric health care providers. The third edition of this manual has been developed to continue to fill the need for which the first was written. The manual has been revised to reflect recent changes in pediatric well child care; protocols for the management of common pediatric problems have been updated and new protocols have been added; and the drug index has been expanded to include some of the new pediatric drugs. The organization of the book is unchanged.

Again, the manual has been written with each of the authors assuming responsibility for a specific section. Part I provides comprehensive guidelines for well child visits from birth through adolescence, which enable the health professional to assist the parent in providing optimal care for the child. A number of child-rearing issues of major concern to parents are included in this section.

Part II of the manual comprises protocols for the management of most common pediatric health problems. This section has been developed according to the SOAP format (Subjective data, Objective data, Assessment, and Plan), which was widely accepted in the first two editions. Each protocol has been researched in current literature from multidisciplinary sources and presents pertinent background information, such as communicability, incubation period, etiology, and incidence; it contains in-depth education along with indications for follow-up and referral.

A concise review of drugs commonly used in pediatric practice is included in Part III. The indications and dosages of all the drugs in this book are recommended in the medical literature and conform to the practices of the general medical community. Because standards for usage change, it is advisable to check package inserts for revised recommendations, particularly concerning new drugs. The drug index includes dosages, side effects, drug interactions, and directions for administration with specific education for the parent.

The authors wish to acknowledge the many people who have contributed to the preparation of the manuscript for the third edition. For the mechanics of Part II, special thanks to Susan and Peter Coker for the use of the computer that enabled the computer illiterate author of Part II to learn a new skill in manuscript preparation; to Dina and Michael Dunn, who provided expert tutelage—hours of on-site instruction and innumerable long-distance telephone consultations—on the intricacies of the formidable computer; to Cate and Dan Arkins, who were always on call for computer questions and consultations; to Sue and Tom Dunn who have used the manual—both as parents and Sue as a nurse and Tom as a resident and intern—and given input into its development; and to Brian Dunn (my very first "guinea pig" as a nurse practitioner) who put my office together. Thank you all for your infinite patience and wisdom.

Charles S. Gleason, M.D., F.A.A.P., has spent many hours as a consultant for Part II, reviewing protocols and answering questions. In addition, his pediatric practice in Wareham, MA has served as a preceptor site and an inspiration and model for practice for many nurse practitioners over the 26 years that we have been a "recognized entity."

Additionally, the author of Part II wishes to acknowledge Manuel L. Brun who has also served as a resource. A registered pharmacist at Jays Drug Store in Wareham, MA, he has responded to the author's many queries regarding pharmaceuticals.

As always, the preparation and production of a book requires assistance. The author of Part III (Drug Index) acknowledges the aid of Jane O'Brien in typing this part of the text. Many thanks for a job well done. And special thanks to Micheline Cignoli and my colleagues in the pediatric department at the Hitchcock Medical Center in Nashua, New Hamshire, for providing a site for preceptorship and teaching of student nurse practitioners and for the positive working environment for other pediatric nurse practitioners.

CONTENTS

Part I: Well Child Care

Geraldine R. Stephens

Part II: Management of Common Pediatric Problems

Elizabeth S. Dunn

Part III: Drug Index

Rose W. Boynton

I

Well Child Care

Geraldine R. Stephens

Part I of this manual develops criteria for individualizing the delivery of well child care. The emotional, intellectual, social, and physical components of development are integrated to show their inseparable interrelationship in the progress of each child toward maturity. Growth periods are divided into three cycles. The first cycle, from birth to approximately 3 years of age, is a period of rapid growth, laying the foundation for the future individual pattern of development. The second cycle, from 3 years through the early school years, is a period of slower physical development but rapidly expanding emotional, social, and intellectual growth. The third cycle, from preadolescence through adolescence, is again a period of rapid physical growth with the drive for maturity affecting social, emotional, and intellectual development.

In each cycle, guidelines have been developed identifying factors to be considered in all of the health supervision visits. Outlines for the initial history and general physical examination are presented to establish the baseline information from which to begin this individualization of a care plan. For each well child visit, specific factors are outlined for maximizing the taking of a broadbased history, and age-specific factors are given to be evaluated during the physical examination. From these, problem lists and appropriate care plans can be established. Also included are outlines of the developmental tasks for each age period. These outlines are to be used for guidance in helping parents reach a positive understanding of the individual path their child is taking toward developing his own capabilities in the maturation process.

INITIAL HISTORY

The initial history is obtained at the child's initial health care visit. Since taking the history is time consuming, allow an additional 30 minutes for that visit. When the appointment is scheduled, the secretary should advise the parent and/or child of the extended visit and request that they have immunization, birth, developmental, and illness records available.

I. Informant's relationship to patient

II. Family history

A. Parents
   1. Age.
   2. Health status.

B. Chronological listing of mother's pregnancies, including miscarriages. List name, age, sex, and health, and consanguinity of children.

C. Familial review of systems (include parents, siblings, grandparents, aunts, uncles).
   1. Skin. Atopic dermatitis, cancer, birthmarks.
   2. Head. Headaches (migraine, cluster).
   3. Eyes. Visual problems, strabismus.
   4. Ears. Hearing deficiencies, ear infections, malformation.
   5. Nose. Allergies, sinus problems.
   6. Mouth. Cleft palate, dental status.
   7. Throat. Frequent infections.
   8. Respiratory. Asthma, chronic bronchitis, tuberculosis.
   9. Cardiovascular. Cardiac disease, hypertension.
   10. Hematologic. Anemias, hemophilia.
   11. Immunologic deficiencies.
   12. Gastrointestinal. Ulcers, pyloric stenosis, chronic constipation, or diarrhea.
   13. Genitourinary. Renal disease, enuresis.
   14. Endocrine. Diabetes, thyroid problems, abnormal pattern of sexual maturation.
   15. Musculoskeletal. Dislocated hips, scoliosis, arthritis, deformities.
   16. Neurologic. Convulsive disorders, learning disabilities, craniosynostosis, mental retardation, mental illness.
   17. General. Obesity, unusual familial pattern of growth, cystic fibrosis.

III. Social history

A. Occupation
   1. Mother.
   2. Father.

B. Housing
   1. Ownership of home.
   2. Age and condition of home.

C. Parents' marital status
   1. Duration of marriage.
   2. Marital relationship.
   3. Single parent, support system.

D. Parents' source of medical care

E. Medical insurance

F. Financial status and source of support

G. Social outlets of parents and family

IV. Pregnancy

A. Prenatal care
   1. Location and duration.
   2. Prenatal classes.

B. Mother's health
   1. Complications: vaginal bleeding, excessive weight gain, edema, headaches, hypertension, glycosuria.
   2. Infection: rubella, urinary tract infection.
   3. Exposure to radiation, drugs (alcohol, medications, smoking).

C. Planning of pregnancy
   1. Methods of contraception.
   2. When contraception discontinued.

V. Birth

A. Location

B. Gestational age in weeks

C. Labor
   1. Induction.
   2. Duration.
   3. Medication, natural birth.
   4. Father present.

D. Delivery
   1. Presentation: vertex, breech, transverse.
   2. Method: spontaneous, forceps, cesarean section (repeat, emergency).

E. Parents' reaction to labor and delivery, including mother's physical and mental recuperation.

F. Complications

G. Neonatal health
   1. Birth weight.
   2. Condition at birth.
      a. Apgar score.
      b. Resuscitation, oxygen.
      c. Special nursery.
      d. Congenital anomalies.
   3. Hospital course.
      a. Respiratory distress.
      b. Cyanosis.

c. Jaundice: physiologic, ABO, Rh, other.
d. Difficulty sucking.
e. Vomiting.
f. Other complications.
   (1) Infection.
   (2) Seizures.
g. Length of stay.
h. Low weight and discharge weight.

VI. Nutrition

A. Feeding
   1. Breast: duration.
   2. Formula: amount, type.
B. Problems
   1. Scheduling.
   2. Vomiting.
   3. Diarrhea.
   4. Colic.
C. Vitamins and fluoride
D. Solids
   1. When introduced—cereal, vegetables, fruits, meats, eggs, juices.
   2. How prepared.
   3. Infant's tolerance.
E. Present diet
   1. Appetite.
      a. Balanced—relate to growth pattern.
   2. Food intolerances and dislikes.

VII. Growth and development

A. Physical
   1. Height and weight at birth, 6 months, 1 year, etc.
   2. Consistent growth rate.
B. Motor
   1. Gross motor
      a. Sits by 6 months.
      b. Crawls by 8 months.
      c. Stands alone by 12 months.
      d. Walks by 16 months.
      e. Undresses, dresses by 2½ years.
      f. Pedals tricycle by 3 years.
      g. Ties shoes by 6 years.
   2. Fine motor
      a. Reaches for objects by 4 months.
      b. Pincer grasp by 1 year.
      c. Holds and drinks from cup by 1½ years.

d. Feeds self by 2 years.
e. Catches ball by 3 years.
f. Uses pencils by 4 years.

C. Language
1. Single words other than "mama" and "dada" by 1 year.
2. Phrases (two to three words) by 1½ years.
3. Sentences by 3 years.

D. Toilet training
1. When started.
2. Technique used.
3. When achieved.

E. School
1. Grade appropriate for age.
2. Academic performance.
3. Social adjustment to school.
a. To teachers.
b. To peers.

F. Personality traits as viewed by parents
1. Relationships with parents: happy, self-actualizing, exhibits self control, takes responsibility for own actions according to developmental stage.
2. Relationships with siblings: cooperative rather than aggressive interaction.
3. Relationships with peers: by school age, able to be a part of a peer group.

G. Behavioral traits
1. Pica, tantrums, thumb sucking, rocking, etc.
2. Sleep patterns.
3. Hobbies, activities.
4. Smoking, drugs, sexual practices.
5. Ability to control behavior.
6. Ability to anticipate and take responsibility for consequence of behavior.
7. Ability to accept and return affection.

VIII. Parental reaction to child's development

A. Proud, understanding

IX. Immunizations and screening tests

A. Types and dates of immunizations, including boosters
1. DPT.
2. Td.
3. TOPV.
4. Measles.
5. Rubella.
6. Mumps.
7. Other (e.g., influenza).

B. Reactions to immunizations

C. Screening and dates of last tests
1. Tuberculin.

2. Sickle cell.
3. Lead.
4. Hearing.
5. Vision.
6. Urine.
7. Hemoglobin, hematocrit.

X. Previous illnesses

A. Contagious diseases
1. Dates.
2. Severity.
3. Sequelae.

B. Infections
1. Dates.
2. Severity.
3. Sequelae.

C. Other illnesses and complications

D. Hospitalizations
1. Illnesses, operations, injuries.
2. Dates.
3. Places.
4. Complications.

XI. Review of systems

A. Skin. Birthmarks, rashes, skin type.

B. HEENT (Head, Eyes, Ears, Nose, Throat)
1. Hair and scalp. Seborrhea, hair loss, pediculosis.
2. Head. Injuries, headache.
3. Eyes. Vision test, glasses, strabismus, infections.
4. Ears. Hearing test, infections, discharge.
5. Nose. Epistaxis, allergies, frequent colds, snoring, sense of smell.
6. Mouth. Dental hygiene, visits to dentist, mouth breathing.
7. Throat. Sore throats, swollen glands, difficulty swallowing, hoarseness.

C. Respiratory. Bronchitis, pneumonia, asthma, croup, persistent cough.

D. Cardiovascular. Heart murmur, cyanosis, dyspnea, shortness of breath, edema, syncope, energy level.

E. Gastrointestinal. Appetite, diet, abdominal pain, vomiting, diarrhea, constipation, type and frequency of stools, jaundice.

F. Genitourinary. Enuresis, urinary tract infection, dysuria, urinary frequency, hematuria, vaginal discharge.

G. Skeletal. Deformities, joint pains, swelling, limp, orthopedic appliances, injuries.

H. Neurologic. Fainting spells, dizziness, tremors, loss of consciousness, seizures, ataxia.

I. Endocrine
1. Sexual maturation.

a. Male: hair, beard, voice, acne.

b. Female: breast development; menarche, duration, regularity, amount of menstrual flow, dysmenorrhea; acne.

2. Growth disturbances.

a. Consistent growth rate.

b. Excessive weight gain.

3. Excessive thirst.

XII. Assessment

A. Problems identified from subjective and objective data.

B. Problem list developed with parent and/or child.

PHYSICAL EXAMINATION

The following outline of the physical examination is to be used, age appropriately, at each well child visit.

I. General appearance and behavior

- **A.** Habitus
  - **1.** Body build and constitution.
  - **2.** Size.
  - **3.** Nutrition.
- **B.** General
  - **1.** Alertness.
  - **2.** Cooperativeness.
  - **3.** Activity level.

II. Measurements

- **A.** Temperature
- **B.** Pulse rate
- **C.** Respiratory rate
- **D.** Blood pressure. Cuff size; examination routine from 3 years of age.
- **E.** Height. Percentile plotted on growth chart.
- **F.** Weight. Percentile plotted on growth chart.
- **G.** Head circumference. Percentile plotted on growth chart.

III. Skin and hair

- **A.** Inspection
  - **1.** Color. Normal, cyanosis, pallor, jaundice, carotenemia, hair color, and distribution.
  - **2.** Eruptions. Macules, papules, vesicles, bullae, pustules, wheals, petechiae, ecchymoses.
  - **3.** Pigmentation. Hemangiomas, nevi.
- **B.** Palpation
  - **1.** Skin texture. Smooth, soft, flexible, moist, rough, dry, scaly, edematous.
  - **2.** Scars.
  - **3.** Hair texture. Fine, coarse, dry, oily.

IV. Head and face

- **A.** Inspection
  - **1.** Size. Normal, microcephalic, macrocephalic.
  - **2.** Shape. Symmetry, bossing, flattening.
  - **3.** Control. Mobility, head lag.
- **B.** Palpation
  - **1.** Fontanelles. Size, shape, bulging, depression.
  - **2.** Suture lines. Separated, overriding, closed.
  - **3.** Craniotabes.
  - **4.** Caput succedaneum, cephalhematoma.

- C. Percussion
    1. Sinuses.
    2. Macewen's sign (cracked-pot sound).
- D. Auscultation. Bruits.

V. Eyes

- A. Inspection
    1. Size and shape. Equal, symmetric.
    2. Control. Ptosis, nystagmus, strabismus, blinking.
    3. Pupils. Shape, equality, size, reaction to light, accommodation.
    4. Conjunctivae and sclerae. Clarity, hemorrhage, color, pigmentation.
    5. Eyelids. Ptosis, blepharitis, sties.
- A. Examination
    1. Ophthalmoscopic. Red reflex, cataract, eye grounds.
    2. Dacryocystitis, dacryostenosis
    3. Visual acuity.

VI. Ears

- A. Inspection
    1. Size and shape. Lop ears, skin tags, dimples, sinus tracts, anomalies.
    2. Position. Low set.
    3. Otoscopic exam
        - a. External canal. Cerumen, discharge, inflammation, foreign bodies.
        - b. Tympanic membrane. Color, light reflex, bony landmarks, mobility, perforation, bulging, retraction, scars.
    4. Auditory acuity. Whisper test, audiometry, Rinnie's test, Weber's test, tuning fork.
    5. Impedance audiometry.
- B. Palpation
    1. Auricle. Pain on retraction.
    2. Mastoid. Tenderness.

VII. Nose

- A. Inspection
    1. Size and shape.
    2. Mucosa. Color, discharge, polyps.
    3. Turbinates. Size, color.
    4. Septum. Deviation, bleeding points.
    5. Foreign bodies
- B. Palpation. Tenderness, crepitus, deformity.

VIII. Mouth: inspection

- A. Lips. Symmetry, color, eruptions, fissures, edema.
- B. Gums. Color, cysts, infection, ulcerations, mucous membranes.
- C. Tongue. Symmetry, tongue-tie, color, anomalies.
- D. Teeth. Number, alignment, caries.

IX. Throat: inspection

- A. Palate. Symmetry, shape, color, cleft, arch, eruptions.

B. Uvula. Symmetry, shape, bifid.

C. Tonsils. Symmetry, shape, size, color, exudate, ulcerations.

D. Epiglottis. Size, shape, color.

X. Neck

A. Inspection. Size, shape, webbing, fistulas, masses, neck veins, cysts.

B. Palpation

1. Trachea. Position.
2. Thyroid. Size, masses.
3. Neck. Masses, mobility, torticollis.

XI. Lymph nodes: suboccipital, postauricular, anterior and posterior cervical, supraclavicular, axillary, epitrochlear, inguinal.

A. Inspection. Size, overlying skin color, lymphangitis.

B. Palpation. Size, consistency, tenderness, mobility.

XII. Chest

A. Inspection

1. Shape. Funnel, pigeon, barrel, precordial bulge, protruding xiphoid, Harrison's groove.
2. Size, symmetry, mobility. Expansion, flaring, retraction.
3. Respirations. Rate, type, tachypnea, dyspnea, hyperpnea.

B. Palpation

1. Tactile fremitus.
2. Breast. Consistency, masses.

C. Percussion. Tympany, resonance, dullness, flatness.

D. Auscultation

1. Breath sounds. Vesicular, bronchovesicular, bronchial.
2. Adventitial sounds. Rales, rhonchi, wheezes, rubs.
3. Vocal resonance.

XIII. Heart

A. Palpation

1. PMI.
2. Thrills.

B. Percussion. Heart border.

C. Auscultation

1. Rate, rhythm, character of first and second heart sounds, third heart sound, splitting.
2. Sinus arrhythmia, gallop, premature beats, murmurs (systolic, diastolic), clicks, rubs.

XIV. Abdomen

A. Inspection

1. Size and shape. Distention, respiratory movements, peristalsis.
2. Umbilicus. Granuloma, hernia.
3. Diastasis recti.
4. Veins.

B. Auscultation. Bowel sounds.

C. Palpation
   1. Tone. Rigidity, tenderness, rebound.
   2. Liver, spleen, kidneys, bladder. Masses.
   3. Femoral pulses.
D. Percussion. Organ size, tympany, fluid.

XV. Genitalia

A. Inspection
   1. Male
      a. Penis. Size, foreskin (phimosis), circumcision, urethral meatus (hypospadias, epispadias, chordee).
      b. Scrotum. Size, testicles (size, shape), hydrocele, hernia.
      c. Hair distribution
   2. Female
      a. Labia, clitoris, vagina. Foreign bodies, adhesions, discharge.
      b. Urethra.
      c. Hair distribution.
B. Palpation (male)
   1. Testicles. Descended, undescended, position.
   2. Hernia. Direct, indirect.
   3. Masses.

XVI. Anus and rectum

A. Inspection
   1. General. Position, fissures, fistulas, prolapse, hemorrhoids.
   2. Sacrococcygeal area
      a. Pilonidal dimple or fistula.
      b. Masses: teratoma, meningocele.
   3. Palpation. Phincter tone, masses, tenderness.

XVII. Musculoskeletal: inspection

A. Hands. Clubbing, polydactyly, syndactyly, nails, dermatoglyphics.
B. Legs and feet. Symmetry, forefoot adduction, pes planus, clubbed feet, knock-knees, bowed legs, tibial torsion, gait, anteversion of femoral head, limp, length, paralysis.
C. Hips. Symmetry of skin folds.
D. Back. Scoliosis, hyphosis, lordosis.

Refer to the well child exam schedule of the American Academy of Pediatrics.

WELL CHILD VISITS

Although the well child visits defined here are labeled for a specific age span, they are intended to be used as a continuum in following each child in his own developmental progress. The broad guidelines for well child visits are as follows:

I. First cycle of growth

- **A.** 0–8 weeks. The neonatal period.
  - **1.** Establishment of the general well-being of mother and baby.
  - **2.** Development of a good working relationship between mother and baby.
- **B.** 2–4 months. Continuing period of symbiosis of mother and baby.
  - **1.** Stabilization of physical systems.
  - **2.** Development of contentment for both parents and baby.
- **C.** 4–6 months. Period of awareness.
  - **1.** Physical system stability and beginning of body control.
  - **2.** Beginning of the separation of the individuality of both mother and baby.
  - **3.** Established reliance of the baby on the goodness/unreliability of his environment.
    - **a.** Primary caretaker.
- **D.** 6–8 months. Becoming the student.
  - **1.** Watching intently what is going on around him.
  - **2.** Progressing from random to purposeful movements.
  - **3.** Building up memory store of people and objects in his environment.
- **E.** 8–14 months. A watershed period.
  - **1.** Past physical and emotional development provides the building blocks for the next stage.
  - **2.** Reaching out into the environment to fashion confidence in his developing skills.
  - **3.** Expansion of his emotional responses.
  - **4.** New physical mobility.
- **F.** 14–18 months. Exploration and self confidence.
  - **1.** Refinement of physical skills.
  - **2.** Beginning to use language as a tool.
  - **3.** Development of self-esteem vs. self-doubt, reflecting encouragement/discouragement by primary caretaker.
- **G.** 18–24 months. Experimenting with establishing independence.
  - **1.** Using "no" as a test of power.
  - **2.** Learning that behavior has consequences.
  - **3.** Safety of primary concern.
- **H.** 24–36 months. Definitive year to complete the development of the physical and emotional tasks of the first period of growth.
  - **1.** Maturation of physical systems.
  - **2.** Establishment of the emotional maturity needed to move away from the security of the family and join his peer group.

II. **Second cycle of growth**

A. 3–5 years

1. Increase in muscle strength, but slower development of endurance.
2. Progressing from fantasy and magical thinking to a world of reality.
3. Sexual identity established.

B. 6–9 years

1. Halcyon years of good health, intellectual curiosity, few responsibilities, and high adventures.
2. Strength and endurance increased (dependent on exercise and use, not on sex).

III. **Third cycle of growth**

A. 9–11 years

1. Physical changes.
2. Transitional period from childhood to adolescence.
3. Need for child and parent to understand and appreciate the individual pattern of each child's development.

B. 12–16 years

1. Physical stability.
2. Establishing independence by making appropriate decisions.
3. Understanding the consequences of and accepting responsibility for one's actions.
4. Learning to accept and appreciate one's own uniqueness.

The general outline used for the presentation of the remainder of Part I is as follows:

I. **Well Child Visit**

A. Developmental process
B. Family status
C. Health habits
D. Growth and development
E. High-risk factors
F. Physical examination
G. Assessment
H. Plan

II. **Anticipatory Guidance**

A. Expectations for development
B. Family status
C. Health patterns
D. Growth and development
E. High-risk factors
F. Child-rearing practices
G. Stimulation
H. Safety

OVERVIEW

2-WEEK WELL CHILD VISIT

I. **Parents**
   - A. Adjustment to new responsibilities.
      - 1. Able to identify and appreciate developing personality of baby.

II. **Baby**
   - A. Physical
      - 1. Quality of care.
         - a. Weight gain.
         - b. Contented baby.
      - 2. Physical problems not already under care identified: Referrals.
   - B. Emotional
      - 1. Quieting easily. Contented baby.
      - 2. Responding to parents by eye contact.
   - C. Intellectual
      - 1. Searching for eye contact with caretaker.

III. **High Risk Factors**
   - A. Apathetic
   - B. Low weight gain.
   - C. Unable to be comforted.
   - D. No consistent, caring caretaker.

IV. **See guidelines for specific factors to be noted in physical exam.**

NOTES

2-WEEK WELL CHILD VISIT

I. Developmental process.

This is the settling-in period for both mother and baby. Adequate physical care and the developing of emotional ties are the essential factors to be evaluated.

- A. Mother
  1. Energy level and general health adequate for demands of family and baby.
  2. Expectations of having and caring for the baby and expectations of physical appearance of the baby fulfilled.
  3. Acceptance of and coping with actual situation.
- B. Baby
  1. Has good sucking instinct, eats and sleeps well, is gaining weight.
  2. Cries appropriately and quiets easily.
  3. Responds to mother's voice, touch, and presence.

II. Family status

- A. Basic needs being met; referrals as needed with follow-up.
- B. Family members
  1. Adjusting to change in family routine.
  2. Appreciation of emotional stress during this adjustment period.
- C. Support system
  1. Father. Giving help and getting pleasure from new role.
  2. Mother. Having time available to regain energy, catch up on sleep, and have free, peaceful periods with baby.
- D. Health status of all family members reviewed.

III. Health habits

- A. Nutrition
  1. Mother. Breast-feeding; see Breast-Feeding Guidelines.
     - a. Adequate diet, weight control, referrals as needed.
  2. Baby. The stomach is approximately 4 oz in size and empties every 3–4 hours. The digestive system is still immature, so formula or breast milk is the only food appropriate at this time.

     Requirement = 50 cal/lb/day or 110 kcal/kg/day

     Standard formulas and breast milk = 20 cal/oz

     10-lb baby = $10 \times 50 = 500$ cal required per day

     4.54-kg baby = $4.54 \times 110 = 500$ cal required per day

     $$\frac{500 \text{ cal}}{20 \text{ cal/oz}} = 25 \text{ oz or } 750 \text{ ml of formula per day}$$

     - a. Number of feedings and amount per 24 hours.
     - b. If reflux occurs, help mother identify whether too many ounces are being given. Advise mother to prop baby up after feedings.
     - c. Projectile vomiting: refer to physician.
     - d. Burping gently accomplished.
     - e. Satisfaction: sleeping after feedings.
     - f. Formula with vitamins, iron, and fluoride per office protocol.

B. Sleep

1. One or two sleep periods of 5–6 hours per 24 hours (individual pattern depends on temperament and energy level).
2. Awake for feedings every ±3 hours.
3. Awake only short periods and seldom awake without fussing.
4. Sleeps through household noises; turns off stimuli around him, so quiet environment is not necessary.

C. Elimination

1. Stools
   - **a.** Breast-fed. Stools with every feeding; not formed; yellow.
   - **b.** Formula-fed. Stools less frequent, less loose, and stronger in odor than if on breast milk; light brown.
2. Urine. Light in color, no odor; wet diaper at each feeding.

IV. Growth and development

A. Physical

1. Central nervous system. This is the most important and fastest growing system, as the brain cells are continuing to develop in both size and number. The effects of nutritional deprivation at this time cannot be reversed.
   - **a.** Holds head up when prone, to side when supine.
   - **b.** Hands fisted—palmar grasp.
   - **c.** Intense startle reaction.
   - **d.** Vision: at 8 weeks, baby is alert to moving objects and is attracted to light objects and bright color. Convergence and following are jerky and inexact.
   - **e.** Movements are uncoordinated but smooth.
   - **f.** Has a lusty cry.
2. Cardiovascular system. The efficiency of this system is identified by the following:
   - **a.** Good color of body and warmth of extremities.
   - **b.** Energy and vigor of activity level.
   - **c.** Increase of color during stress.
3. Respiratory system. Breathing is still rapid and irregular.
4. Immune system
   - **a.** The antigen-antibody response is present by 6–8 weeks, so the immunization program can be started at that time.
   - **b.** Maternal antibodies, which help protect the baby from infection, are present.

B. Emotional development—Erikson: basic trust vs. mistrust. The quality of care that is provided can form the basis for the baby's feelings and attitudes toward himself and the world.

1. Mother
   - **a.** Obtaining gratification from child care.
   - **b.** Feels adequate to care for baby.
   - **c.** Adequate support system; basic needs being met.
2. Baby
   - **a.** Adequate physical development.

b. Searching for mother's face; making eye contact.
c. Contented baby.

C. Intellectual development—Piaget: sensorimotor response. The stimuli to the five senses are the tools through which the baby responds to his environment.
1. Mother. Understanding crying as an instinctive response to other discomforts besides hunger.
2. Baby. Individuality of response pattern becoming evident. Innate reflex responses guide spontaneous behavior.

D. High-risk factors
1. Mother
a. Overload of responsibilities and no adequate support system.
b. Low energy level and health problems.
c. Distressed by child care.
2. Baby
a. Poor feeding habits and low weight gain.
b. Lags in physical development.
c. Unable to be comforted.

V. Physical examination

A. Growth
1. Weight gain of l oz/day.
2. Fontanelles: measure and record.
3. Developing consistent growth curve.

B. Appearance and behavior
1. Activity level and smooth movements.
2. Intensity of startle reaction—with quieting easily.
3. Alert when awake and falls asleep easily.
4. Good color, rapid change in color with activity and crying.

C. Specific factors to note while doing routine physical examination
1. Head. Configuration and smooth movement, bulging or depressed anterior fontanelle, seborrhea.
2. Eyes. Red reflex, discharge, reaction to light.
3. Mouth. Thrush (unremovable while spots on tongue). Tongue should be able to protrude beyond lips.
4. Chest. Respirations—abdominal, irregular rate present.
5. Heart. Refer to physician if abnormal sounds present that have not been previously diagnosed. Sinus arrhythmia continues to be present; normal rate of 100–130/minute.
6. Abdomen. Navel, liver, spleen, femoral pulses, hernias.
7. Extremities. Range of motion. Hips: check for leg folds and abduction.
8. Skin. Rashes, hemangiomas (measure and record).

D. Mother–child interaction
1. Mother. Expression of fatigue and nervousness in handling baby; ability to quiet baby.
2. Baby. Positive response to mother's attention.

VI. Assessment

A. Physical

B. Developmental

C. Emotional

D. Environmental

VII. Plan

A. Immunization at 8 weeks per office protocol.

B. Fluoride, vitamins, and iron per office protocol.

C. Problem list (devised with parent); SOAP (Subjective data, Objective data, Assessment, and Plan) format for each.

D. Appropriate timing for office, home, and/or telephone visits.

BREAST-FEEDING GUIDELINES

Breast-feeding is the most natural way to feed a baby. It should be something a mother does because she wants to, because she and the baby find it satisfying. If, for any reason, it does not work out, there is no cause for feelings of guilt. The method of feeding is of much less importance than the general quality of the relationship between mother and baby.

I. Mother

A. Bras should fit well and provide support without causing pressure on any part of the breast. Most women are more comfortable if they wear a bra around the clock during the early postpartum weeks.

B. Food and drink. There may be an increase in appetite and thirst during lactation. It is recommended that 500 cal be added to the prepregnant diet.

1. Control weight by eliminating sweets and cutting back on fatty foods. Do not skimp on fruits, vegetables, meat, fish, poultry, cereals, and breads. Do not diet. Breast-feeding aids maternal weight loss.
2. Drink at least 3 quarts of liquid a day, including some milk. Other milk products include yogurt, ice cream, cheese, and custards. Coffee/teas consumed should be decaffeinated, since caffeine is excreted in breast milk. Avoid colas with caffeine.
3. Rarely does a food that agrees with the mother cause a problem for the baby; however, onions and garlic may affect the taste of the mother's milk, causing the baby to protest. Be aware of this as a possible cause of the baby's fussiness.
4. Beer and other alcoholic drinks should be eliminated from the diet, since they are excreted in breast milk.

C. Drugs. Check with the doctor before taking *any* medication. Most doctors discourage the use of birth control pills during lactation, because these often decrease the milk supply and possibly its nutrient value. Since many drugs do pass into the milk, one must always question their effect on the baby. Nicotine should be avoided, since it accumulates in breast milk and can limit the amount of milk produced.

D. Menstruation. The return of periods may be delayed for as long as breast-feeding is continued without supplementation with formula or solids. However, this does not mean that the mother cannot get pregnant; breast-feeding is not a reliable form of birth control. Menstruation has no effect on the quality of milk.

E. Fatigue and discouragement. The mother will probably be surprised at how tired and on edge she feels during the early postpartum weeks. She will get little else done besides meeting the baby's needs. Fatigue and emotional stress not only decrease milk supply but also affect the way mother and baby get along. If the mother is upset, the baby will be too. Do not feel guilty about the following:

1. Admitting fatigue and accepting (or demanding) help from others.
2. Napping when the baby sleeps (curl up together).
3. Cutting activities down to bare essentials, ignoring the dust and resorting to simple dinners for a while.

F. Sore breast. The usual cause is a blockage of one of the milk ducts due to engorgement, a tight bra, or poor or delayed emptying of that breast. There will probably be a lump or two in the tender area. Because an infection is possible, treat immediately.

1. Nurse very frequently on the sore side to "empty" it; offer it to the baby first.
2. Gently massage the area while taking a hot shower; make sure no crusted milk is covering a portion of the nipple.
3. Try different nursing positions to change pressure areas.
4. Remove the bra if it is too tight, or get a bra extender.
5. Extra fluids and rest help.
6. If the lump does not disappear after two or three feedings, if the area becomes red and more tender, and/or if a fever is present with flulike aches, call the doctor; an antibiotic may be necessary.
7. Do not stop nursing; the milk will not harm the baby.

G. Sore nipples. Some discomfort is usual during the first week or two of nursing. This soreness is temporary and should not be a reason to stop nursing or resort to nipple shields. To reduce soreness:

1. Always
   - **a.** Get the milk flow started manually before putting the baby to the breast. This prevents irritation from the initial "dry" sucking necessary to draw the milk down.
   - **b.** Nurse frequently for short periods (5–10 minutes on each side every 2–3 hours).
   - **c.** Break the suction before removing the baby.
   - **d.** Offer both breasts at each feeding (if 10 minutes on one side fills the baby up, nurse for 5 minutes on each side).
   - **e.** Make certain the baby takes the nipple and most of the areola into his mouth. The mother should be able to see the brown area "pucker" slightly as baby nurses.
   - **f.** Wash breasts with water only.
   - **g.** Rotate pressure areas by experimenting with different positions for both mother and baby.
   - **h.** Begin on the less painful breast; then switch to the sore side after let-down has occurred and baby's hunger has eased a bit.
   - **i.** Take a hot shower to help relax and to get the milk flowing before nursing.
   - **j.** Expose nipples to sunlight for brief periods.
2. Never
   - **a.** Skip a feeding or avoid nursing on the sore side.
   - **b.** Use a nipple shield. This only postpones the toughening process and often adds to the irritation, since the baby must get the milk by suction alone.
   - **c.** Use excessive amounts of cream on nipples. A thick layer of cream tends to trap moisture and also makes the nipples slipper, which forces the baby to clamp down repeatedly in an effort to stay on.
   - **d.** Use plastic-covered bra pads.
   - **e.** Use soap or drying agents on nipples.
3. When the soreness diminishes, increase the nursing time to meet the baby's needs.

II. Baby

A. Feeding schedules. Nurse 10–15 minutes on the first side, then allow the baby to nurse until satisfied on the second. At times the baby may fall asleep, yet by reflex his lower jaw will move rhythmically without effective sucking. After a minute or two of this, he will usually remain asleep when removed from the breast. Follow the baby's signals rather than the clock. Most breast-fed babies want to nurse every 2–3 hours during the early weeks. Human milk is easier to digest than formula, so a breast-fed stomach empties sooner than a formula-fed one. As the mother's milk supply increases, the number of feedings will decrease. If the baby is small and consistently sleeps 4–5 hours between feedings, the mother should attempt to nurse him at least every 3 hours during her waking hours.

B. Indications that the baby is getting enough milk

1. Six to eight wet diapers over a 24-hour period (not a good indication if the baby is also getting a lot of water).
2. Contented, vigorous, frequent (every 2–3 hours) nursing periods of at least 5 minutes per side.
3. An alert, responsive baby.
4. Do not test for hunger by offering the baby a bottle after feeding. Often a baby will take an extra ounce or two just because it is there, because he likes to suck, and because he is not used to a nipple that allows milk to flow so fast and easily.
5. Adequate weight gain.

C. Supplementary feeding. Although frequent bottles can interfere with the mother's milk supply, an occasional bottle of breast milk or formula can be given without creating a problem.

1. Formula. The most convenient kind of substitute is ready-to-feed formula that comes in a bottle and requires only attaching a sterile nipple, but powdered formula (mixed with boiling water) is more economical.
2. Breast milk. Mother can express milk before or after feedings to freeze for supplementary feedings.
   - **a.** Manual expression. Baby gets milk by squeezing the areola with his gums and not by direct suction. To imitate this action, grasp the edge of the areola with a thumb and forefinger, and gently squeeze the fingers together while pressing inward toward the chest. Never pull or squeeze just the nipple itself. Since there are many ducts arranged around the nipple somewhat like the spokes of a wheel, change the position of the fingers often.
   - **b.** Hand or electric pump (bulb type). While taking a hot shower, gently massage each breast, starting at the chest wall and working toward the nipple. Immediately afterward, moisten the pump's cone with warm water, compress the bulb only halfway, and apply the cone to the breast so the nipple points toward the bulb. Gently and rhythmically apply and release pressure on the bulb. It probably will take a minute or two before the milk starts flowing.
   - **c.** Collecting milk. Cleanliness is essential when collecting milk.
     - (1) Take apart and wash all equipment in hot, soapy water, rinse well.
     - (2) Place parts in a covered pan, and cover with water.
     - (3) Boil for at least 5 minutes.
     - (4) Turn off heat, and allow pan to cool on burner.

(5) Drain water, and store parts in the covered pan until ready to use.

(6) Wash hands before reassembling equipment; be careful not to touch parts that will come in contact with the milk.

(7) Repeat step (1) immediately after use.

d. Storing milk

(1) Plastic or glass bottles may be used for freezing; disposable bottle liners may be frozen in the outer case and then sealed with a twist-tie.

(2) Label the container with the date if it is to be frozen.

(3) Breast milk should be used within a day after it is refrigerated. It will stay fresh up to two weeks in the freezer, at 0°F or below.

(4) Milk separates into layers as it cools but will mix again when thawed.

e. Thawing milk

(1) Do not thaw milk slowly at room temperature.

(2) Place bottle in pan of cold water, and bring water to a boil.

(3) Remove pan from heat, and take bottle out when milk is warm.

(4) Refrigerate leftover milk, but discard if not used within 2–3 hours.

D. Weaning

1. The baby's age or the appearance of teeth should not be the reason to stop breast-feeding. The decision should be based on the mother's feelings and needs, as well as on the baby's cues and needs. Although there is no right time to wean, there is a wrong time. Delay weaning if the baby is irritable from teething or sick or if some other stress is present.
2. Weaning can be accomplished in a matter of days if absolutely necessary, but doing it so rapidly can be extra hard on both mother and baby. The weaning process should be spaced over a period of weeks so there is time to adjust gradually.
3. Choose the feeding in which there is the least milk or in which the baby is least interested, and replace it with a cup or bottle of formula or milk, depending on the baby's age and nutritional and sucking needs. If the breasts become uncomfortably full, nurse (or express) a short time to relieve the discomfort.
4. When "supply with demand" is again balanced, skip another feeding; continue this pattern until the baby is completely off the breast.

OVERVIEW

ANTICIPATORY GUIDANCE FOR THE PERIOD OF 2–8 WEEKS

I. Parents

- **A.** Aware of baby's reactive pattern and the interactive relationship of mother and baby.
- **B.** Check breast-feeding protocol.

II. Baby

- **A.** Physical
  1. Smoother muscular movement.
  2. Hands reaching out.
- **B.** Emotional
  1. Settling in to a feeding and sleeping schedule.
  2. Responding appropriately to type of care being given.
  3. A fussy baby needs careful investigation. See guidelines.
- **C.** Intellectual
  1. Curiosity shown by searching with eyes and reaching out with hands.
  2. Responding by smiles and eye contact.
     - **a.** Stimulation. See guidelines.

III. See guidelines for Safety and Accident Prevention

NOTES

ANTICIPATORY GUIDANCE FOR THE PERIOD OF 2–8 WEEKS

I. **Expectations of this period.**

This is a quiet period of settling into a scheduled daily routine. It is also a time for parents to become sensitive to the individuality of the baby's reactive pattern and to the interactive relationship that is being established between mother and baby.

A. Mother

1. Developing confidence in her ability to interpret baby's needs.
2. Enjoying and satisfied with care.
3. Understanding and coping with own physical and emotional status.

B. Baby

1. Developing a daily pattern of sleeping, feeding, and wakefulness.
2. Quieting easily when needs are met.

II. **Family status**

A. Basic needs being met; referrals as needed with follow-up.

B. Mother and father adjusting to their new roles as parents.

C. Appropriate support systems available.

III. **Health patterns**

A. Nutrition

1. Formula or breast milk the only food necessary, owing to immaturity of the GI tract and the slow development of digestive enzymes.
2. Supplements of vitamins, iron, and fluoride per office protocol.

B. Elimination

1. Stools continue to be loose.
2. Urine light in color and odorless. If this changes, identify the cause, as this change can be an early indication of dyhydration.

IV. **Interpreting baby's signals**

A. Crying following feeding and diapering

1. Physical discomforts
   a. Bowel movement: it is helpful to have something for the infant's feet to push against; hold the baby over the shoulder with one hand, and place the other hand on the soles of his feet.
   b. An air bubble in the stomach takes up space, is uncomfortable, and prevents the baby from eating as much as desired. Lay the infant across the mother's folded knees with his head resting on the mother's arms; hold one hand on the baby's abdomen, and gently rub back in an upward motion.
   c. Diaper rash: leave diapers off as much as possible; try another brand of disposables; if using cloth diapers, change soaps, rinse well, and use vinegar in the final rinse. Call the office if there is no improvement, and report any vaginal irritation.
2. Missing physical contact and sounds heard in utero
   a. Warmth and snugness: wrap blankets tightly around the baby, and provide body support.
   b. Music: lullabies are important; tapes and recordings make it easy to supply music.

c. Rocking: cradles and rocking chairs have proved effective over the years.

3. Need for stimulation. Fussing can be a way of baby's saying he is not ready to go back to sleep.

   a. Use a baby chest carrier; the baby enjoys his mother's heart sounds and motion.

   b. Take a bath with the baby.

   c. Air baths allow freedom of movement; change the baby's position from back to stomach.

   d. Take the baby outdoors for a change of colors, sounds, and temperature.

   e. A car ride is often used by harassed parents.

   f. A change of caretaker to walk him, talk to him, etc. is helpful.

B. Continued fussing

   1. Check clothes—they may be uncomfortable; the baby may be too hot or too cold.

   2. Colic

      a. Breast-feeding: more frequent feedings for smaller amount at each feeding.

      b. Mother's diet: restrict to simplest foods; no colas, coffee, tea; no medications or vitamins; add one food back at a time and see if there is any change in behavior.

      c. Formula-feeding: smaller and more frequent feedings; eliminate vitamins and fluoride for a few days.

      d. Return for medical check if no improvement.

      e. Obtain extra caretakers so mother can get adequate rest.

V. Stimulation

A. Stimulation depends on the energy level and individuality of the baby.

B. Baby reacting to stimulation of all the senses—taste, touch, smell, sight, and hearing.

C. Mother/caretaker interpreting baby's signals for rest and quiet.

D. Parents can provide proper stimulation by spending time feeding, holding, rocking, changing the baby's position, establishing eye contact, and talking and singing to the baby.

E. Suggested crib toys

   1. Noisy clocks, music (radio or tapes).

   2. Paint a happy face on a paper place, and hang approximately 10 in. from the baby's face or attach to the side of the crib.

VI. Safety

A. Accidents happen most frequently

   1. When routine changes (holidays, vacations, illness in the family).

   2. Following stressful events for caretakers.

   3. When caretakers are tired or ill.

   4. Late in the afternoon.

B. Accident prevention

   1. Crib: slats no more than 2 in. apart; firm mattress; no plastic used as mattress cover.

2. House: fire alarm system; fire escape plan; no smoking in nursery. Baby should never be left alone in the house for even one minute.
3. Carrying: football carry—baby on hip with hand holding and protecting head; other hand free to prevent caretaker from falling.
4. Car: approved baby carrier in the back seat.
5. Baby seat: sturdy, broad based; place in safe, protected spot.

C. Not all injuries are accidents. Investigate possible child abuse and neglect.

D. Instructions to baby-sitters

E. Emergency telephone numbers posted

VII. Asking for help

A. Appreciation of the importance of establishing a good working relationship with the baby.

B. Concerns and problems need to be evaluated.

C. Telephone contact available with pediatric nurse practitioner; home visits, office visits, referrals made as needed.

D. Resources

1. Parent groups: community or church related; social service referrals as needed.
2. Information on child care: library provides reading list.

OVERVIEW

2-MONTH WELL CHILD VISIT

I. **Parents**
   - A. Evaluation of their new role.
   - B. Identifying baby's developing skills and reactive patterns.

II. **Baby**
   - A. Physical
     1. Baby's growth pattern, eating, and sleeping schedule evaluated.
        - a. Health problems identified.
   - B. Emotional
     1. Contented baby. Reacting to caretaker with enthusiasm.
   - C. Intellectual
     1. Curiosity
     2. Watching more intently.
     3. Reaching out to feel and touch.

III. **High Risk Factors**
   - A. Fussy or apathetic baby needs further investigation.

IV. **Check Safety protocol**

NOTES

2-MONTH WELL CHILD VISIT

I. **Developmental process.**
The continued close symbiotic relationship of mother and baby is characterized by the stabilization of physical systems and feelings of contentment and pleasure for both mother and baby.

A. Mother
1. Deriving pleasure and satisfaction from care of the baby.
2. Developing confidence in her ability to understand and fulfill the needs of the baby.
3. Establishing a consistent schedule.

B. Baby
1. Establishing a normal developmental pattern.
2. Cries appropriately and quiets easily.

II. **Family status**

A. Life-style. Adequate housing and finances to meet needs.
B. Parental roles. Establishing responsibilities; feeling gratification and pride in these new roles.
C. Siblings. Parental understanding of siblings' reactions to changes.
D. Concerns and problems. Ability to identify problems and to cope; referrals as needed.
E. Mother
1. Physical status. Energy level; postpartum examination; family planning.
2. Emotional stability. Satisfactory support system; pride and pleasure with baby.

III. **Health habits**

A. Nutrition
1. Mother
   a. Breast-feeding: understanding of dietary requirements.
   b. Weight control.
   c. Establishing a feeding schedule.
2. Baby. Formula or breast milk continues to be adequate nutrition, as immaturity of the GI tract and the slow development of digestive enzymes can cause difficulties if other food is added.
   a. 0.25 mg of fluoride per office protocol. Check with physician about Vitamin D supplementation at 3 months.
   b. Feedings: showing satisfaction, sucking strength; beginning to establish a schedule.
   c. Requirement = 50 cal/lb/day or 110 kcal/kg/day

      Standard formulas and breast milk = 20 cal/oz

      10-lb baby = 10×50 = 500 cal required per day

      4.54-kg baby = 4.54×110 = 500 cal required per day

$$\frac{500 \text{ cal}}{20 \text{ cal/oz}} = 25 \text{ oz or } 750 \text{ ml of formula per day}$$

B. Sleep

1. Mother needs at least one sleep period of 6 hours for sufficient deep sleep.
2. Baby
   a. Has one sleep period of 6–7 hours and sleeps a total of 16–20 hr/day.
   b. Filters out household noises.
   c. Awake for longer periods without fussing.

C. Elimination

1. Bowel movements at each feeding; continue to be loose.
2. Urine. Light in color; little odor; strong odor and dark color indicate need to investigate for dyhydration.

IV. Growth and development

A. Physical

1. Central nervous system
   a. Head not held at midline.
   b. Arms have random movements.
   c. Hands are fisted, thumbs inside.
   d. Startle reflex less intense.
2. Gastrointestinal system. Sucking reflex continues to be strong. Satisfaction is important; if not met by frequent feedings, a pacifier is helpful.
   a. Swallowing from a spoon is difficult because tongue thrust still occurs.
   b. Drooling and taste buds are not present until 3 months of age.
   c. Stomach is somewhat larger; now holds 4–6 oz and empties every 3–4 hours.
   d. Frequent watery stools continue, since intestinal tract is immature and unable to absorb fluids well.
3. Excretory system. Immature kidney structure affects stability of fluid and solute balance.
   a. Wet diaper at each feeding.
   b. Urine. Light in color.
4. Immune system
   a. Antigen-antibody response present by 2 months of age; immunization program can be started.
   b. Maternal antigens still present in bloodstream.

B. Emotional development—Erikson: basic trust. The close symbiotic relationship of mother and child continues to envelop the baby in an environment without stress. His needs of food, warmth, and human contact must be met to continue the establishment of security and trust in his new world.

1. Mother
   a. Ability to quiet baby.
   b. Making eye contact with baby.
2. Baby
   a. Consistent physical growth.
   b. Sleep pattern being established.
   c. Self-quieting.
   d. Cries appropriately.

C. Intellectual development—Piaget: The baby is learning through the sensorimotor response to his bodily needs. Eye contact and a responsive smile are early indications of the baby's taking in the world around him.

1. Mother
   a. Understanding of crying: as the instinctive response to discomfort.
   b. Taking time and interest to understand baby's signal of distress.
   c. Spoiling is not an issue at this age—a crying baby needs attention.
2. Baby
   a. Low patience level; unable to postpone need satisfaction; does not anticipate, so cannot "wait."
   b. Language begins with random vocalizing other than crying.
   c. Begins to make different crying sounds for different needs.

D. High-risk factors

1. Mother
   a. Lack of pride in baby.
   b. Unresponsive/overresponsive to baby.
   c. Low energy level.
   d. Inadequate support system.
2. Baby
   a. Poor feeding habits; weak sucking reflex.
   b. Lethargy.
   c. Unable to be comfortable.
3. Child abuse indicators
   a. Mother
      (1) Unable to quiet baby.
      (2) Overwhelmed by child care and dissatisfied with maternal role.
   b. Parents
      (1) Isolated from friends and relatives.
      (2) History of child abuse in their own lives.
      (3) Drug abuse.

V. Physical examination

A. Growth

1. Measurement of length and weight: coordinate within 2 standard deviations on growth chart.
   a. Weight gain: 1 oz/day.
   b. Length increase: 1 in./month.
2. Fontanelles: measure and record.

B. Appearance and behavior

1. Alertness: eye contact, responsive smile.
2. Activity level: smooth, coordinated movement with less vigorous movements in legs than in arms.
3. Color: pink; color changes quickly with activity level and temperature of environment.

C. Specific factors to note while doing routine physical examination

1. Head. Check for configuration and smooth movement; bulging or depressed anterior fontanelle; check scalp for seborrhea.
2. Eyes. Check for smooth tracking, reaction to light, dacryostenosis, discharge; tears present from 2–3 months.
3. Mouth. Check for thrush (unremovable while spots on tongue). Tongue should be able to protrude beyond lips.
4. Chest. Respirations: abdominal; irregular rate.
5. Heart. Shunts closed. Refer to physician if abnormal sounds are present that have not been previously diagnosed.
6. Abdomen. Check navel, femoral pulses, hernias.
7. Extremities. Check for range of motion, smooth movements. Hips: check leg folds and abduction.
8. Skin. Check for rashes, hemangiomas (measure and record), bruises, burns.
9. Neurologic. All reflexes present but less intense.

D. Mother–child interaction

1. Mother. Expression of fatigue and nervousness in handling baby; ability to quiet baby.
2. Baby. Responsive to mother's attention.

VI. Assessment

A. Physical

B. Developmental

C. Emotional

D. Environmental

VII. Plan

A. Immunization series per office protocol; discuss importance of completing and recording series.

B. Problem list (devised with parent); SOAP for each.

C. Appropriate timing for office, home, and/or telephone visits.

OVERVIEW

ANTICIPATORY GUIDANCE FOR THE PERIOD OF 2–4 MONTHS

I. **Parents**

A. Understanding and keeping records of development and description of baby's moods and reactions to care.

II. **Baby**

A. Physical

1. Increase in activity level and strength. Muscular movements more defined.
2. Reach out and hold on but not letting go at will.
3. Eating and sleeping schedule being established.

B. Emotional

1. Becoming upset at mother's going out of sight (see this guideline for details).
2. Importance of a primary caretaker.

C. Intellectual

1. The baby's crying at mother's going out of sight is the beginning of memory development and baby's striving to control his world. Parents' need to understand that this is a necessary step toward reaching out of himself and not hindering this development with over-indulgence.

III. **High Risk Factors**

A. No consistent caretaker to whom he can develop a relationship.

IV. **See guidelines for Safety and Accident Prevention**

NOTES

ANTICIPATORY GUIDANCE FOR THE PERIOD OF 2–4 MONTHS

I. Expectations of this period

The responsive smile is one of the first important evidences that the baby is beginning to take the outside world into account. As his physical systems stabilize and mature, his energies are freed, enabling him to become aware of what is going on around him. Although he continues to respond instinctively, he is developing a reactive pattern to his world. He reacts joyfully and energetically to care that is consistent and loving. He reacts with crying and irritability when his basic needs are not met. By 4 months of age his reactions arc less instinctive, and he begins to respond in a manner that will best serve his own purpose.

A. Mother
   1. Responsive to baby's rhythms and signals.
   2. Able to define and appreciate baby's individuality.

B. Baby
   1. Responding to primary caretaker with responsive smile, extended eye contact, turning to voice.
   2. Comforted and quieted easily.
      a. Increased awareness of separation from mother causes distressful crying.
      b. Need of parents to understand and appreciate this first clash of wills.
      c. Playing music and keeping baby around family activities may help dispel this feeling of desertion.
      d. Too frequent changes of caretakers may inhibit the development of this first important step toward attachment.

II. Family status

A. Basic needs being met
   1. If referrals made, follow up to be sure that appropriate help is received.
   2. Adequate support system available.

B. Parents
   1. Adjustment to and enjoyment of new roles.
   2. Understanding of symbiotic role of mother and baby and that both will have a broadened emotional base by 4 months.
   3. Knowledge and appreciation of childhood developmental tasks.

C. Child abuse indicators
   1. Maladjustment to new roles and responsibilities.
      a. Fatique and poor health in parents.
      b. Crankiness in baby.
   2. Unrelieved social and emotional pressures.
   3. Aggressive pattern of behavior.
   4. Parents abused in their childhood.

III. Health patterns

A. Nutrition
   1. Formula or breast milk continues to be adequate nutrition.
   2. Do not substitute with cow's milk.
   3. Water offered between feedings, particularly in warm weather, as baby loses fluids quickly; color and odor of urine indicate state of hydration.

4. Baby beginning to develop pattern of eating 5–6 times/day; night feedings continue until larger amount taken during day; stomach has 4- to 6-oz capacity.
5. Baby held for bottle-feeding to continue development of close mother-baby relationship. Baby should never be given a bottle in bed. He will fall asleep with the bottle in his mouth. Sleeping this way can lead to tooth decay, due to prolonged exposure to lactose, the sugar in milk.
6. If baby continues fussing after and between feedings, investigate other areas of need satisfaction. Schedule office visit if problem continues.

B. Sleep
   1. Sleeps for longer periods (8 hours); total of 15–16 hr/day.
   2. Night feedings discontinued when able to take larger feedings during day.
   3. Sleeps through family noises—being kept within family activity area or having music played during naps continues ability to sleep through normal sound levels.
   4. By 4 months of age, baby is aware of separation from mother and may have difficulty falling asleep.

C. Elimination
   1. Stools. Maturation of GI tract allows better fluid absorption, so stools firmer and less frequent.
   2. Urine. Kidneys not functioning at mature level until 4 months of age; dehydration still a concern.

IV. Growth and development

A. Physical
   1. Central nervous system. Myelination continues in a cephalocaudal direction.
      a. Fastest growing system; adequate nutrition essential for maximum development.
      b. Head: from resting on crib to being held at midline.
      c. Arms: from random to purposeful movements.
      d. Hands: baby opens and closes hands; thumbs held in grasping position.
      e. Extremities: legs more vigorously active, held off crib.
      f. Vision: bifocal vision develops when head held at midline. Mother observes "finding" hands, scrutiny of faces, attraction to colors.
      g. Hearing: sound discrimination (recognizing voices). Mother observes baby turning toward sound of her voice.

B. Emotional development. Basic trust continues to be established.
   1. Primary caretaker provides consistent loving care. Too many different caretakers can interfere with the establishment of basic trust.
   2. Baby responds to caretaker by vocalizing, making eye contact, and smiling.

C. Intellectual development
   1. Reactive patterns becoming more stable and consistent—quiet or noisy, energetic or passive, joyful or somber.
   2. Awareness of and attachment to primary caretaker established, but object permanence (memory) not yet present, so there are distress signals if baby observes mother/primary caretaker leaving.

3. Language: experimenting with making sounds; pays close attention to mother's mouth as she talks to him.

D. High-risk factors
   1. No loving primary caretaker.
   2. A cranky, inconsolable baby.

E. Child-rearing practices
   1. A consistent schedule; few changes for visits or visitors.
   2. Touching, rubbing, rocking needed in addition to food and sleep.
   3. Early intervention for concerns and problems.

F. Stimulation
   1. Communication and sounds
      a. Sing to child.
      b. Encourage smiling, laughing.
      c. Use music and rhythms only as a quiet background.
      d. Introduce sounds—running water, rattles, household noises.
   2. Touch and smell
      a. Cuddling, holding, kissing, stroking,
      b. Feed and change from both sides.
   3. Sight
      a. Single bright object such as mobile 12 in. from eyes—change frequently.
      b. Move objects in arcs and circles for eyes to follow.
   4. Gross motor
      a. Exercise arms and legs while bathing.
      b. Place baby on stomach on a firm surface (preferably the floor, if safe from siblings and animals).
      c. Help baby roll over—first from stomach to back.
      d. Use bounce chair for increasing leg strength and enjoyment of body movement.
   5. Fine motor
      a. Give objects of various textures to handle.
      b. Bring hands together around bottle or toy.
      c. Provide bright objects for eyes to follow.
   6. Feeding. Make feeding a relaxed and pleasant time, staying within scheduled time of every 3–4 hours.
   7. Schedule. A consistent daily routine helps establish body rhythms and anticipatory responses.
   8. Watch for baby's cues of over stimulation.

G. Safety
   1. Accidents happen most frequently
      a. When usual routine changes (holidays, vacations, illness in the family).
      b. Following stressful events for caretakers.
      c. When caretakers are tired or ill.
      d. Late in the afternoon.

2. Accident prevention
   a. Crib should be away from window and curtain cords.
   b. Fire: baby should never be left in house alone.
   c. Have house equipped with smoke alarms.
   d. Baby should never be in car without proper car seat; never held in adult's lap; all adults should be in seat belts.
   e. Baby seat: baby strapped in; set in safe, protected area.
   f. All objects smaller than 2 in. should be kept out of baby's reach.
   g. Not left alone on bed or couch. Developing strength makes it possible to roll over or hitch himself to edge and roll off.
3. Not all injuries are accidents. Investigate possible child abuse and neglect.
4. Instructions to baby-sitters
5. Emergency telephone numbers posted

OVERVIEW

4-MONTH WELL CHILD VISIT

I. **Parents**

A. Able to describe the effects of the new baby on all the family members.

B. Show appreciation for baby's increasing physical skills, individual temperament, and his way of reaching out and getting attention from those around him.

II. **Baby**

A. Physical

1. Weight and height continues on previous pattern on growth chart.
2. Holding head in mid-line. Purposeful reaching out.

B. Emotional

1. Turning to mother when distressed.
2. Fussing when mother goes out of sight.

C. Intellectual

1. Purposeful repetition of activities.

III. **High Risk Factors**

A. Mother-Parents' dissatisfaction with new role of parenting.

B. Baby difficult to comfort.

IV. **See guidelines for specifics of physical exam.**

NOTES

4-MONTH WELL CHILD VISIT

I. **Developmental process.**

The close symbiotic relationship of mother and child is changing in the direction of individualization for both of them.

A. Mother

1. Return to prepregnant health pattern (weight and energy level).
2. Coping with family responsibilities.
3. Relating to other family members.
4. Developing or returning to outside interests.
5. Appreciation of importance to baby of one primary caretaker.

B. Baby

1. Schedules for feeding and sleeping established.
2. Investigating environment: reaching out with arms; grasping with hands; searching with eyes.
3. Social awareness: smiling and vocalizing for reaction from mother; crying at separation from family.

II. **Family status**

A. Concerns and problems. Ability to identify problems and to cope; understanding of problem-solving techniques.

B. Siblings. Parents' understanding of siblings' adjustment to family changes.

C. Adequate support system for all members.

III. **Health habits**

A. Nutrition

1. Mother
    a. Breast-feeding: understanding of dietary requirements.
    b. Weight control. Adequate diet.
    c. Use of drugs, cigarettes, stimulants.
2. Baby
    a. Breast milk or formula with iron per office protocol; five feedings daily; amount depends on weight and correlation of weight with length (as shown on growth chart); no other foods needed.
    b. Water offered between feedings if strong odor and color of urine indicate need for more fluids.

B. Sleep

1. One long sleep period of 6–8 hours; total of 15 hours/day.
2. Awake for ±2-hour periods with less fussing.
3. Crying when put to bed, as baby is aware of separation from parent.

C. Elimination

1. Bowel movements are not formed but are now less frequent.
2. Urine. Important to note color, odor, and amount.

IV. **Growth and development**

A. Physical

1. Central nervous system. Increased myelination.
    a. Holds head at midline while prone; lifts head and chest while supine.

b. Body: rolls from front to back.
c. Extremities: arms beginning purposeful reaching; hands open, beginning to grasp; legs held off crib, vigorous kicking.

2. Vision. Bifocal, staring, searching.
3. Speech. Experimenting with sounds; attempting to imitate.
4. Hearing. Localizing sound; quieted by pleasant sounds (voice and music).

B. Emotional development—Erikson: basic trust—adaptation through experience. An environment providing adequate physical care and consistent, loving attention fosters the feeling that the world is a safe and dependable place.

1. Appropriate physical growth.
2. Baby relaxed, easily quieted.
3. Baby turns to caretaker when distressed.

C. Intellectual development—Piaget. From 4–6 months of age, automatic and random reactions are progressing to purposeful repetition of activities to form patterns of intentional action. Baby now begins to adapt his behavior through the following experiences:

1. Anticipating and waiting (for feeding, to be picked up).
2. Fascinating caretakers with sparkling eyes, vigorous body activity, gurgles, and smiles as a repetitive response to loving care.

D. High-risk factors

1. Mother
   a. Dissatisfaction with role of motherhood.
   b. Unresponsive/overresponsive to baby.
   c. Unable to tune into baby's signals.
2. Baby
   a. Feeding problems; failure to thrive.
   b. Excessive activity and crying.
   c. Difficult to comfort; unresponsive.
3. Child abuse indicators: parents
   a. Inability to quiet baby; feeding problems.
   b. Fatigue; overload of responsibilities.
   c. Inadequate support system.
   d. Aggression as a reactive pattern.

V. Physical examination

A. Growth

1. Length commensurate with established pattern.
2. Weight varying with caloric intake, energy level, and illnesses. Weight within 2 standard deviations of length.
3. Genetic factors should be considered.

B. Appearance

1. Color still easily affected by environment and activity.
2. Movements smooth and coordinated.
3. Legs: alternate flexing.

C. Specific factors to note while doing routine physical examination

1. Anterior fontanelle measurements. Bulging, depressed.

2. Skin. Seborrhea, rashes, bruises, burns.
3. Heart sounds. Refer to physician if murmur present.
4. Hips. Equal leg folds, full abductions.
5. Extremities. Forefoot adduction.
6. Reflexes. Still present but of diminished intensity; check for head lag and poor muscle tone.

D. Mother-child interaction
1. Mother. Holding baby close to her body, making eye contact when baby responds; able to quiet baby.
2. Baby. Responsive to mother's attention.

VI. Assessment

A. Physical
B. Developmental
C. Emotional
D. Environmental

VII. Plan

A. Immunizations
B. Screening. Laboratory tests and developmental screening as indicated.
C. Problem list (devised with parent); SOAP for each.
D. Appropriate timing for office, home, and/or telephone visits.

OVERVIEW

ANTICIPATORY GUIDANCE FOR THE PERIOD OF 4–6 MONTHS

I. **Parents**

A. Responsive to baby's needs.

B. Asking for help if concerned.

II. **Baby**

A. Physical

1. Increased vigorous body movements.
2. Appropriate weight and height gain.
3. Eating and sleeping with schedule established.

B. Emotional

1. See guidelines for discussion of separation anxiety.
2. Responding to attention with smiles, gurgles, reaching out.

C. Intellectual

1. Beginning of object-permanence (memory). Will begin to accept that mother's absence is not permanent.

III. **High Risk Factors**

A. Low growth rate.

B. Apathetic. Difficult to comfort.

C. No loving primary caretaker

IV. **See guidelines for Child-Rearing Practices and Accident Prevention**

NOTES

ANTICIPATORY GUIDANCE FOR THE PERIOD OF 4–6 MONTHS

I. Expectations of this period

A. A delightful period of a now physically well-organized baby who is turning outward to his caretakers and environment and finding that his activities can influence the outside world.

1. Parents
   - **a.** Responding to baby's overtures for approval and attention.
   - **b.** Concerned at negative behavior—investigating and asking for professional help if unsuccessful in understanding and coping.
   - **c.** Providing loving, approving primary caretaker.
2. Baby
   - **a.** Gurgles, smiles, vigorous body movements, and sustained eye contact get responses of approval and attention.
   - **b.** Increased fussing, wakefulness, and poor feeding also get attention and will become a pattern of response if that is the only way attention is obtained.

B. Separation anxiety. Baby has an increased awareness of primary caretaker, and object permanence (memory) is not sufficiently developed for baby to realize that disappearance of caretaker is not permanent.

1. Mother. Understanding problem of separation anxiety; keeping crib in family area; family noises not diminished for baby. Voice contact and music may help this transitory problem.
2. Baby. Fussing at being left at bedtime; even mother's walking out of a room causes tears of anguish.

II. Family status

A. Parents providing adequate environment for each family member.

B. Parents understanding developmental needs of each child.

C. Sufficient support system for parents' needs; not using children as only means of gratification.

III. Health patterns

A. Nutrition

1. Baby continues to require 50 cal/lb or 100 kcal/kg daily.
2. Breast milk or formula only food needed until ±6 months of age.
3. Vitamins and fluoride continued per office protocol.
4. A consistent growth pattern is one of the indicators of the state of nutrition.
5. Continued fussing or crying after feeding: investigate reasons other than hunger (discomfort, unsatisfied sucking instinct, need for comfort or cuddling). Schedule office visit if problem continues.

B. Feeding

1. Stabilized schedule: sleeping through the night (8 hours); as size of stomach increasing, larger feedings possible during the day.
2. Tongue thrust diminishing.
3. Taste buds mature; taste discrimination present.
4. Solid foods not needed for proper nutrition; add rice cereal with iron only if food is to be introduced.

5. Be alert to overfeeding. A healthy baby is best able to regulate when and how much to eat. Parents should pay attention to signals and not force extra formula.

C. Drooling
1. Increased activity of salivary glands—not an indication of teething.
2. Up to 2 years before automatic swallowing is present.

D. Sleep. Fussy at bedtime.
1. Try leaving dim light or music on.
2. Keep baby in crib, but bring to where family is; baby is self-quieting with the security of being near others.

E. Elimination
1. Bowel movements less water, better formed as GI tract matures.
2. Distention caused by undigested foods or illness: limit diet by eliminating all foods but formula; if it continues, dilute formula with water; call office if no improvement.
3. Urine. Watch color and amount; if there is a change, increase fluids; call office if no improvement.

IV. Growth and development

A. Physical
1. Central nervous system still the fastest growing system; adequate nutrition mandatory for its development.
2. Gross motor skills. Able to sit with support; rolling over; putting weight on feet; enjoying bounce chair.
3. Fine motor skills. Reaching out and grasping; bringing hand to mouth at will.

B. Speech
1. Experimenting with making sounds; trying to repeat them.
2. Paying attention to mouth action of caretaker; attempting to imitate.
3. Listening to own sounds; attempting to repeat.

C. Emotional development—Erikson. This period is the beginning of the baby's establishment of trust in himself. By his beguiling ways, he enchants his caretakers into providing him with attention, and he learns to repeat the activities that bring him this attention.
1. Smiling, vocalizing, making good eye contact.
2. Has a loving, approving primary caretaker with whom a positive response pattern can be developed.

D. Intellectual development—Piaget. developing object permanence (memory) by finding consistent results from his own activities and from those of others.
1. Beginning to realize that if mother leaves, she will return.
2. Anticipating events of daily routine.
3. Spends much time repeating simple activities.
   a. Reaching out and touching: has awareness of sizes, shapes, textures.
   b. Listening: shows recognition of familiar voices and sounds; responds to rhythms.
   c. Looking: is fascinated by faces (even his own reflection), varied colors and shapes.

d. Large muscle development: enjoys free activity, bounce chair, and swing; hitches body to reach out and grasp toys.

e. Body confidence: enjoys being tossed, swung high (swinging or lifting by arms can dislocate elbows).

4. Language: parents respond to baby's vocalizing; baby attempts to imitate and repeat sounds.

E. High-risk factors

1. Parents

a. Inability to cope with problems.

b. Lack of pleasure and satisfaction in child care.

c. Not understanding importance of child development principles.

2. Baby

a. Physical developmental lag.

b. Nutritional deprivation and inadequate growth pattern.

c. Emotional immaturity: unresponsive; no eye contact; dominant mood of fussiness.

d. Inadequate child care; no one significant person as caretaker.

F. Child-rearing practices

1. Regular schedule with as few interruptions as possible; baby's learning to anticipate events is helped by consistency of schedule.

2. Demanding of attention. Respond within reason; provide other stimulations, such as variety in toys, sounds, things to look at (as putting crib in another part of house).

3. Weaning. Separation awareness at 4–5 months is a difficult period for baby, so weaning is more easily accomplished at 3 months or at 6 months.

4. Day-care centers. Ratio of caretakers to infants is 1:3; visual and auditory stimulation provided; opportunity to exercise (not kept in crib all the time); time for caretaker to hold and cuddle.

5. Baby-sitter. Careful selection; know personally or get references; set up job description, pay schedule, telephone contacts.

G. Stimulation

1. Communication and sounds

a. Call child by name.

b. Tell child what you are doing; name objects.

c. Point out various sounds—whispering, the wind, cars, animals.

d. Keep background of soft music. Too loud music prevents learning from usual sounds of environment.

2. Touch and smell

a. Rub baby with different textures—silk, feather, wood, yarn.

b. Play touching games such as "this little piggy."

c. Point out various odors—flowers, cloths, foods.

3. Sight

a. Move crib around room; move infant to different rooms and near windows.

b. Use bright sheets, blankets, clothing.

c. Hold baby up to a mirror to see his reflection.

4. Gross motor
    a. Sitting position for short periods.
    b. Sits up on a mat on the floor.
5. Fine motor
    a. Colorful plastic keys on a ring.
    b. Cradle gym.

H. Safety

1. Accidents happen most frequently
    a. When usual routine changes (holidays, vacations, illness in family).
    b. Following stressful events for caretakers.
    c. When caretakers are tired or ill.
    d. Late in the afternoon.
2. Accident prevention
    a. Crib should be away from open window and curtain cords.
    b. Fire: baby should never be left in house alone. Have house equipped with smoke alarms.
    c. Baby should never be in car without proper car seat; never held in adult's lap; all adults should be in seat belts.
    d. Baby seat: baby strapped in; set in safe, protected area.
    e. All objects smaller than 2 in. should be kept out of baby's reach.
    f. Caretakers should be alert to baby's developing ability to become self-propelled.
3. Not all injuries are accidents. Investigate possible child abuse and neglect.
4. Instructions to baby-sitters
5. Emergency telephone numbers posted.

OVERVIEW

6-MONTH WELL CHILD VISIT

I. **Parents**
   - A. Appreciation of baby's developing personality and skills.
   - B. Providing safe environment for increased mobility of baby.

II. **Baby**
   - A. Physical
     1. Sitting without support.
     2. Transfers objects from one hand to the other.
     3. Teething.
        - a. Making for cranky baby.
        - b. Increased incidents of U.R.I.
   - B. Emotional
     1. Keen observer of what is going on around him.
     2. Responding to music and motion.
     3. Turns to caretaker for support and comfort.
   - C. Intellectual
     1. Random activities replaced by purposeful actions.

III. **High Risk Factors**
   - A. Poor weight gain.
   - B. Frequent illnesses.
   - C. Check safety guidelines.

IV. **See Guidelines for specifics of Physical Examination**

NOTES

6-MONTH WELL CHILD VISIT

I. **Developmental process.**

Less vibrant personality, becoming the student, concentrating on what is going on around him, repetitive activities replace random movements.

A. Mother
1. Understanding developmental principles and appreciation of the baby's accomplishments.
2. Developing a philosophy of child-rearing practices.
3. Providing adequate stimulation and a safe environment.

B. Baby
1. Sitting propped up or in a baby seat, scrutinizing all that can be touched and seen.
2. Particularly scrutinizing his primary caretaker.

II. **Family status**

A. Basic needs being met.

B. Marital stability

C. Single parent
1. Needs being identified and goals established.
2. Referrals: provide with follow-up.
3. Visits scheduled to provide support and help in establishing healthy child-rearing practices.

D. Parents
1. Concerns and problems: ability to identify problems and to cope.
2. Realistic assessment and appropriate expectations of baby's development.
3. Deriving satisfaction and pleasure from parental role.
4. Mother's role defined—student, working, special interests, adequate support system.
5. Child care arrangements—day-care centers, baby-sitters.

III. **Health habits**

A. Nutrition—diet history
1. Breast-feeding: supplementary formula, weaning.
2. Formula: number of feedings and amount.
3. Vitamins and fluoride per office protocol.
4. Other foods: rice cereal with iron the first food.

B. Sleep
1. Sleeps for 8-hour period at night.
2. Awake for 4-hour periods.
3. Less fussing when put to bed.

C. Elimination
1. Bowel movements less frequent, better formed; distention and flatulence with diet change.
2. Urine better concentrated; color and odor used as indicators of hydration.

IV. **Growth and development**

A. Physical

1. Central nervous system
   a. Vertical position possible, with ability to sit and hold head erect.
   b. Puts weight on legs; stands with support.
   c. Grasping with both hands; transfers from one hand to another.
2. Teething
   a. Usually the first teeth cause physical discomfort; succeeding eruptions are less difficult.
   b. Importance of night bottle syndrome understood.
3. A period of low immunity, causing susceptibility to infections.
4. Vision. Improved distance vision and depth perception; staring at objects or movement at distance.
5. Speech
   a. One-syllable babbling; attempts to imitate sounds.
   b. Watches intently the mouth of someone speaking to him.

B. Emotional development—Erikson. Establishment of basic trust is evident by the baby's now turning out to explore his environment. He is eager to touch, feel, and taste all within his reach. He watches his caretakers in particular. Establishing a close attachment to one person who can give support to his explorations is a preliminary step toward the next developmental task of beginning the path toward independence.
   1. Eager to touch, feel, and mouth all things within his reach.
   2. Watches results of activity with surprise and pleasure.
   3. Responds to mood of caretaker.
   4. Keen observer of activities of caretaker.

C. Intellectual development—Piaget. development of object permanence (memory). The repetition of activities and the finding of a consistency of results replace random movements with purposeful activity. Baby attempts to repeat the kind of activity that affects the care and attention he receives.
   1. Anticipating events of daily schedule.
   2. Responding to familiar voices and sounds.
   3. Crying and fussing more selectively.
   4. Delight at return of primary caretaker.
   5. Language: may be less vocal, as main concern is observing his environment and his caretakers.

D. High-risk factors
   1. Mother
      a. Unresponsive to baby's cues.
      b. Restlessness at confinement of parental role.
      c. Overprotective: keeping as "baby"; giving little stimulation or opportunity for physical activity or new adventure.
      d. Not providing one consistent caretaker.
   2. Baby
      a. Not attempting to reach out.
      b. Lack of body confidence; rigid body movement.
      c. Unsatisfied needs; whininess.
      d. No loving, approving primary caretaker.

E. Child abuse indicators: parents
   1. Low self-esteem—lack of confidence and competence in managing their world.
   2. Rigid response pattern.
   3. Marital conflict.
   4. Fatigue; overload of responsibilities.
   5. Inadequate support system.
   6. Child abuse in own childhood.

V. Physical examination

A. Growth. Continues on established pattern; check for excess or inadequate weight gain.

B. Appearance and behavior
   1. Chubby.
   2. Sits with support.
   3. Good head control.
   4. Happy, bright-eyed; a delightful member of the family; not generally fussy or fearful.

C. Specific factors to note while doing routine physical examination
   1. Anterior fontanelles. Bulging, depressed.
   2. Skin. Check for seborrhea, rashes, bruises, burns.
   3. Eyes. Check for equal tracking.
   4. Teeth. May be erupting; gums swollen.
   5. Heart sounds. Refer to physician if murmur present.
   6. Hips. Equal leg folds, full abductions.
   7. Extremities. Forefoot adduction.
   8. Reflexes. Disappearance of tonic neck reflex, Moro reflex; sucking and rooting (when awake), palmar grasp still present.

D. Mother–child interaction
   1. Mother
      a. Holding baby less close.
      b. Willing to have others care for baby.
   2. Baby
      a. Responding to others.
      b. Turns to mother for comfort.

VI. Assessment

A. Physical
B. Developmental
C. Emotional
D. Environmental

VII. Plan

A. Immunizations and laboratory tests as needed.
B. Problem list (devised with parent)—SOAP for each.
C. Appropriate timing for office, home, and/or telephone visits.

OVERVIEW

ANTICIPATORY GUIDANCE FOR THE PERIOD OF 6–8 MONTHS

I. **Parents**

A. Understanding physical changes.

B. Asking for help as needed.

C. Show pride and affection for baby.

II. **See Guidelines for specifics of "stranger anxiety."**

III. **Baby**

A. Physical

1. Increased activity. Losing chubbiness.
2. Rolling over and reaching out to obtain what he wants.
3. Teething and illnesses less a problem by 8 months.
4. See Guidelines for introduction of new foods and homemade baby food.

B. Emotional

1. Illnesses, new activities, and adventures broadening emotional responses.
2. Needs primary caretaker for comfort and support.

C. Intellectual

1. Watch persistence in trial and error to accomplish new skills. Frequent failures can cause frustrations and fussiness.

IV. **High Risk Factors**

A. Safety.

B. Frequent illnesses.

V. **See Guidelines for specifics of Child-Rearing Practices and Safety Protocols**

NOTES

ANTICIPATORY GUIDANCE FOR THE PERIOD OF 6–8 MONTHS

I. Expectations of this period

A. Baby

1. Increased awareness.
   a. Insatiable desire to investigate; reaching out to touch, taste, and scrutinize.
2. Baby is increasingly fussy, since s/he wants to reach out and experiment and is frustrated when unable to do so.

B. Parents

1. Positive reinforcement of baby's accomplishments.
2. Provide stimulating but safe environment.

C. Stranger anxiety

1. By 8 months of age, object permanence (memory) is present. Baby can now identify from whom he most often receives attention and comfort, and he appears to concentrate his attention on this one person. Other adults seem to interfere with his efforts to form a close attachment to this primary caretaker and so are rejected.
2. This attachment is the beginning of the baby's forming the emotional capability for future relationships of trust and love.
3. Lack of stranger anxiety can indicate that the baby has no one significant caretaker.

II. Family status

A. Basic needs being met; assess coping ability; refer as needed.

B. Problem-solving techniques used.

C. Parents

1. Appreciation and evaluation of child's developmental progress.
2. Understanding of the individuality of each child.

III. Health patterns

A. Nutrition

1. Breast-feeding. Solids should be introduced by 6 months; breast milk is low in iron and may not contain enough protein for the baby's needs.
2. Weaning. There is no right time for weaning; it depends on the mother's schedule and feelings and the baby's cues. Delay if the baby is fussy from teething or ill; do it slowly, over a week or more. Follow office protocol for change from breast to formula.
3. Vitamins and fluoride continued per office protocol.

B. Introduction of new foods

1. Add one new food at a time (per week) so an allergic reaction can be identified.
2. Cereal is the first new food; start with iron-fortified rice cereal, which is the least allergic cereal; use dry cereal mixed with apple juice, formula, or breast milk. Begin with 1–2 tbsp once a day, increasing gradually to $1/3$–$1/2$ cup, total, fed twice a day. If this is tolerated, barley or oatmeal can be tried.
3. Vegetables or fruits are the second food; 1 tsp at a time working up to 3–4 tbsp of fruits and vegetables by 1 year of age.

a. Vegetables should be introduced first, since they are harder to "learn" to like than fruits, which are sweeter. Begin with green ones, then yellow.

b. Fruits. Bananas and applesauce are constipating; pears, peaches, and prunes are bowel softeners.

4. Egg yolk can be given at 6 months of age; hard boil and strain over foods. Delay introduction of egg whites until all other foods have been introduced.

5. Meats. Introduce last. Try all kinds. Buy the jars of meat; mixed dinners have only small amounts of meat.

6. Do not feed from the jar unless the whole jar is to be used, since saliva from the spoon stays in the jar and can cause spoilage. Refrigerate any food not used.

7. Most commercially prepared baby foods contain no preservatives and are acceptable. *Do not* season with salt or sugar. These are not necessary and can lead to poor eating habits.

C. Homemade baby foods

1. Equipment needed

a. Electric blender, food processor, or food mill.

b. Clean pans for cooking.

c. Utensils: vegetable brush, spatula, peeler, knife.

d. Ice cube trays, preferably those that have separate "pop-out" cubes.

2. Freezing and serving

a. After food is prepared and pureed, pour into the pop-out ice cube trays.

b. Freeze quickly.

c. Pop out frozen cubes, and put into plastic freezer bags; label and date.

d. Each cube contains about 3 tbsp.

e. Before a meal, take out food cubes and thaw in the refrigerator or warm in a warming dish or in an egg poacher over hot water.

f. Cubes travel well for short trips; they defrost quickly.

3. Food preparation

a. Fruits

(1) Fresh fruits retain the best nutritional value; however, juice-packed canned or frozen fruits may also be used.

(2) Cooked fresh or canned fruits blend very well into a fine puree.

(3) Do not add sugar; babies prefer the natural sweetness in fruits.

(4) Pureed fruits can be added to cottage cheese or plain yogurt (a good source of protein, calcium, and riboflavin).

b. Vegetables

(1) Fresh vegetables have the best nutritional quality; frozen vegetables are more convenient; canned vegetables are already cooked and need only be pureed.

(2) Use canned vegetables that have no salt.

c. Meats, poultry

(1) Meats tend to shred in the blender rather than puree; if ground first, they are easier to puree; add 1 cup of liquid per pound of ground meat.

(2) Chicken livers puree very well.

(3) Meats should be cooked by braising or roasting; not frying; no seasoning is necessary.

d. Fish

(1) Should be poached or baked; preferably cod, haddock, or flounder.

(2) Do not give shellfish to infants—can cause allergies.

(3) One pound of fish yields about eight food cubes.

e. All foods can be combined to make stewlike dinners; meat, potato, and vegetable, for example, can be pureed together; seasoning is not necessary.

4. Freezer life of home-prepared baby foods

a. Temperature must be 0°F or below; use a true freezer or a separate-door freezer/refrigerator combination; freezer compartment inside refrigerator does not stay cold enough.

b. Timetable for keeping foods

Fruits	6 months
Vegetables	4 months
Meats	3 months
Liver	1 month
Fish	1 *week*
Poltry	3 months
Dried beans, peas, etc.	3 months
Combination dinners	2 months

5. Suggested readings

a. Castle, S. *The Complete Guide to Preparing Baby Foods at Home.* New York: Bantam, 1992.

b. Lansky, V. *Feed Me! I'm Yours.* New York: Bantam, 1994.

c. Satter, E. *Child of Mine: Feeding with Love and Good Sense.* Palo Alto, CA: Bull, 1991.

d. Sturtz, George S., & Zabriskie, Susan L. *Common Sense Guide to Growth and Nutrition.* Hojack Publishing Company, 1991.

e. *Boston Children's Hospital. Parents' Guide to Nutrition.* Reading, MA: Addison Wesley, 1987.

D. Establishing good eating habits

1. Baby will take sufficient food for his needs. When satiated he does not take food from spoon, pulls back—do not force food.

2. Babies are messy—will spit out food, throw food, upset dish, not sit still.

3. Establish *always* a quiet, matter-of-fact manner.

4. Nutritional patterns established during infancy can have lifelong effects.

a. Feeding is a learned experience; each child develops at his own rate.

b. Food preferences are acquired.

c. Ethnic patterns influence food preferences.

E. Sleep

1. Less fussing at bedtime; may need favorite toy or blanket.

2. Sleeps through the night; awakes early, does not cry; can amuse himself for a short period.
3. Still needs two naps.

F. Elimination

1. New foods are usually no problem if added slowly; if a problem does occur, eliminate the new food and try again later in small amounts.
2. Urine. Continue to check amount, color, and odor for indication of hydration.

IV. Growth and development

A. Physical

1. Teething. Baby's first experience with pain; usually the first tooth is the most bothersome. Reduce gum swelling and pain by providing a cold, wet cloth to chew on.
2. Low immunity. Susceptible to infections; own immune system still immature, and protection from maternal antigens diminished.

Table 1-1. Schedule of teeth eruption

Teeth	Age
Primary	
Lower central incisors	5–10 months
Upper central incisors	8–12 months
Upper lateral incisors	8–12 months
Lower lateral incisors	12–14 months
Lower & upper first molars	12–14 months
Lower & upper canines	16–22 months
Lower & upper second molars	24–30 months
Secondary	
First molars	5–7 years
Central incisors	6½–8 years
Lateral incisors	7–9 years
First bicuspids	9–11 years
Second bicuspids	10–12 years
Canines	10–12 years
Cuspids	11–14 years
Second molars	11–13 years
Third molars	16–21 years (or later)

3. Gross motor skills. Progressing from immobile to self-propelled; sitting → creeping → crawling → standing is a long period of trial and error.
4. Fine motor skills. Use of hands to reach out, grasp, and let go at will; touching as a means of investigating; reaching out as a perceptual motor skill.

5. Speech
   a. Attempting to duplicate sounds; repeats syllables such as dada, mama.
   b. Babbles contentedly to himself on waking.

B. Emotional development—Erikson. Establishment of basic trust gives the baby the assurance to investigate his environment. This is done tentatively with looking back at or returning to mother for reassurance. A significant caretaker is needed to provide encouragement for these new adventures.
   1. Increased awareness of movement, color, sounds.
      a. Keen observer of movement, color, sounds.
      b. Reaching out to touch and hold.
      c. Fascinated by looking at and picking up small objects.
   2. A dangerous period, since the baby is physically able to get to more places and cannot be trusted "not to do it again."

C. Intellectual development—Piaget. Object permanence (memory) is becoming better developed, and the baby is using repetitive actions to establish purposeful activity.
   1. Repetitive actions are building up memory of cause and effect.
   2. Developing control by persistent trial and error; gets to sitting position unaided; uses legs to get around in a walker; manages to crawl in the right direction and around obstacles. Frequent failures cause increase in frustration and fussiness.
   3. Language
      a. Enjoys being talked and sung to; responds to rhythms.
      b. Attention to goings-on around him supersedes concentration on vocal development.
      c. Responds to caretaker's tone of voice.

D. High-risk factors
   1. Mother
      a. Unable to cope with baby's periods of frustration.
      b. Not providing stimulating environment; baby given no opportunity to move about freely.
      c. Child abuse indicators present.
   2. Baby
      a. Physical developmental lag.
      b. Passivity—does not attempt to reach out and investigate.
      c. No loving, approving, consistent caretaker.

E. Child-rearing practices
   1. Increased fussy periods can be due to frustration at not being able to get at or have what he wants.
   2. The baby's being persistent and difficult to distract makes life more complicated for both caretakers and baby.
   3. Use tone of voice to show approval or disapproval of baby's activities.
   4. Environment important.
      a. Area large enough to satisfy new skill of crawling.
      b. Safety the main factor.
         (1) Baby cannot be trusted to control behavior.

(2) Eliminate all small objects, since everything possible is put in mouth.

(3) Almost constant surveillance is necessary; siblings and baby-sitters need careful instructions.

F. Stimulation

1. Communication and sounds

a. Praise language attempts, but do not overemphasize.

b. Provide toys that make noise or music.

c. Sing and talk to baby; demonstrate rhythms.

2. Touch and smell

a. Provide various motions, such as swinging, water play, dancing.

b. Tickling and touching games.

c. Textured and patterned objects to handle.

d. Identify different odors.

3. Sight

a. Alternate toy selection—divide into groups, change groups frequently.

b. Mirror play.

c. Indicate outdoor objects in motion—trucks, cars, birds, airplanes.

4. Gross motor

a. Rock back and forth on beach ball on stomach.

b. Support while sitting—sitting alone.

c. Water play.

d. Rides on parents' shoulders.

e. Jumper swing—feet supported.

f. Open, safe area for crawling.

5. Fine motor

a. Blocks, lids, pans to bang.

b. Various-sized containers to fill and empty.

c. Small objects of various shapes to handle (large enough not to be swallowed).

6. Feeding

a. Offer cup.

b. Finger foods—crackers or hard toast (i.e., zwieback), especially when baby is teething.

c. Baby dips fingers into foods, brings them to mouth.

G. Safety

1. Accidents happen most frequently

a. When usual routine changes (holidays, vacations, illness in family).

b. Following stressful events for caretakers.

c. When caretakers are tired or ill.

d. Late in the afternoon.

2. Accident prevention

a. Baby-proof house.

b. Mobility: be prepared for unexpected mobility of baby; new skills make constant surveillance necessary.
c. Beware that all objects picked up go into the mouth.
d. Choking: first aid instruction per office protocol.
e. Water safety: never leave baby alone in tub or wading pool.
f. Provide safe spot for baby when caretaker is out of sight (e.g., playpen, crib).
g. Use proper car seat at all times.

3. Investigate possibility of child abuse and neglect if many bruises or burns are present.
4. Instructions to baby-sitters
5. Emergency telephone numbers posted

OVERVIEW

8-MONTH WELL CHILD VISIT

I. **Parents**

- A. Understanding baby's new needs of a safe environment to explore and investigate.
    - 1. Understand the baby's frustrations and anxiety from these new adventures.
- B. Rejecting all other adults, turns only to parent for comfort.

II. **Baby**

- A. Physical
    - 1. Increased mobility. Persistent in exploring.
    - 2. Increased interest in food.
    - 3. Difficulty in falling asleep.
- B. Emotional
    - 1. Developing confidence in his own capabilities.
    - 2. Finding ways to gain control of his world, such as refusing food, crying at parents' leaving, staying awake at night.
- C. Intellectual
    - 1. Increase in memory, helping him to rely on his world and repeat activities that get him attention.

III. **High Risk Factors**

- A. Mother's unrealistic expectations of baby.
- B. No primary caretaker to rely on.

IV. **See Guidelines for specific factors of the Physical Examination.**

NOTES

8-MONTH WELL CHILD VISIT

I. Developmental process.

This is a watershed period in which the physical and emotional patterns developed over the past 8 months provide new skills. With his increased physical abilities and the establishment of basic trust, the infant begins, in his own way, to test out and develop his capabilities. Erikson defines this process as moving from the stage of basic trust to the new stage of autonomy.

- A. Mother
  1. Has understanding of baby's new needs.
     - a. Provides adequate, safe environment for exploring.
     - b. Accepts baby's periods of frustrations and anxiety caused by his new adventures.
     - c. Develops a philosophy of child rearing to promote positive behavior patterns.
- B. Baby
  1. Eager to move about; frustrated at confinement.
  2. Persistent, less destructible.

II. Family status

- A. Parental concerns and problems. Ability to identify problems and to cope.
- B. Parental and sibling roles redefined to accommodate the increased activity and safety needs of the baby.
- C. Child care arrangements adequate to provide safety and promote development.

III. Health habits

- A. Nutrition
  1. Diet history. Tolerance and acceptance of new foods. Minced foods (including meat), enriched breads, potatoes, rice, and macaroni should be introduced, as well as cottage cheese, soft cheese, and egg yolks.
  2. Eating habits. Battleground for mother and baby; mother accepting and outwitting the uncooperative, independent baby. Baby can begin to sit with family at mealtime.
  3. Nutritional needs. Decrease in amount of cow's milk, breast milk, or formula to 12–16 oz/day; introduction of cup.
- B. Sleep
  1. Difficulty "turning off" to fall asleep.
  2. Awake for periods during the night.
  3. Fretful sleep—carrying over of daytime activities.
- C. Elimination
  1. General curiosity includes curiosity about feces.
  2. Parents' understand the physical and emotional components of toilet training techniques (see Anticipatory Guidance for the period of 14–18 months).
- D. Dental care
  1. Importance of night bottle syndrome understood.
  2. Teething: number of teeth; problems during eruptions.

E. Safety. This age is a dangerous period, since baby cannot be expected to control behavior. Safety checks:
   1. Lead paint. Check if in older house or apartment.
   2. Gates on stairs. Give time to climb stairs under surveillance.
   3. Electrical outlets capped.
   4. Cleaning fluids, soaps, medicines behind secured doors.
   5. Appropriate car seat used at all times.
   6. Safe place to put baby while not in caretaker's sight, such as playpen or crib.
   7. Constant surveillance of baby's activities by reliable caretaker.

IV. Growth and development

A. Physical
   1. Central nervous system. Myelination to extremities (giving strength and control).
   2. Immune system. Maternal antigens decreased; baby developing own immunity; particularly susceptible to upper respiratory infections.
   3. Hematopoietic system. Maternal red blood cells decreased; baby now developing sufficient red blood cells for his own needs. Iron fortified food.
   4. Vision. Eye/hand coordination, as well as depth perception, improving.
   5. Hearing. Reacts to whisper test; localizes sounds.

B. Emotional development—Erikson. With the security of basic trust the baby is now free to do the following:
   1. Become aware of the differences in people and sense their importance to him. For babies with strong support from a specific adult, other adults do not provide the same feeling of security; hence stranger anxiety.
   2. Move physically out into the environment with eagerness to use new physical skills to explore.
   3. Develop a sense of his own capabilities.
   4. Expand his emotional responses to new experiences.
      a. *Frustration* in the long process of learning new skills.
      b. *Anxiety* in leaving the safety of physical and emotional supports: walking without mother's hand, watching mother put on her coat to leave him with someone else.
      c. *Affection.* Returning to parent for encouragement and support.

C. Intellectual development—Piaget. Progressing from equilibrium to disequilibrium as new physical and emotional development produces new challenges.
   1. Intentional behavior replacing random responses with increasing ability to recall past experiences.
   2. Much practice in learning new skills.
   3. Language
      a. Repeats definitive sounds; beginning to understand the meanings of words (although unable to use them).
      b. Regularly stops activity when his name is called.

D. High-risk factors
   1. Mother

a. Unrealistic expectations of baby's control of behavior: over- or under-protective; coerces baby to perform desired behavior.
b. Dissatisfaction with role of parenting in this new phase (end of baby's complete dependency).
c. History of child abuse in her own family.

2. Baby
a. Not exhibiting drive to investigate surroundings.
b. A "too good baby"—shallow emotional responses.
c. Dull personality; irritable; nonloving.
d. No primary caretaker with whom to form loving relationship.

V. Physical examination

A. Growth. Continuing on established pattern; length, weight, and head circumference within 2 standard deviations.

B. Appearance and behavior
1. Less rotund; beginning to lengthen out.
2. Activity level: difficult to keep baby lying down on examination table, quieter on mother's lap.
3. Serious scrutiny of strangers; difficult to establish eye contact.

C. Specific factors to note while doing routine physical examination
1. Skin. Check for excessive bruising and burns, carotenemia.
2. Eyes. Equal tracking without strabismus.
3. Teeth. Central incisors present.
4. Ears. Check for mobility of tympanic membrane, ability to locate voice.
5. Musculoskeletal. Bearing weight on legs; hips—Ortolani's click, equal gluteal folds; check for tibial torsion, genu varum, externally rotated hips; check stance, gait.
6. Genitalia. Female—irritation, discharge; male—phimosis, descended testes.
7. Reflexes. Presence of parachute reflex; sucking and rooting no longer present.

D. Mother–child interaction
1. Baby turning to parent for support when frightened.
2. Cheerful, pleasant rapport between mother and child.

VI. Assessment

A. Physical
B. Developmental
C. Emotional
D. Environmental

VII. Plan

A. Screening. Hematocrit/lead/urine/developmental as indicated.
B. Problem list (devised with parent); SOAP for each.
C. Appropriate timing for office, home, and/or telephone visits.
1. Continue close contact during this critical period.
2. Visits planned according to the individual needs of the family and the developmental and physical needs of the baby.
3. Home visits to assess environment as indicated.

OVERVIEW

ANTICIPATORY GUIDANCE FOR THE PERIOD OF 8–14 MONTHS

I. **Parents**

A. Need to learn of the importance of this period so that they can continue their appreciation and understanding of their baby's free-wheeling activities. During this period, a quiet, consistent schedule is important.

II. **Baby**

A. Physical

1. Needs safe environment but with opportunity to investigate, examine, and use stored-up energy.

B. Emotional

1. Slowly beginning to accept behavior control for kind support and gentle reinforcement of appropriate behavior.

C. Intellectual

1. Recall of previous results of a particular activity.
2. Responds to caretaker's voice. Upset by disapproval.

III. **High Risk Factors**

A. Parents lack of understanding and unrealistic expectations.

B. Baby's lack of energy and curiosity in his environment.

IV. **See Guidelines for specific factors on Caretaking Arrangements.**

NOTES

ANTICIPATORY GUIDANCE FOR THE PERIOD OF 8–14 MONTHS

I. **Expectations of this period.**
These 6 months are a critical period for both parents and baby, since it is during this time that a cooperative working relationship between parent and child needs to be established. The baby, with his new skills of moving about, is eager to investigate his surroundings in his own way, at his own pleasure, without any interference. As it is necessary for the parents to protect him during these adventures, so is it necessary for them to help him learn that only acceptable behavior will receive rewards and praises. In turn, he is learning that his need for approval and affection may be worth the effort of accepting these constraints. It is through this willingness to compromise that the baby experiences the wonderful feelings of self-worth and self-confidence.

- A. Parental tasks
  1. Provide a safe environment that gives baby the opportunity to use his new motor skills of crawling and walking and also satisfies his need to investigate by touching, tasting, and manipulating.
  2. Provide a reliable and consistent caretaker who will be aware of the baby's activities at all times.
  3. Provide a routine schedule that the baby can anticipate; this will help him accept daily events and develop his sense of consistency in his world.
  4. Provide freedom of activity within this environment and schedule so that there is as little opportunity for rebellion and frustration as possible.
  5. Understand the developmental stages so that unattainable tasks are not expected (such as toilet training, table manners, sharing, reliable behavior control).
  6. Understand that attention given to a particular activity will cause this activity to be repeated. Rewards and praise for a behavior will help establish this behavior as a pattern. Unacceptable behavior will also be repeated if that is the only way that attention is gained.
  7. Provide a primary caretaker who will give encouragement and comfort and who will accept the baby's attempts to express affection.
- B. Baby's developmental tasks
  1. Master the physical skills of walking and using the hands to carry and manipulate objects.
  2. Use new physical skills and self-confidence to investigate surroundings.
  3. Learn by repetition of an activity to anticipate its result.
  4. Develop a close relationship with and affection for someone outside himself through consistent interaction with that person.
- C. The nurse practitioner can now plan extended office visits, or preferably home visits, so as to be a resource and support to the parents in understanding and coping during this critical period of growth.

II. **Family status**

- A. Basic needs being met
  1. Referrals: if made, follow up to be sure that appropriate help is received.
  2. Adequate support system available.
- B. The family unit
  1. Mother

a. Satisfaction with life-style; is confident, cheerful, energetic.
b. Support system intact; outside interests present.
c. Maturation level: own needs being met; can view baby objectively and not as the only means of satisfying own needs.
d. Coping with confusion of women's role in today's society—women's rights, career planning, divorce, separation, men's changing role.

2. Working mother
   a. Satisfaction with child care arrangements.
   b. Adjustments to physical stress of two jobs.
   c. Ability to express and work through emotional reactions, such as guilt for leaving home, distress if going to work is a necessity, and satisfactions from new role.
3. Single parent
   a. Needs being identified and goals established.
   b. Referrals: provide with follow-up.
   c. Visits scheduled to provide support and help in establishing healthy child-rearing practices.
4. Mother and father
   a. Developing a unified philosophy of child-rearing.
      (1) Evaluating their own upbringing as to disciplinary practices and cultural influences.
      (2) Identifying how these influence their child-rearing practices.
      (3) Gaining knowledge of developmental principles.
   b. Interactive patterns and communication skills:
      (1) Reactive pattern when under stress.
      (2) Knowledge and application of problem-solving techniques.
5. Siblings. Their goal is to develop positive feelings toward each other.
   a. Each child should have the opportunity to develop at his own pace without interference.
   b. Separate planning for each child (bedtimes, activities, play, schools).
   c. Playing together and sharing takes about 6 years to develop. Children need to learn to respond to disagreements with positive behavior patterns.
   d. Parents reinforce positive behavior and demonstrate gentleness.
   e. Parents appreciate children's attempts to show concern for one another.

III. Health patterns

A. Nutrition
1. Baby showing less interest in food; is too busy investigating his world.
2. Growth rate slowed, so smaller intake is normal.
3. Anemia. Be sure hematocrit is done.
   a. High-iron diet.
   b. Cut back on milk intake to 12–16 oz.
4. Balanced diet to include the following:
   a. Finger foods—fruit, vegetables, meat.
   b. Protein—eggs, fish, whole-grain cereals, meat.

c. Milk 12–16 oz. Office protocol.

d. Water—offer frequently. Avoid all soda pops; give fruit juices, not fruit "drinks."

B. Sleep

1. Baby often needs help slowing down. Establish bedtime routine, with quiet time with parent reading or music; not the time for roughhousing.

2. Waking during the night; needs reassurance often; when further along in establishing autonomy, he will sleep soundly all night.

a. Develop routine for these periods such as diapering, playing soft music, singing to him from parents' room; use night-light.

b. This is part of his developmental pattern; needs careful consideration and consistent response.

3. Crib: watch carefully for attempts to climb out of crib; safety is the prime consideration.

a. If baby is climbing out, leave sides down so he can get out without a serious fall.

b. Put a mattress on the floor or get a regular bed.

c. Babyproof room, particularly ensuring that window screens secured and bureau drawers hooked closed.

d. Put gate on baby's room door so he cannot roam the house while parents sleep.

C. Elimination

1. Muscle control of sphincters not sufficiently developed to begin toilet training.

2. Bowel movements and urinary output can help in evaluation of dietary and liquid intake.

3. Constipation (cow's milk can cause problems); to prevent, include in diet large amounts of water, whole-grain cereals, dried fruits; ask for professional help if problem continues.

IV. Growth and development

A. Physical

1. Motor development

a. Gross motor. The joys and perils of learning to creep → crawl → walk; getting direction straightened; moving forward or backward at will; negotiating body around obstacles; pulling to standing; learning to get back down; hands and arms used as balancing pole; need to carry something in hands.

b. Fine motor. Manipulating objects; turning knobs; pulling, opening, poking; pincer grasp.

2. Reaction to pain

a. Inability to locate.

b. Continues activity level.

c. Irritability the usual indicator.

3. Reaction to illness

a. Skill development halted.

b. Return to earlier developmental stage.

c. Separation from primary caretaker is overwhelming.

B. Emotional development—Erikson: progression from basic trust to stage of autonomy. This is a transitional period that, if successful, shows the amazing progress from a stationary, happy baby to a mobile, impatient, energetic investigator. Baby is beginning to realize through the encouragement of his caretakers that he has the ability to be all right—most of the time—out on his own.

1. *Affection:* returns hugs and kisses.
2. *Joy:* excitement at parent's return, at accomplishing a task, at rhythm of body movement.
3. *Ambivalence of feeling:* returning to earlier behavior patterns when tired, distraught, or ill.
4. *Obstinacy:* persistent in solving problems by trial and error.
5. *Anger:* at body constraint, at interruptions during play.
6. *Fear and anxiety:* natural response to new adventures, so reassurance from primary caretaker is important.
7. *Distress:* irritable, apathetic, unlovable (a high-risk factor if this is dominant mood).

C. Intellectual development—Piaget: development of causality. Baby is progressing from random activities to intentional activities by observing and recalling the previous results of a particular activity.

1. Steps in learning self-control
   - **a.** Watches responses of caretaker to his efforts to conform.
   - **b.** Delayed gratification: waiting for meals to be served; waiting to be picked up when first awake, etc.
   - **c.** Amuses himself for longer periods.
   - **d.** Comforts himself.
2. Memory
   - **a.** Recognizes himself in mirror (reaches up to touch something on himself that he sees in mirror).
   - **b.** Anticipates sequence of daily routine.
   - **c.** Object permanence: will search for an object after it is out of sight.
   - **d.** Recognizes sounds—daddy's car or footsteps; individual voices.
   - **e.** Repeats actions: plays pat-a-cake, waves bye-bye.
   - **f.** Recognizes foods and demonstrates likes and dislikes.
3. Language
   - **a.** Word development: repeats definitive sounds (dada, mama).
   - **b.** Understands words before being able to use them (commands, names, body parts).
   - **c.** Listens to own voice.
   - **d.** Attends as caretaker names objects around him.
   - **e.** May subordinate language development while attending to new motor skills.

D. High-risk factors

1. Parents. Identify child abuse precursor:
   - **a.** Mother's dissatisfaction with role.
   - **b.** Parents' own child-rearing experiences.

c. Emotional poverty (low self-esteem, rigid response patterns, marital conflict).

2. Baby
   a. Developmental and physical lags.
   b. Irritable, apathetic, overcautious.

E. Child-rearing practices
   1. Parents have confidence in coping with the reality of their spontaneous feelings of frustration, boredom, anger; appreciate the need for ingenuity, patience, and positive ways of expressing these emotions.
   2. Honest responses: baby soon learns which of his behaviors bring hugs and which bring unpleasant feelings.
   3. Reinforce positive behavior; set up environment so few opportunities for negative behavior.
   4. Identify individuality of baby's capabilities and reactive patterns.
   5. Provide cheerful, fun-loving environment.
   6. Let him try to solve his problems. Help only when necessary.

F. Caretaking arrangements
   1. Baby-sitter
      a. Able to be regular caretaker.
      b. Personality: cheerful and energetic but gentle.
      c. Responsible: follows daily schedule; provides safety precautions; responds appropriately to baby's cues; enjoys child care.
   2. Day-care centers. Parents need to investigate and observe day-care centers before choosing appropriate one.
      a. State approved, with professional, educated personnel.
      b. Environment: attractive, quiet; sufficient space for activity needs; sufficient equipment for stimulation; safety precautions observed.
      c. Caretaker: consistency in baby's caretaker; responds to individual needs, has time to give individual attention.
      d. Health services
         (1) Safe and sanitary conditions.
         (2) Nutritious food.
         (3) Identification of sick child: appropriate plans for care.
         (4) Health education services to parents—group meetings, regular health bulletins to families.
      e. Evaluation of facility
         (1) Observe children enrolled (relaxed, happy children).
         (2) Watch responses of caretakers to children's requests.
         (3) Get assessment from other parents.

G. Stimulation
   1. Communication and sounds
      a. Provide toy phone; let baby listen to real phone.
      b. Use single names for toys, foods, names, animals.
      c. Name and point to body parts.
      d. Play blowing games—bubbles, horns.

   - e. Provide noisy push-and-pull toys.
   - f. Read books with simple, repetitive themes and rhymes.
2. Touch
   - a. Encourage baby to return affection by hugs and kisses.
   - b. Bathtub toys—boats, various-sized containers, colored sponges.
3. Sight
   - a. Texture pictures: encourage touching, change often.
   - b. Change of environment: trips to the store, out in the car; point out distant objects such as birds, planes, clouds.
4. Gross motor
   - a. Removing clothes.
   - b. Fetching and carrying.
   - c. Climbing.
   - d. Walking backward.
   - e. Walking on variety of surfaces—grass, mattress, sidewalk.
   - f. Using wading pool with supervision.
5. Fine motor
   - a. Puts things in and out of boxes.
   - b. Plays in sandbox with spoons, cups, cars, strainer.
   - c. Transports objects.
   - d. Builds tower with cubes.
   - e. Opens, shuts cupboard doors.
6. Feeding
   - a. Feels food—raw, cooked, dough, vegetables, liquid.
   - b. Splashes, stirs, pours.
   - c. Feeds self; uses cup.
   - d. Can use meal time to demonstrate he can get his own way.

H. Safety

1. Accidents happen most frequently
   - a. When usual routine changes (holidays, vacations, illness in family).
   - b. Following stressful events for caretakers.
   - c. When caretakers are tired or ill.
   - d. Late in the afternoon.
2. Accident prevention
   - a. Increased mobility: baby needs freedom to investigate, but must also have constant surveillance.
   - b. Safe place to put baby while caretaker is out of sight.
   - c. Falls and burns: first aid instructions per office protocol.
3. Investigate frequent injuries for possible child abuse and neglect.
4. Instructions to baby-sitters
5. Emergency telephone numbers posted

OVERVIEW

14-MONTH WELL CHILD VISIT

I. **Parent**

A. A quieter period as a more relaxed cooperative toddler. A more consistent schedule can be established with new activities and outside excursions giving the toddler a wider view of the world.

II. **Baby**

A. Physical

1. Eating and sleeping habits improve.
2. Improving coordination and large muscle strength.

B. Emotional

1. Showing more confidence in using new skills. Reflecting caretaker's attitude toward him of acceptance and affection or disapproval and mistrust.

C. Intellectual

1. Concentrates on one thing at a time. Language of interest but may be subordinated to his improving physical capabilities.

III. **High Risk Factors**

A. Unresponsive or over-active toddler.

B. Frequent illness or accidents.

C. No consistent caretaker.

IV. **See Guidelines for specific factors of physical examination.**

NOTES

14-MONTH WELL CHILD VISIT

I. **Developmental process.**

This is a period of consolidation. New-found physical skills are being refined, and the progression from dependence toward independence is becoming a smoother path, though frequent backsliding is still seen. The excitement of mastering physical skills and the courage to do it myself now make for a happier and more relaxed baby.

- A. Mother
    1. Showing pride and pleasure in each new step of the baby's growth and development.
    2. Establishing consistent family schedule.
    3. Setting realistic limits for acceptable behavior.
- B. Baby
    1. Behavior characterized by playfulness and good humor.
    2. Testing his own power by frequent use of "no."
    3. More selectivity and control in activity.

II. **Family status**

- A. Parental concerns and problems. Ability to identify problems and to cope.
- B. Baby now meshed happily into family circle.
- C. Adequate child care arrangements.

III. **Health habits**

- A. Nutrition
    1. Diet history
        - a. Being offered and accepting a balanced diet. Servings should be small. Good rule of thumb: a measuring tablespoon of each food for each year of age or one quarter of an adult serving.
        - b. Accepting new foods.

          High-protein and high-iron foods essential.
    2. Eating habits
        - a. Self-feeding of finger foods.
        - b. Drinking from cup and attempting to use spoon.
        - c. Mealtimes are short and matter-of-fact.
        - d. No forcing of unwanted foods.
        - e. Food should never be used as a reward or punishment.
- B. Sleep
    1. Sleeps total of 10–15 hr/day.
    2. Improvement in sleeping all night.
    3. Falling asleep more quickly.
    4. Long afternoon nap; morning nap short or discontinued.
    5. Crib: baby attempting to climb out; safety factors assessed.
- C. Elimination/Toilet Training
    1. Baby developing awareness of soiling.
    2. "Catch" bowel movements in potty chair if consistent pattern established.
    3. Potty chair used only if baby cooperates to sit on it at time of bowel movement.

4. Avoid praise or threat; a matter-of-fact attitude to prevent putting too much importance on something the baby may not yet be able to control.

IV. Growth and development

A. Physical

1. Smooth, coordinated movements.
2. Gross motor. Increase in strength; climbs stairs on hands and knees; throws ball overhand.
3. Fine motor. Good pincer movement; improving eye/hand coordination.
4. Speech
   a. Uses phrases, but cannot use individual words out of the phrases.
   b. Uses about seven true words.
   c. Has developed phrasing and sounds into jargon talk.
5. Vision
   a. Smooth ocular movements.
   b. Good eye/hand coordination being established.
   c. Improved depth perception: dropping and watching objects fall.
6. Hearing
   a. Reacts to soft sounds (likes to be whispered to).
   b. Traces source of sound.
   c. In a loud, shouting, noisy environment, baby "turns off" sounds; this decreases his natural response from stimuli around him and can result in undeveloped language skills.

B. Emotional development—Erikson. Completing the passage from basic trust to that of autonomy is to work toward establishing self-esteem. Baby's improving physical skills push him to new and daring feats. He turns from such adventures to those around him for admiration and reflects their feelings that he is someone special. Without this response, he learns nothing positive about himself.

1. Cheerful, playful *vs.* irritable, destructive.
2. Energetic, curious *vs.* apathetic, fearful.

C. Intellectual development—Piaget: period of consolidation or equilibrium. The baby is comfortable with his new skills and beginning to appreciate his own competencies. This confidence allows him to take the next step of observing the consequences of his actions, called causality.

1. General mood of self-satisfaction.
2. Attends specifically to one toy rather than being distracted by other toys around him.
3. Attempts to solve a problem before turning to parent for help.
4. Language
   a. Development may still be subordinated while the baby is attending to new motor skills and explorations.
   b. Attends to objects and people named by caretaker.

D. High-risk factors

1. Mother
   a. Lack of pride in baby, which is reflected in her attitude and actions toward baby.

b. Lack of confidence in her own child care ability.

c. Unrealistic expectations of baby, such as behavior control and successful toilet training.

d. Overwhelming personal problems.

2. Baby

a. Frequent health problems.

b. Not "settling" into family circle.

c. Destructible, tense.

d. Not moving out to investigate surroundings.

V. Physical examination

A. Growth. Continuing on established pattern; use growth chart to help mother understand that although she states baby not eating, he is eating enough to maintain his normal growth.

B. Appearance and behavior

1. Has lost roundness of babyhood.
2. Energetic but better able to sit still and concentrate on one toy.
3. Less fearful of strangers.

C. Specific factors to note during routine physical examination

1. Skin. Check for excessive bruising, burns, scratch lines.
2. Teeth. Central incisors present.
3. Ears. Check for mobility of tympanic membrane.
4. Hair. Texture, nits.
5. Musculoskeletal. Bearing weight on legs; hips—Ortolani's click, equal gluteal folds; check for tibial torsion, genu varum, externally rotated hips; check stance, gait.
6. Reflexes. Presence of parachute reflex.

D. Mother–child interaction

1. Mother understands child's behavior patterns.
2. Baby shows recognition of parents' commands.
3. Cheerful, pleasant rapport between mother and child.

VI. Assessment

A. Physical

B. Developmental

C. Emotional

D. Environmental

VII. Plan

A. Screening. Hematocrit, lead, urinalysis as indicated.

B. Problem list (devised with parent); SOAP for each.

C. Appropriate timing for office, home, and/or telephone visits.

1. Continue close contact during this critical period.
2. Visits planned according to the individual needs of the family and the developmental and physical needs of the baby.
3. Home visits to assess environment as needed.

OVERVIEW

ANTICIPATORY GUIDANCE FOR THE PERIOD OF 14–18 MONTHS

I. **Parents**

A. Understanding their toddler's progress and their appreciation of his new skills and needs. Father's role is important to give toddler broader experiences and support.

II. **Toddler**

A. Physical

1. Decrease in appetite as a slower growth rate.
2. Falling asleep more easily.
3. Increase strength. Needs opportunity to use large muscles.
4. Toilet training—see guideline.

B. Emotional

1. Attempting to set balance between doing things his way and accepting necessary constraints on his behavior. Using "no" as an experimental tool.
2. See Guidelines for specific factors of development of self-esteem, temper tantrums, and child-rearing practices.

C. Intellectual

1. Returns to fascination of language.
2. Needs a listener but not one that over-corrects.

III. **High Risk Factors**

A. See safety protocols.

B. Frequent illnesses with slow recovery.

NOTES

ANTICIPATORY GUIDANCE FOR THE PERIOD OF 14–18 MONTHS

The previous outlines need to be reviewed to identify the parental and toddler tasks that have been accomplished. Development is such an individual process that the stages cannot be closely related to a specific age period. Office or home visits still need to be set up on an individual basis.

I. **Expectations of this period.**

The baby has now become a toddler, and with this new title comes, fortunately for his family, the skills to settle down. Physically he has better coordination and muscle control, and his energy is now not wasted on random activities but can be used to accomplish specific tasks. He is better able to pay attention to his caretakers and more willing to respond with the type of behavior that gets him the most attention. Continuing to satisfy his need for attention and approval through behavior control, he is becoming a more cooperative member of the family.

- A. Parental tasks
    1. Encourage with attention and reward (love pats, not food) the type of behavior expected.
    2. Continue to provide a safe environment and regular schedule.
    3. Stimulate new activities and then leave toddler to carry on (but without pressure to complete activity).
    4. Provide a loving, caring caretaker.
- B. Toddler tasks
    1. Settling into household routine.
    2. Developing behavior pattern that receives the most attention from a primary caretaker.
    3. Turning to caretaker for encouragement and affection.

II. **Family status**

- A. Basic needs being met through the following:
    1. Adequate finances, security of environment, stability of life-style.
    2. Knowledge of where to obtain aid.
- B. Parents
    1. Good interactive pattern; problem-solving skills.
    2. Cooperation in establishing child-rearing practices.
- C. Working mother
    1. Adequate child care arrangements.
    2. Acceptance of sharing child care with others.
    3. Communicating philosophy of child-rearing practices to caretaker.
    4. Health maintenance.
- D. Single parent
    1. Adequate support system.
    2. Good health habits maintained.
    3. Career goals being implemented.
- E. Father: important to child's well-being.
    1. Broadens emotional response of toddler.
    2. Serves as a role model for boys.

3. Helps girls develop the ability to form a close relationship with the opposite sex.

F. Siblings

1. Independent activities and separate schedules.
2. Positive behavior patterns established toward toddler.

III. Health patterns

A. Nutrition

1. Emotional and physical factors may increase difficulty of maintaining adequate nutrition.
   a. Physical factors: slower growth rate; appetite and need for food decreases.
   b. Emotional factors: distractibility and negativism; using refusal to eat as a means of showing power.
2. Eating habits: will sit still longer; enjoys feeding self finger foods; still a poor family dinner companion.

B. Sleep

1. By 18 months of age, falls asleep more easily.
2. Able to amuse and talk to himself; will turn off outside stimuli.
3. Sleeps through the night; awakens early and can amuse himself for a longer period.
4. Naps: changing from two naps to one longer one during the middle of the day.
5. A regular daily schedule is important.

C. Elimination

1. Regular pattern established; new foods less irritating.
2. Distention and flatulence: return to simpler diet.
3. Dry for longer periods, as bladder is larger.
4. Toilet training
   a. "Catch" bowel movement if pattern established.
   b. Have toddler practice sitting on potty chair (regular toilet too frightening) with diaper on, then finally with it off.
   c. Do not expect success too early; pressure to comply only adds to confusion for toddler.
   d. Girls train earlier than boys; small children train more easily than big ones.
   e. Play it cool; if toddler realizes he can get a lot of attention from this, he will prolong the process.

IV. Growth and development

A. Physical

1. Ability to "get to" most places; practices getting back down.
2. Increased strength. Needs to use large muscles; pushes or carries around large objects.
3. Fine motor. Established pincer movement; delights in handling small objects, poking, pushing, turning.
4. Grasping and releasing at will. If well established, may indicate the time to begin toilet training.

5. Spatial relations. Spends much time working this out, doing things such as putting toys in and out of boxes, dropping and throwing objects, climbing up and down, steering self around obstacles.

B. Emotional development—Erikson. Development of autonomy. The toddler is setting a balance between the drive for independence and the necessity to become a member of society. This means being able to accept constraints on his self-will and impulses. This he will learn to do through the expectations and approval of his caretakers.

1. Development of self-esteem being established through the following:
   - **a.** Negativism: testing power to affect others.
   - **b.** Challenging physical activities: climbing higher, carrying heavier objects.
   - **c.** Taking initiative for actions: self-amusement.
   - **d.** Demanding: is showing off, mischievous, joyful.
   - **e.** Attempting more than he has the ability to do.
   - **f.** Absorbing the attitudes and feelings shown by others toward him; beginning to select behavior that fits into these expectations.
   - **g.** Child-rearing practices
     - (1) Treat with respect; attempt to see the world from his perspective.
     - (2) Avoid battles over "no" when possible, and do not try to win them all.
     - (3) Provide enough freedom for him to try new activities.
     - (4) Constructively reinforce accomplishments.
2. Development of self-control
   - **a.** Identified by the following:
     - (1) Accepting and anticipating daily routine; being less impulsive; fitting into family plans more easily.
     - (2) Learning that his behavior has consequences; parental reaction teaches what is "right" and what is "wrong."
   - **b.** Child-rearing practices
     - (1) Understand that control of impulses will continue to take time and much reinforcement.
     - (2) Provide a safe environment, since a toddler of this age cannot be completely trusted not to act on impulse.
3. Development of aggression
   - **a.** Frustrations from too many commands and unrealistic expectations lead to stored-up energy; the toddler has few ways of releasing this energy constructively.
   - **b.** Frustrations are also caused by siblings, fatigue, hunger, illness, and changes in routine, in caretaker, etc.
   - **c.** Releasing of this stored-up energy in a way destructive to himself and others, such as temper tantrums, breath-holding, biting, hitting.
   - **d.** Child-rearing practices
     - (1) Temper tantrums
       - (a) Provide firm but soothing restraints (hold under arm); do not leave alone, as child is frightened by loss of control.
       - (b) Keep record of the events preceding the incident, the intervention, and the results.

(c) Seek professional help if such destructive behavior continues.

(d) Provide a quiet, gentle, consistent environment.

(2) Negativism

(a) "No" used as a means of learning which behaviors are acceptable: caretaker must demonstrate that acceptable behavior has more power to get attention and approval than unacceptable behavior.

(b) Avoid opportunities for toddler to use negative response—*do not ask him to make a choice;* state what is to be done, such as: "This is what we will have to eat." "Now, it is time for bed."

(c) Set limits; do not give in to unreasonable requests.

(d) Maintain cheerful, fun-loving, well-organized daily routine.

(e) Provide large, stimulating, safe environment.

4. High-risk factors

a. Parents. Demanding coercive behavior that is beyond toddler's developmental ability to comply.

b. Toddler. Excessive negativism; frequent temper tantrums; dominant mood of irritability or apathy; frequent illnesses.

C. Intellectual development—Piaget. The toddler is learning intuitively about his environment with the increase in physical agility and memory development. He is also taking the first steps in symbolic thinking but needs concrete symbols first (drink for teddy bear requires a cup).

1. Independent actions; beginning to observe actions of others and to imitate caretakers, siblings, peers.

2. Studying

a. Experimenting (things in motion, difference in weights).

b. Varying a pattern and observing the results.

c. Varying a response to an activity and observing the results.

3. Language

a. Returns to fascination with words; is word hungry.

b. Articulation lags behind vocabulary; carries on "jargon" conversations with himself and toys.

c. Experiments with using words to affect those around him.

d. Child-rearing practices

(1) Talk to child; name objects, feelings, odors, textures, sounds; sing to him.

(2) Listen; pay particular attention as he attempts to "talk" to you.

(3) Accept his strivings to express himself; do not overcorrect, do not overload; let him take the lead in how much he wants.

(4) Look at pictures and name things; do not expect the child to sit still for "story hour."

D. Stimulation

1. Communication and sounds: parents

a. Read short, simple stories.

b. Give simple directions.

   - **c.** Say words for objects child desires.
   - **d.** Provide books with cardboard pages, simple colorful pictures, rhymes, songs.
2. Touch. Water tubs; sandboxes.
3. Sight. Bulletin board in child's room, using large single picture; point at things at a distance.
4. Gross motor
   - **a.** Walks up and down stairs.
   - **b.** Balances on one foot.
   - **c.** Jumps.
   - **d.** Rides kiddie car.
   - **e.** Does somersaults.
5. Fine motor
   - **a.** Uses paper and crayons to scribble. Provide large paper such as old newspapers.
   - **b.** Enjoys finger paints.
   - **c.** Puts on shoes.
   - **d.** Washes and dries hands.

E. Safety

1. Accidents happen most frequently
   - **a.** When usual routine changes (holidays, vacations, illness in family).
   - **b.** Following stressful events for caretakers.
   - **c.** When caretakers are tired or ill.
   - **d.** Late in the afternoon.
2. Accident prevention
   - **a.** Most dangerous age, since the child is mobile but has little ability to control behavior and poor depth perception (may step off high step, etc.).
   - **b.** Safety-proof house, yard, porches.
   - **c.** Constant surveillance necessary.
   - **d.** Insist on child's remaining in car seat.
3. Investigate possibility of child abuse and neglect
4. Instructions to baby-sitters
5. Emergency telephone numbers posted

OVERVIEW

18-MONTH WELL CHILD VISIT

I Parents

A. Understanding toddler's self-centered world and his growing willingness to conform by controlling his behavior. This he does for the return of support and affection to him, or if his misbehavior is the only behavior to get attention, he will continue that behavior.

II. Toddler

A. Physical
  1. Walking alone
  2. Manipulating small objects
  3. Slower growth rate
  4. Falling asleep more easily

B. Emotional
  1. Struggle toward independence can lead to excessive use of "no." He is a keen observer of how this word affects his caretakers.

C. Intellectual
  1. Increased interest and use of language can begin the development of "pretending" or symbolizing.

III. High Risk Factors

A. Parents letting the use of "no" develop into battleground of wills.

B. Whiny child needs investigation.

C. Illness becoming a way to gain attention.

NOTES

18-MONTH WELL CHILD VISIT

I. **Developmental process.**

For the last few months the toddler has been concentrating on mastering and perfecting physical skills. Now that his physical skills take less concentration and energy, he turns to the next developmental task of language acquisition.

- A. Parents
    1. "Listen" to toddler's expostulations.
    2. Talk to child about child's world.
- B. Toddler
    1. Attends to speech of others.
    2. Assertive; gives two-word commands.
    3. Physical agility and coordination.

II. **Family status**

- A. Basic needs being met.
- B. Stability of family structure.
- C. Siblings receiving appropriate care and age-specific activities. Relationships evaluated and referrals given as needed.
- D. Parental concerns and problems. Ability to identify problems and to cope.

III. **Health habits**

- A. Nutrition
    1. Diet history.
        - a. Variety of foods.
        - b. Amount of milk.
        - c. Adequate caloric intake. Relate to pattern on growth chart.
    2. Eating habits.
        - a. Self-feeding, manages spoon.
        - b. Reasonable time spent on meals.
        - c. Atmosphere pleasant; no attention given to rejected foods.
- B. Sleep
    1. Sleeps total of 10–15 hours/day.
    2. Contented in crib for longer periods; practicing jargon and new words.
    3. In a bed if able to climb out of crib; gate on the door of room.
    4. Room unstimulating to promote restfulness.
    5. Accepting bedtime routine.
    6. Daytime naps: parental awareness of type of behavior child will display when he runs out of steam.
    7. Ability to turn off stimulation and relax.
- C. Elimination
    1. Toilet training not usually accomplished by 18 months.
    2. Parents understand principles of toilet training.
    3. Regularity of bowel movements established.
    4. Longer periods between urinating.
- D. Dental. Teeth cleaned with soft brush.

IV. Growth and development

A. Physical

1. Gross motor. Testing strength; pushes and carries heavy and large objects.
2. Fine motor. Handedness; scribbling.
3. Speech
   a. Uses two- to three-word phrases but is unable to use the words separately.
   b. Gives two-word commands.
   c. Follows one-step directions.
   d. Perfects inflections and rhythms of speech in his jargon.

B. Emotional development—Erikson. Feelings of autonomy and self-esteem continue to grow through the child's mastery of the physical control of both his body and his activities. Language acquisition will continue to add to his feeling of self-esteem by giving him a new tool with which to understand and control his environment.

1. Physical agility, good coordination, high energy level.
2. Playing with putting together a string of sounds.
3. Experimenting with words and observing their effect on caretaker.
4. Contented to play by himself for longer periods.
5. Instigates own activities.

C. Intellectual development—Piaget. Sensorimotor learning is progressing to the beginning of preoperative or intuitive learning, which is the ability to store mental images (as in memory) and to symbolize (as in words being substituted for the actual object, feeling, or event).

1. Attends carefully to activities of peers, but does not play interactively.
2. Shows interest in names of things and people.
3. Remembers where possessions belong.
4. Simple "pretending."

D. High-risk factors

1. Mother
   a. Too helpful; fearful of providing physical challenges.
   b. Too busy/uninterested to spend time listening to or talking with child.
   c. Unhappy, frustrated.
2. Toddler
   a. Physical cautiousness.
   b. Not initiating activities for himself; sits doing nothing for long periods.
   c. Clinging to caretaker; whiny or irritable.
   d. Not attempting to use words to get what he wants.

V. Physical examination

A. Growth. Continuing on established pattern; periods of illness will affect the pattern, but growth should be made up within a period of months.

B. Appearance and behavior

1. Good physical coordination.
2. Energetic, playful.

3. Cautious in relating to strangers, but more trustful than at previous visit.
4. Eye contact possible.

C. Specific factors to note while doing routine physical examination
1. Skin. Check for excessive bruising, burns.
2. Head. Anterior fontanelle usually closed.
3. Eyes. Smooth tracking; no strabismus.
4. Teeth. Lateral and central incisors present; first and second molars may be present.
5. Cardiovascular system. Heart rate: 90–100/minute.
6. Musculoskeletal. Check coordination and gait.

D. Mother–child interaction
1. Mother understands child's behavior patterns.
2. Toddler shows recognition of parents' commands.
3. Rapport between mother and child appears cheerful, pleasant.

VI. Assessment

A. Physical
B. Developmental
C. Emotional
D. Environmental

VII. Plan

A. Immunizations. DPT/polio booster; H. Flu—check office protocol.
B. Screening. Hematocrit, urinalysis as indicated.
C. Problem list (devised with parent); SOAP for each.
D. Appropriate timing for office, home, and/or telephone visits; continue individual scheduling.

OVERVIEW

ANTICIPATORY GUIDANCE FOR THE PERIOD OF 18–24 MONTHS

I. **Parents**

A. Able to discuss their understanding of discipline vs. punishment and to establish realistic goals for the toddler.

B. Parents who are unable to provide adequate support need referrals or more frequent visits.

II. **Baby**

A. Physical

1. Better able to concentrate on meals. Milk intake. No more than 16 oz. (too much milk will curb appetite for other foods).
2. Enjoys strenuous activities. Needs appropriate and safe environment.
3. Toilet training— see Guidelines.

B. Emotional

1. Increased feeling of competence so has less need for "no." Continues to be egocentric (selfish, stubborn, and assertive).
2. See Guidelines for child rearing practices and high risk factors.

C. Intellectual

1. Learning words important to him first. Careful "listening" by caretaker encourages use of language.
2. Able to "symbolize" a thing by using words so can now begin to "pretend."

D. Social Development

1. Egocentric. Unable to share.
2. Amoralistic. Will show signs of guilt if found doing something wrong.

III. **High Risk Factors**

A. See safety protocol.

B. Frequent illness.

C. No interest in using language.

D. No primary caretaker to help establish behavior control through positive reinforcement.

NOTES

NOTES

ANTICIPATORY GUIDANCE FOR THE PERIOD OF 18–24 MONTHS

Review previous guidelines for a reference point as to the toddler's developmental level. It is important to identify a family whose environment does not support or facilitate the toddler's optimal development. The proper intervention at this time can be of lasting benefit.

I. Expectations of this period.

These months continue the long road of establishing a balance between an individual's needs and society's expectations. A very tentative beginning has been made by the toddler's experiencing and anticipating the results of controlling a behavior. However, the toddler's impulses and drive for independence rule most of his activities. It is the parent/caretaker's task to persuade him, through attention and affection, that it is worth the effort to conform. The acquisition of language is now an added tool that can make this development an easier task.

- **A.** Parental tasks
  1. Continue to provide a safe environment.
  2. Provide child opportunities to develop physical strength and agility.
  3. Provide a variety of experiences.
  4. Provide a caring adult to encourage and praise child's efforts, to talk with him, and to listen to his efforts to use language.
- **B.** Toddler tasks
  1. Bargaining for behavior control.
  2. Attempting to use language to control activities.
  3. Increasing socialization; delights in being with and watching others.

II. Family status

- **A.** Basic needs being met; referrals providing needed help with follow-up of these referrals.
- **B.** Parents
  1. Health and resources sufficient to maintain satisfactory life-style.
  2. Appreciation of the importance of this age period.
  3. Wholesome child-rearing practices established.
- **C.** Mother
  1. Deriving satisfaction and pride from role.
  2. Content with life-style.
- **D.** Working mother
  1. Health and energy level sufficient for daily schedule.
  2. Satisfactory child care arrangements.
  3. Arranging some time each day to be alone with toddler.
- **E.** Single parent
  1. Receiving satisfaction from child care, but not depending on this care for only emotional support.
  2. Adequate parenting skills developed.
  3. Adequate support system.
  4. Career goals being implemented.

F. Siblings
   1. Older siblings demonstrating caring and gentleness with toddler.
   2. New baby in family
      a. Toddler will show crude reactive patterns to hold parents' attention; regressive behavior should be understood and not punished.
      b. New emotion of jealousy is experienced, and toddler must learn another step in coping with his world.

G. Toddler
   1. Basic physical and emotional needs being met.
   2. Learning that needs, but not all wants, are met.

H. High-risk factors
   1. Reaction of parents to children during divorce or separation: lack of attention, overprotection, use as emotional crutch, broken routine, abandonment.
   2. Siblings: teasing or aggressive acts; frustrating toddler into destructive action toward himself or others.

III. Health patterns

A. Nutrition
   1. Sufficient calories for toddler's high energy level; include high-value food (potatoes, dark bread, peanut butter, yogurt, honey, molasses).
   2. Avoid junk food (if such foods are not bought, they will not be available).
   3. Food variety: keep menus and seasoning simple; add new foods in small amounts.
   4. The following foods must not be given to toddlers: potato chips, coconut, nuts, popcorn, whole kernel corn, hot dogs, and raw carrots. They are difficult to chew and swallow and can cause choking or aspiration.
   5. Eating habits
      a. Improved attention to food, as now less destructible.
      b. Expects to feed himself, so finger foods are best.
      c. Offer simple, bland foods; no substitutes offered, no snacks between meals if food refused at mealtimes.
      d. Watch milk intake, and offer only after or between meals.
      e. Keep mealtime a short, matter-of-fact event; give no attention to rejected food.
      f. Do not offer food as a reward or withhold it as a punishment.

B. Sleep
   1. Sleeps 10–15 hr/day.
   2. Definite schedule and routine established.
   3. Now better able to "turn off" stimulation around him, so falls asleep more easily.
   4. Enjoys talking to himself, and wants a bedtime companion such as a teddy bear.
   5. Returns to sleeping through the night.
   6. Naptime: one long nap in the middle of the day.
   7. Fatigue: watch for behavior when tired; help child establish a "quiet place."

C. Elimination: toilet training
   1. Girls train earlier than boys; small children train earlier than big children.
   2. Treat as a matter-of-fact event; special attention will encourage delaying the training for continued attention.
   3. Attempt training if
      a. Regular pattern of bowel movement established.
      b. Connection of physical awareness of bowel movement and parental request to use toilet has been made by toddler (heads for potty at time of bowel movement).
      c. Toddler is willing to sit still on potty chair.
   4. Bladder control usually not accomplished until at least 3 years of age.

D. High-risk factors
   1. Frequent illnesses.
   2. Divergence from expected growth pattern.
   3. Child irritable, whiny, destructible.
   4. Exaggerated feeding or elimination problems.

E. Dental
   1. Clean teeth with soft brush.

IV. Growth and development

A. Physical
   1. Improved coordination and agility.
      a. Needs large area to expend energy.
      b. Improved agility; running and jumping.
   2. Spatial relations: exploring possibilities by climbing up and down, crawling in and out, dropping toys over and over again; fascination with balls rolling and bouncing.

B. Emotional development—Erikson. Continued development of self-esteem. The acquisition of language is a new tool that can be used to increase this feeling of self-worth by helping the toddler control his own activities and influence his environment.
   1. Less negativism; developing feeling of competence, which diffuses need for testing power.
   2. Shallower mood swings; words help others understand his needs and wishes.
   3. Continues to demonstrate affection.
   4. Fewer frustrations, since learning to put problems into words.
   5. Continues to be egocentric—selfish, stubborn, assertive.
   6. Destructive feelings of defiance, willfulness, and combativeness need careful investigation of what is wrong in the child's environment.
   7. Child-rearing practices
      a. Overexaggerated praise can be detected as insincerity.
      b. Expect compromises to be accepted.
      c. Provide different environments for toddler to observe.
      d. Play games (hide and seek, etc.) to use memory skills.
      e. Avoid putting toddler in situations where more is expected of him than he can perform.

f. Overstimulation can reduce desire to learn.
g. Provide a regular, quiet schedule most of the time.
h. Provide a caring adult to listen to toddler.
i. Begin to identify learning style (an observer, a toucher, a talker).

8. High-risk factors
   a. Temper tantrums, breath-holding, irritability, crying.
   b. Problems with eating, sleeping, elimination.
   c. Developmental lag; continues characteristics of 14-month-old (destructible, no interest in naming objects, extreme negativism).
   d. Overdependent; lack of initiative.
   e. Excessive crying; whining; appears lazy (be sure no physical problem exists).

C. Intellectual development—Piaget. Language allows for the use of words to symbolize actions, objects, and feelings. This skill develops by repetition of activities, object permanence, and vocabulary development.

1. Language opens a new world; labeling and categorizing the world is a difficult job. "What's that?" is toddler's favorite question.
2. Improved problem-solving techniques, works out alternative solutions.
3. Increase in memory; knows own possessions and where they belong.
4. Spends time observing the world around him; increased interest while looking out the window, riding in the car, going shopping.
5. Mimics actions of those around him—tone of voice, facial expressions, mannerisms.
6. Periods of apparently doing nothing—taking time to "catch up" (a high-risk factor if this becomes a dominant mood).
7. Language
   a. Learns best what he needs to know when he needs to know it; remembers first the words that are important to him:
      (1) Words that gain him attention (me do, watch).
      (2) Words that express feelings (tired, hungry).
   b. Uses own name and "I," which indicates an increased awareness of self.
   c. Reaction of caretakers to efforts of toddler to express himself gives/takes away motivation to acquire language.
8. Child-rearing practices
   a. Minimum of instruction and correction; toddler turned off if expectations are beyond his capacity.
   b. Watch errors, since they demonstrate method of learning.
   c. Caretakers describe in simple terms what they are doing, their reactions and emotions—help child develop appropriate vocabulary.
   d. Caretakers maintain eye contact when toddler is attempting to tell them something.
   e. Books: simple action books; toddler has short attention span and cannot be expected to sit still and listen to a story.
   f. Fascinated with rhymes and music; enjoys nursery rhymes, recordings; have toddler sing with caretaker.

g. Listening: identify various sounds and point out new ones; observe if child can pick up faint sounds.
h. Handle toddler's commands with gentleness, humor, and diversion.

9. High-risk factors
a. Not responding to speech with speech.
b. No primary caretaker to listen to and talk with toddler.

D. Social development

1. Autonomy: uses own name; is possessive about own things; shows hostility to older siblings and fights back; is bossy with younger siblings.
2. Self-control: less impulsive; beginning to comprehend effect of his actions.
3. Egocentric: unable to share; sees the world only from his perspective.
4. Amoralistic: beginning to appreciate what is acceptable behavior through parental teaching; will eventually accept cultural and moralistic code of parents in return for security, respect, and love; will show signs of guilt if found doing something he knows is wrong.
5. Child-rearing practices
a. Provide opportunity for toddler to observe other children.
b. Do not expect toddler to share or play cooperatively with others.
c. Emphasize acceptable behavior through attention and affection.
d. Ignore unacceptable behavior as far as safety will allow.

E. Stimulation

1. Communication and sounds
a. Child fills in words of stories and rhymes.
b. House and small people dolls.
c. Naming games.
d. Listening—naming sounds; music, poetry.
e. Books—nursery rhymes.
2. Sight
a. Identifies colors.
b. Identifies shapes.
c. Points out and identifies things at a distance.
3. Gross motor
a. Dressing with help.
b. Walking games—well-defined track to follow.
c. Large riding toys.
d. Wooden blocks.
4. Fine motor
a. Busy board.
b. Clay.
c. Simple puzzles.
d. Play to enjoy, not to accomplish a task.
e. Parents interact in enjoyment.

F. Safety

1. Accidents happen most frequently

   a. When usual routine changes (holidays, vacations, illness in the family).
   b. Following stressful events (either for caretakers or for toddler).
   c. When caretakers are tired or ill.
   d. Late in the afternoon.
2. Accident prevention
   a. Negativistic period makes toddler seem disobedient.
      (1) Save severe tone of voice for emergency.
      (2) Develop a method for emergency compliance (use of whistle, hand clap); practice and use rewards.
   b. Do not trust child's training; lack of behavior control and little memory will not stop child from dangerous activity.
3. Investigate frequent injuries as possible child abuse and neglect
4. Instructions to baby-sitters
5. Emergency telephone numbers posted

OVERVIEW

24-MONTH WELL CHILD VISIT

I. **Parents**

A. Understanding and appreciation of toddler's personality and capabilities.

B. Providing a stimulating and varied environment.

II. **Baby**

A. Physical

1. Continuing on usual growth curve. Short illnesses will not affect this.
2. Needs a "quiet place" of his own to use during the day.
3. Walking with confidence.
4. Using hands to carry toys while walking.

B. Emotional

1. Dominant mood of cheerfulness and cooperation.
2. Responds to parents' tone of voice and will act sorry if found doing something wrong.

C. Intellectual

1. Enjoying experimenting with language and using it to get what he wants.
2. Can symbolize words for things so can now enjoy "pretending."

III. **High Risk Factors**

A. Not attempting to use speech.

B. Using aggressive behavior to get what he wants.

IV. **See Guidelines for specific factors of Physical Exam**

NOTES

24-MONTH WELL CHILD VISIT

I. **Developmental process.**

The acquisition of a few important words has given the toddler a new sense of power. It is of great help to be able to name what he wants and tell how he feels. With amazing rapidity he is labeling and categorizing his world. This makes for an easier and more pleasant rapport between toddler and family.

A. Parents
1. Give simple, concise, gentle commands, but still do not attempt to reason with child.
2. Demonstrate understanding of toddler's capabilities.

B. Toddler
1. Vocabulary of about 25 words.
2. Half of speech intelligible to other than family members.
3. Responds to parents' requests.

II. **Family status**

A. Basic needs being met.

B. Parental concerns and problems. Ability to identify problems and to cope.

C. Illness in family since last visit; course; resolution.

D. Parental assessment of child's development.

III. **Health habits**

A. Nutrition
1. Diet history. Food intake, including snacks; balanced diet being offered.
2. Eating habits, appetite. Regular schedule of meals and snacks; self-feeding; pleasant atmosphere at mealtime; limited time for eating; no attention paid to unwanted foods; food not used as a reward or punishment.

B. Sleep
1. Well-established bedtime routine.
2. Sleeping all night.
3. Danger of climbing out of crib: put child in a bed or leave sides of crib down; make room safe, and put a gate on the bedroom door.
4. One nap period.
5. Quiet place for rest periods.

C. Elimination
1. Regularity of time of bowel movements; effects of new foods; periods of constipation or diarrhea.
2. Urinating less frequently as bladder capacity increases.
3. Color of urine used as indicator of state of hydration.
4. Toilet training only if regularity of bowel movements.
   a. Practicing with potty chair with or without diapers on.
   b. Too much pressure on toilet training can be seen by regressive behavior patterns such as eating problems, waking during the night, and increased negativism.

IV. **Growth and development**

A. Physical

1. Gross motor
   a. Improved coordination and agility.
   b. Increased muscle strength.
   c. Rides kiddie cars.
2. Fine motor
   a. Hand/eye coordination improved.
   b. Observes and handles small objects such as pebbles and crumbs.
   c. Traces patterns and designs.

B. Emotional development—Erikson. Toddler is reaching a plateau of physical and emotional development for first period of growth. Language acquisition will lead him to the next developmental task of using words to help control his environment and his own actions. The toddler is now willing to accept compromises in his behavior for affection and attention from those important to him. Without this positive reinforcement, he will reflect the negative feelings of discouragement and shame. Positive and negative reinforcement are the origin of the basic values of optimism and pessimism.
1. Physical well-being.
2. Dominant mood of cooperation and cheerfulness.
3. Using words appropriately.

C. Intellectual development—Piaget. Being able to symbolize thoughts and actions through words opens up a new world of imagination and fantasy.
1. Vocabulary development.
2. "Pretending" without actual object present (can pretend to give a teddy bear a drink without needing an actual cup).

D. High-risk factors
1. Mother
   a. Unrealistic demands on child for self-control.
   b. Harsh vocal commands.
   c. Too busy or distracted for a quiet, gentle approach to child.
2. Toddler
   a. Frequent illnesses.
   b. Not responding to speech with speech.
   c. Exhibits behavior of earlier period (destructible, nonobservant, pronounced negativism).

V. Physical examination

A. Growth. Continuing on established pattern; use this as a guide for parents for toddler's continued growth and caloric intake.

B. Appearance and behavior
1. High energy level, but a degree of ability to control actions (sit still, follow directions).
2. Losing cherubic look; taller and thinner.

C. Specific factors to note while doing physical examination
1. Skin. Check for excessive bruising, burns; birthmarks fading.
2. Eyes. Equal tracking; no strabismus.
3. Teeth. Complete set of 20 teeth by 2 1/2 years of age.
4. Musculoskeletal. Smooth coordination and gait; check hips.

D. Mother–child interaction
   1. Child turning to mother for support.
   2. Mother's ability to quiet child following painful experiences such as immunization or blood test.
   3. Child's ability to separate from mother.

VI. Assessment

A. Physical
B. Developmental
C. Emotional
D. Environmental

VII. Plan

A. Immunization. Complete schedule as needed.
B. Screening. Hematocrit, urinalysis as indicated.
C. Problem list (devised with parent); SOAP for each.
D. Appropriate timing for office, home, and/or telephone visits; continue individual scheduling.

OVERVIEW

ANTICIPATORY GUIDANCE FOR THE PERIOD OF 24–36 MONTHS

I. **Parent**

A. Some characteristics of the "terrible twos" can be eliminated if the parents can appreciate the toddler's attempts to give up his comfortable baby ways to accept a new world of adjusting to playing with peers, going off without mother to play school, complete toilet training, and often a new baby in the family. This is a time of great fluctuation of independence and over-dependence.

II. **Baby**

A. See Guidelines for expectations of this period for toddler and family.

B. Physical

1. Increase in agility and eye-hand coordination.
2. Diet. Provide various foods to choose from, but no pressure to eat. Food not used as a reward.
3. Sleep. Change of pattern needs investigation.
4.. Speech. Two- to three-word sentences intelligible to family.

C. Emotional

1. Greater range of emotional responses. See Guidelines for development of personality traits.

D. Intellectual

1. By 3 years, can "symbolize" using words for objects so the world of "pretend" becomes a part of his play.
2. Listening carefully to toddler is a way to understand how he is beginning to see his world and the things that are important to him.

E. Social

1. Separates from family easily.
2. Enjoys being with peers.
3. Needs external controls for "being good."
4. May have an imaginary friend he uses as scapegoat.
5. Sexual identify
   a. Selects type of behavior that society has accepted for each sex.
6. See Guidelines for child-rearing practices and high risk factors.

III. **High Risk Factors**

A. Not using speech as a tool.

B. Regressing to earlier behavior patterns.

NOTES

NOTES

ANTICIPATORY GUIDANCE FOR THE PERIOD OF 24–36 MONTHS

Review previous guidelines for a reference point as to the toddler's developmental level, and schedule future visits as needed.

I. **Expectations of this period.**
In this most important year, the toddler completes the tasks of the first period of growth. By 3 years of age the successful completion of these developmental tasks can be expected.

- A. Stability of bodily processes and mastery of physical skills.
- B. Toddler sees himself as an individual with ability and value.
- C. Appears confident in his activities and curious to investigate his world.
- D. Uses language as a tool to influence his own actions and affect his environment.
- E. Able to compromise his activities for attention from a meaningful caretaker.
- F. Shares affection with a primary caretaker.

II. **Family status**

- A. Basic needs being met; self-direction in coping with problems.
- B. Parents
    1. Stability of life-style; family routine established that allows the child to predict what is going to happen and gives him a feeling that his life has some consistency.
    2. Cooperating in and understanding their child-rearing practices.
    3. Understanding that the child will begin to move away from them and become interested in peers and the outside world.
    4. Identifying and implementing a plan for their own life goals.
    5. Appreciating their role as family coordinators and standard-bearers for the family's behavioral patterns, mores, and spiritual foundation.
    6. Set example of a gentle, caring attitude.
    7. Understand the importance of child spacing.
- C. Working mother
    1. Adequate health practices and satisfaction with life-style.
    2. Scheduling sufficient time with toddler to ensure the implementation of her philosophy of child-rearing.
    3. Counseling available for career goals and personal support.
- D. Single parent
    1. Ability to assess child-rearing practices of caretakers and to coordinate with own.
    2. Support group intact; not using child as only means of emotional satisfaction.
- E. Siblings
    1. Parents providing opportunity for each child to pass through each developmental stage without undue interference from siblings.
    2. Identify whether one child is overdominant/submissive.
    3. Prohibit teasing; teach alternative ways of interacting.
    4. Older siblings seen as role models.

5. Initiate use of communication skills as a way of expressing feelings and resolving conflicts.

III. Health patterns

A. Nutrition

1. Good appetite; will eat most foods offered.
2. Adequate diet being offered.
   a. Adequate nutrients and calories can be supplied by simple, easily eaten finger foods; rely on foods of high-caloric concentration, such as bread, potatoes, peanut butter, cheese.
   b. Sufficient intake of fluids can be identified by the color and odor of urine. Avoid sweetened drinks such as chocolate milk, drinks containing colored sweeteners, and soda drinks; encourage frequent drinks of water and diluted fruit juice.
   c. Periods of crankiness and fatigue need to be investigated.
      (1) Offer quickly absorbed foods such as fruit juice and a cookie.
      (2) If food is helpful, attempt to avoid such periods by scheduling meals and snacks at more frequent intervals.
3. Eating habits. There are so many developmental tasks going on in this period that putting too much attention on food and eating can become an unnecessary burden to the toddler.
   a. Asking him what he wants to eat or giving him a choice can be too confusing to a toddler busy with his own affairs of experimenting with the things around him and learning a language.
   b. Using food as a reward can begin the establishment of the need for oral satisfaction throughout life—as seen in the obese, the chain-smoker, and those who have inverted the process and have difficulty eating and enjoying foods.
   c. Children mimic the world around them and will adopt the attitudes and habits about foods and the use of food of those around them.

B. Sleep

1. Regular pattern
   a. Sleeps 10–12 hours/night; one nap period.
   b. Falls asleep quickly.
   c. Sleeps all night.
2. Disturbances in pattern indicate health or emotional problems.
   a. Review previous anticipatory guidance outlines to identify unaccomplished tasks.
   b. Identify environmental changes.
   c. Check physical examination and laboratory tests.
3. Safety
   a. Out of the crib and into a bed.
   b. Room and windows checked for safety; gate placed on the bedroom door to keep toddler from roaming the house while the rest of the family sleeps.

C. Elimination

1. Regular pattern; little effect with new foods; continued problems need special investigation.

2. Toilet training. Expectation of control of bowel movements and daytime wetting by 3 years of age.
   a. Schedule regular periods for sitting on potty.
   b. Clothing should be easy to remove; use training pants.
   c. Carefully watch the child's reaction to training.
      (1) If using as a means of getting attention, look for dissatisfactions in other areas.
      (2) Successful training provides a feeling of self-control and adds to feeling of self-worth.

D. High-risk factors
1. Frequent illnesses; overattention to illnesses by parents.
2. Poor appetite; inadequate nutrition.
3. Regressive behavior.

IV. Growth and development

A. Physical
1. Gross motor. Good coordination, smoothness of movements, agility, increase in muscle strength.
2. Fine motor. Improved eye/hand coordination; can do large buttons; scribbles with some intent.
3. Enjoys physical activity; has body confidence—enjoys being tossed in the air, rolling down a hill, splashing in water, etc.
4. Stability of body systems.
5. Growth rate leveling off.
   a. 3 in./year in length.
   b. 5 lb/year in weight.
   c. Legs growing faster than the rest of the body; head slows in growth rate.
   d. Child loses top-heavy appearance.
6. Speech
   a. Vocabulary development: ±50 words; discards jargon.
   b. Articulation
      (1) Half intelligible to people outside family.
      (2) Omits most final consonants.
      (3) Uses all vowels.
   c. Sentence structure
      (1) Two- to three-word sentences, grammatically correct.
      (2) Uses pronouns and prepositions correctly.
      (3) Uses simple adjectives (big, little, short, long).
      (4) Verb tense denotes sense of time—not always used correctly until 5 years of age.

B. Emotional development—Erikson. By 36 months autonomy—or self-worth—has been established and the child is ready to move on and use his physical abilities to learn new skills and interact with others. Without this confidence the child turns inward, feeling guilty and shameful of himself. However, from 2–3 years of age is a time of great fluctuation of independence and overdependence. Personality traits that come into focus during this year are as follows:

1. *Temperament*
   a. Assertiveness: accomplishing tasks without using destructive acts toward himself or others.
   b. Aggressiveness: child has inadequate controls for the pressures put on him.
      (1) Substitutes actions such as bed-wetting, temper tantrums.
      (2) Watch to whom child is aggressive and identify the reasons.
   c. Stubbornness: ascertain whether caused by giving up a pleasure or being overcome by some fear—an expected reaction to the drive for autonomy and the egocentric outlook he has on his world.
2. *Fears and anxiety*
   a. These develop now, since memory and fantasy are working well enough to distort reality.
   b. Demand for impulse control provides fear of failure; child copes by projecting failure on others or on things, and can even conjure up an imaginary friend to take the blame.
   c. Help needed if fears interfere with normal functions of age.
3. *Affection*
   a. Forming attachment to others besides parents.
   b. Fond, helping relationship with siblings; constant aggression or teasing between siblings needs further investigation.
4. *Ambivalence*
   a. Despite urge to "do it myself," turns frequently to parents for reassurance.
   b. Changes in environment and periods of illness cause regression to earlier behavior patterns.
5. *Cooperation.* Continues to develop ability to postpone gratification and accept compromise.
6. *Competence.* Wants to try new activities, and shows pride in his accomplishments.
7. *Wariness.* Keen observer of the goings-on around him.
8. *Joy.* Good health combined with the feeling of the value of himself and others can make joyfulness his dominant mood.
9. Child-rearing practices
   a. Continue to engage in conversation with child; help him express feelings and ideas.
   b. Provide opportunities for companionship of peers.
   c. Careful supervision necessary to avoid one child's becoming overdominant/oversubmissive.
   d. Variety of friends gives child opportunity to observe wide range of behaviors.
   e. "Playing" at 3 years of age consists of enjoying being with and watching each other, with little interchange. When they talk, each talks on a different topic with little relevance to the other.
   f. An adult is needed as a middleman.
   g. As much as possible, provide a consistent, gentle environment.

h. Begin enlarging the environment for wider experiences.
i. Stretch expectations, but do it with an understanding of the child's individual developmental patterns and capabilities; be aware of regressive reactions.

C. Intellectual development—Piaget. The progression from sensory to intuitive learning continues, as shown by the development of memory and symbolic play. Memory is used to recall what has happened in previous incidences and to predict the outcome of the present situation. In symbolic play, by using symbols (words) for actual objects, the child frees himself from reality to be able to take off into fantasy or to take reality apart and put it together in a different manner. By 3 years of age, the following characteristics are present:

1. Uses toys to represent different things (blocks become bridges).
2. Anticipates consequences of actions; expects parental reaction when caught doing something wrong and is more cautious in attempting new physical activities.
3. Symbolizes and pretends; make-believe becomes part of play.
4. Dramatic play, usually imitating those around him.
5. Concentrates on his projects, but keeps an eye on what is going on around him.
6. Understands time—before, after, yesterday.
7. Language
   a. Increased vocabulary; perfects sentence structure and grammar.
   b. Continues labeling and categorizing.
   c. Can make most of wants known verbally.
   d. Makes statements about feelings (I like/hate you; I'm mad at you).
   e. Understands most of what is said to him.
   f. Follows three-step directions.
   g. Can relate experiences from the recent past.
8. Child-rearing practices
   a. Stimulation
      (1) Play equipment for large-muscle use and agility—climbing gyms, balance beam, swings.
      (2) Fine motor: scribbling, puzzles, variety of textures to handle, toys with various shapes and sizes.
      (3) Spatial relations: sandboxes, water tubs.
      (4) Language: simple stories and picture books; being listened to, talked with, and given a minimum of instruction and correction; child is turned off if expectations are beyond his capacity.
      (5) Not burdened with choices and reasoning.
   b. Anticipating consequences
      (1) Talk about plans for the day.
      (2) Have child take as many plans forward as possible ("After breakfast we do. . ." "After Daddy comes home . . .").
      (3) Discuss "if I do this, then I will have this to do."
      (4) Expect and insist on occasional delayed gratification.
      (5) Get child started on projects, but let him carry on as he wishes.

(6) Show approval for child planning out an activity; also help him anticipate the results and consequences.

c. Dramatic play

(1) Simple make-believe helps stretch the imagination.

(2) Help child act out and talk about areas of pressure (sibling rivalry, dominating peers, toilet training, fear of abandonment, punishment, abuse).

d. Needs individual attention for personal rewards and exchange of affection.

9. High-risk factors

a. Poor motor coordination.

b. Delayed speech development (investigate possible hearing loss); inability to use language as a tool.

c. Inability to initiate activities for himself; play is random, without plan or make-believe.

d. No primary caretaker to turn to for help, comfort, and positive reinforcement.

D. Social development

1. Showing initiative to go off on his own.

a. Most of the time, will separate from his mother easily.

b. Enjoys being with peers, but can play by himself and initiate his own activities.

2. Can show affection to others.

3. Practicing self-control; learning to accept realistic limits.

4. Continues to need external controls for "being good."

a. Approval and affection of parents is the incentive, but child needs consistent limit setting before self-control will be dependable.

b. Shows guilt *only* if found out "doing wrong."

c. Acceptance of self-criticism and of responsibility for his actions takes much gentle insistence on behavior standards.

d. Will blame others and even use an imaginary friend as a scapegoat.

5. Confidence in turning to adults; good eye contact.

6. Cooperative, affectionate; eager to please.

7. Enjoys small group of peers; keenly observant of their behavior; little sharing; no "conversation"—each talks about his own interest.

8. Sexual identity established.

a. Ability to look beyond self; observes physical differences.

b. Selects the typed behavior that society has accepted for each sex.

(1) Girls: given positive reinforcement, indulgence, and protectiveness.

(2) Boys: given negative reinforcement and less sympathy; toys and play are of aggressive nature.

c. Role model of female caretaker: girls rewarded for following role model; boys punished for it—approved behavior is a trial-and-error situation for boys, demanding ingenuity and creativeness.

d. Masturbation: a natural result of increased body awareness; a concern if used as a major form of self-satisfaction.

9. Child-rearing practices
   a. Safety is greatest concern; caretakers' expectations of impulse control can be unrealistic.
   b. Stretch expectations, but be aware of signs of overpressuring.
   c. Provide friends; watch and listen to interaction; be available as a middleman.
   d. Attempt to equalize sex behavior expectations.
      (1) Treat boys positively and gently.
      (2) Treat girls with greater expectations of independence and self-assertiveness.
   e. Accept masturbation as a normal occurrence; ask for help if concerned.
   f. *Discipline* consists of positive actions toward promoting self-control, in contrast to *punishment*, which consists of aggressive actions by caretakers, leading to self-degradation of child.
   g. Limit setting: provide consistent routine and safe environment; give attention to any and all acceptable behavior; correct unacceptable behavior with as little attention and show of emotion as possible.
   h. Parental role: setting exemplary standards with which child can identify.
10. High-risk factors
   a. Limit setting not providing establishment of impulse control.
      (1) Overindulgence: child does not lose parents' affection, so has no motive to bargain appropriate behavior for approval and attention.
      (2) Overstrictness: child is fearful of rejection by parents, so does not admit naughtiness done by himself—blames others or a mythical friend; becomes unsure of being able to control behavior in a new situation, so refuses to try.
   b. Child identified as mean and cruel to others—unable to feel or give affection; i.e., unable to understand the feelings of others, so feels no remorse for his actions toward others.
   c. Mother
      (1) Overanxious, overstrict, or overpermissive.
      (2) Has exacting standards above the child's ability to conform.
      (3) Unable to accept child's sex; fosters inappropriate behavior.
   d. Child
      (1) Immature behavior of negativism; distractible and impulsive.
      (2) Unable to relate to adults or peers with affection; appears furtive, aggressive or shy, unhappy.

E. Safety
   1. Accidents happen most frequently
      a. When usual routine changes (holidays, vacations, illness in family).
      b. Following stressful events (either for caretakers or for child).
      c. When caretakers are tired or ill.
      d. Late in the afternoon.

2. Accident prevention
    a. Increased energy and curiosity with little behavior control continue to make this a dangerous period.
    b. When in car, child should always remain in car seat.
    c. Accidents—check environment.
    d. Constant surveillance.
3. Investigate possibility of child abuse and neglect.
4. Instructions to baby-sitters
5. Emergency telephone numbers posted

OVERVIEW

3-YEAR WELL CHILD VISIT

I. A special visit to review the accomplishments of these three years. The health and personality patterns are well established. The investigation of any concerns or problems will have better results now than ever again.

II. **Parents**

- A. Assessment and appreciation of child's accomplishments.

III. **Child**

- A. Physical
  1. Following growth chart.
  2. Accepting simple balanced meals.
  3. Sleep
     - a. Dreams and nightmares may frighten child from wanting to follow usual bedtime routine.
  4. Toilet training accomplished. Girls earlier than boys.
  5. Systems review. See Guidelines.
- B. Emotional
  1. Increasing confidence and independence.
- C. Intellectual
  1. Using language for things important to him.
- D. Social
  1. Enjoys peers. Carefully watches their activities but with little interaction.
  2. Plays equally well with either sex.

IV. **High Risk Factors**

- A. Frequent illnesses and slow recovery.
- B. Impulsive behavior/excessive shyness.
- C. No eye contact.
- D. No primary caretaker to help establish behavior control.

NOTES

NOTES

3-YEAR WELL CHILD VISIT

I. Developmental process.

This visit can be planned as a special review session to assess the growth and development that have taken place during the past 3 years. Identifying both accomplished and unaccomplished tasks will provide a guide for the next critical period of growth: the preschool years, ages 3–6.

II. A review outline

A. Parents

1. Providing basic physical and emotional needs.
2. Self-direction in identifying and coping with problems.
3. Appreciating their role in setting standards for the family's behavioral and cultural patterns.

B. Children

1. Each child having the opportunity to pass through his own developmental stage without undue interference from siblings.
2. A caring, cooperative, interactive pattern of behavior.

C. Toddler

1. Stability and maturation of his physical systems.
2. Sees himself as a person of worth and competence.
3. Identifying his sexual identity.
4. Beginning to use language as a tool.

III. Health habits

A. Nutrition

1. Accepting simple, balanced menus.
2. Pleasure in eating, but not emphasized as a way of gaining attention or a substitute for emotional needs.

B. Sleep

1. Accepts bedtime as another pleasant part of his daily routine.
2. Sleeps 10–12 hours at night, with one nap or rest period.
3. Dreams are beginning to become real, as the ability for magical thinking develops; the inaccurate assessment of reality can be frightening.

C. Elimination

1. Daytime control usually by 3 years of age.
2. Nighttime control accomplished later.
3. Takes pride in accomplishment of this control.

D. Speech

1. Adequate vocabulary to express needs.
2. Not all consonants are articulated.
3. Labeling and categorizing.

IV. Review of systems

A. Growth

1. Growth pattern is consistent with the influencing factors of genetics, nutrition, and illnesses.
2. Rate of growth decelerating—height 3 in./year, weight 5 lb/year.

3. Weight is now four times birth weight; length is half of adult size.
4. Head is 80% of adult size; rate of growth slowing.
5. Legs growing faster than other body parts.

B. Skeletal
1. Bones are becoming stronger as percentage of cartilage to bone is decreasing; long bones first to be ossified, joint bones last.
2. Craniofacial development gives facial features more definition.
3. Skeletal age can now be used as an indication of overall body maturity.
4. Bone functioning as a reservoir for calcium and bone marrow, providing adequate production of red blood cells.

C. Muscle
1. Muscle tissue development influenced by hormones, nutrition, and exercise.
2. Muscle strength depends on amount of tissue, age, and exercise.
3. Because endurance relates to maturation of the cardiac and respiratory systems, which supply oxygen to the muscle tissue, children often have less endurance than expected.

D. Teeth
1. The complete set of 20 deciduous teeth is present; important for mastication and prevention of malocclusion. Dental care now is important.
2. Permanent teeth are being formed in the jaw.
3. Dental age is an indication of overall body maturation.

E. Skin
1. Functioning more efficiently to maintain temperature control.
   a. Number of sweat glands developing.
   b. Maturity of function of the capillaries.
   c. Development of adipose tissue, which decreases evaporation of body fluids.
2. Increased acidity of skin aids in resistance to infection.
3. Increase in melanin production provides better protection from sun's rays.
4. Sebaceous glands are less active, so skin may become dry.
5. Subcutaneous fat decreasing now until ±6 years of age.

F. Vision. Normal acuity of 2–3 years is 20/80.
1. Hyperoptic until ±8 years.
2. Astigmatism may still be present because of immaturity and distortion of lens.
3. Depth perception not complete until ±6 years.

G. Hearing
1. Acuity at adult level.
2. Aware of pitch and tone.

H. Central nervous system
1. Continuation and refinement of myelinization gives increasing neuromuscular coordination.
2. Intellectual abilities increasing because of continued development of cerebral cortex.

3. Location of sensations possible; better able to locate and describe pain.

I. Cardiovascular

1. Body temperature, pulse, and blood pressure more stable.
2. Heart size increasing.
3. Sinus arrhythmia still present; heart murmur in 30–50% of children.

J. Respiratory

1. Increasing lung capacity, as number and size of alveoli increase and muscles of chest are stronger.
2. Diaphragmatic breathing still present until ±6 years of age.

K. Digestive

1. Digestive juices all present and functioning; all types of simple foods can be handled.
2. Peristalsis less sensitive, so assimilation and absorption of food is more efficient.
3. Less frequent and firmer stools.
4. Habit of swallowing saliva established; drooling no longer occurs.

L. Excretory

1. Maturation of kidney function provides more stable solute levels and less danger of dehydration.
2. Increase in bladder size and sphincter control makes toilet training possible.

M. Immune

1. Ability to produce antibodies improving, but immunoglobulin levels are unstable.
2. Lymphoid tissues growing rapidly; provide protection from infection until immunoglobulin production is mature.
3. Developing own set of antibodies as infections are overcome; slowly increasing resistance to infection.

N. Endocrine

1. Growth hormones are well developed.
2. Pituitary gland regulating growth rate.
3. Thyroid gland involved in regulating metabolism and skeletal and dental growth.
4. Adrenal gland regulating blood pressure, heart rate, and glucose metabolism.
5. Islets of Langerhans regulating blood sugar levels. Immaturity of this system can cause periods of low blood sugar; nutrition and timing of food intake need to be evaluated.

V. Growth and development

A. Emotional

1. Sufficient confidence to participate in activities away from home and mother.
2. Resourceful in managing to get his own way.
3. Able both to give and to receive affection.
4. Dominant mood of cheerfulness and self-satisfaction.

B. Intellectual

1. Beginning to anticipate and verbalize consequences of actions.
2. Attempts to solve problems through trial and error.
3. Distorts reality with make-believe.
4. Beginning to use language as a tool.

C. Social
1. Still separates from mother with some apprehension.
2. Enjoys being with peers, but has little interaction with them.
3. Plays well by himself.
4. Aware of sexual identity, but plays equally well with members of his own and of the opposite sex.
5. Indicates awareness of right from wrong, but shows guilt only if found doing something wrong; anxious to please.

D. High-risk factors
1. Inadequate environment to provide basic needs.
2. Inconsistent growth pattern and poor coordination.
3. Health problems not under medical supervision.
4. Impulsive, aggressive/passive behavior patterns.
5. Inability to use language as a tool.
6. Inability to show affection or accept affection from others.
7. No primary adult with whom to establish a caring relationship.

VI. Physical examination

A. Growth. Continuing on established pattern; "catch up" if there was severe or prolonged illness.

B. Appearance and behavior
1. Color.
2. Posture.
3. Body proportion.
4. Energy level, alertness, attention to instructions, ability to control activity.
5. Good eye contact, confident manner, interaction with adults other than parent.

C. Specific factors to note while doing routine physical examination
1. Skin. Check for bruising, burns.
2. Eyes. Strabismus.
3. Ears. Mobility of tympanic membrane.
4. Throat. Enlarged tonsil tissue.
5. Neck. Lymph nodes.
6. Chest. Increased breath sounds; diaphragmatic breathing.
7. Heart. Sinus arrhythmia; heart murmurs—refer to physician if not previously evaluated.
8. Abdomen. Muscle tone; femoral pulses; hernias.
9. Genitalia. Irritation, discharge; testes.
10. Musculoskeletal. Muscle development and tone; range of motion.
11. Central nervous system. Gait; more refined coordination; balance; stands on one foot; hops on one foot; buttons up; beginning control in using crayons.

D. Mother-child interaction.

1. Mother. Pride and affection evident.
2. Child. Attention to mother for support and control of activity.

VII. Assessment

A. Physical

B. Developmental

C. Emotional

D. Environmental

VIII. Plan

A. Immunization. Complete schedule as needed.

B. Screening. Hematocrit, urinalysis as indicated; check blood pressure; hearing and eye test; dental visit.

C. Problem list (devised with parent); SOAP for each.

D. Appropriate timing for office, home, and/or telephone visits; continue individual scheduling.

OVERVIEW

ANTICIPATORY GUIDANCE FOR THE PERIOD OF 3–6 YEARS

I. The guidelines for this period are to be used as a continuum as each child passes through these developmental stages at his own pace. Chronological age may not be applicable.

II. **Parents**

A. Their interest, support, and affection will help to guide the child from the 3-year-old and his world of magic to a realistic 6-year-old ready for school and friends.

III. **Child**

A. Physical

1. Health

a. Following growth pattern.

b. Frequent colds as associating with other children and slowly building up his own immunity.

c. Eating

(1) Selective and independent about food. A wide variety of foods offered with no choices or discussion. Food not to be used as a threat or reward.

d. Sleeping

(1) See Guidelines. Nightmares common from 3 to 4 years of age. By 6 years, if still frequent, investigation is necessary.

B. Emotional

1. These years are continuing development of self-esteem and confidence to turn from the security of home to the outside world of peers and school.

2. This may be a difficult path with frequent regressive or aggressive behavior.

3. Able to maintain expected behavior.

4. Beginning to distinguish right from wrong.

5. A consistent caretaker is needed to turn to for guidance and encouragement.

6. See Guidelines for child-rearing practices of each age.

C. Intellectual

1. Learning through increased memory of experiences and their consequences.

2. Initiating own activities and creative play.

3. TV watching inhibits these creative activities.

4. See Guidelines for each age's expectations.

D. Social

1. Enjoys being with peers but watching each other rather than interactive play. (Listening to children's conversations is a way to observe how each child is carrying on his own independent conversation.)

2. Sex Identity

a. Will play equally well with either sex.

b. See Guidelines for each age's expectations and child-rearing practices.

IV. High Risk

- **A.** Poor health or serious illness.
- **B.** Overly shy or overly aggressive behavior.
- **C.** Poor language development.
- **D.** No appropriate role model.

NOTES

ANTICIPATORY GUIDANCE FOR THE PERIOD OF 3–6 YEARS

I. Expectations of this period.

These 3 years provide the time needed to expand physical and psychosocial skills. By age 6 the child will be a competent, self-assured, friendly first-grader.

- A. Physical maturity
  1. Increasing muscle strength and endurance.
  2. Developing immunity to infectious disease.
- B. Magic and fantasy will give way to reality.
- C. Language skills developing. Beginning to attend to what others are saying. By six years can have interactive speech.
- D. Values of the environment being internalized, and actions being guided by these standards.

II. Family status

- A. Parents
  1. Providing basic physical and developmental needs.
  2. Responsible for adequate child care arrangements.
  3. Household tasks scheduled and responsibilities for each family member defined.
  4. Emergency planning—accidents, illness, fire, telephone contacts.
  5. Family group meetings to share experiences, plan activities, and give support to each other.
- B. Children
  1. Each developing according to his own capabilities without being overpowered by parents or siblings.
  2. Demonstrating tolerance, affection, and support for each other.
  3. Developing interactive techniques without teasing or aggression.

III. Health patterns

- A. Nutrition
  1. Child is selective and more independent about food.
  2. Encourage some involvement in food preparation and shopping.
  3. Encourage good breakfast habits in anticipation of school years.
  4. Offer small amounts of nutritious foods often during the day.
  5. Encourage eating of vegetables and fruits (children often prefer these raw).
  6. Child should not be forced to eat; poor appetite needs further investigation.
  7. Food should not be used as a bribe, threat, or reward.
- B. Health. Frequent "colds" can be expected due to child's associating with other children and still building up immunity to infections. If recovery prolonged, evaluation of basic health pattern needed.
- C. Sleep
  1. Regular pattern established (10–12 hours at night).
  2. Naps: help child become aware of periods of fatigue, and provide a "rest area."

3. Dreams can be frightening, since child is still learning to distinguish dreams from reality; investigate overstimulation, anxiety, exhaustion.
4. Teeth grinding: correlates with frequency of nightmares; can be a way of releasing unrelieved emotional pressures.

D. Elimination
1. Regular pattern established; learning to manage himself.
2. Occasional accidents, usually due to illness, changes in his world, or some traumatic experience.
3. Continued soiling or a return to bed-wetting needs further investigation.
4. Enuresis: see Enuresis in Part II.

E. Child-rearing practices
1. No rewards for illness.
2. Responsibility for "wellness" becoming part of child's learning.
3. Provide openness to talk about unusual discomforts, body functions, and maltreatment.

F. High-risk factors
1. Basic health patterns not becoming routine.
2. Somatic complaints being used for emotional support.

IV. Growth and development

A. Physical
1. Growth rate slows to ±3 in./year.
   a. Legs growing the fastest.
   b. Facial bones developing and fat pads disappearing, so by age 5 child looks as he will as an adult.
   c. Muscle development and strength increasing through activity; not sex dependent.
2. Gross motor. Improving coordination makes hopping, skipping, and dancing possible.
3. Fine motor. By 5–6 years, able to draw recognizable objects.
4. Speech
   a. Vocabulary
      (1) Increasing seemingly without any effort.
      (2) By 5–6 years of age, child uses verb tenses and plurals correctly.
   b. Articulation
      (1) Stuttering occasionally present, as ideas come faster than words can be found.
      (2) Lisping until 5–6 years is a matter of maturation.

B. Emotional development—Erikson. initiative vs. guilt. This stage sees the progression from activities motivated merely by responses to stimuli or imitative actions to purposeful activity. Initiating activity, both physical and intellectual, continues the development of competence and feelings of independence. Without either the opportunity or the physical skills to explore, manipulate, and challenge the environment, the competencies and independence that could have been attained are delayed or never developed. These experiences become the basic values determining the ratio of self-confidence to feelings of inferiority.

1. Emotions become more stable as the child develops.
   a. Feelings of competence in doing things for himself.
   b. The ability to manage away from home.
   c. The ability to make friends and relate to adults other than parents.
   d. An increase in intellectual capacity so he can understand events and plan activities.
2. Temperament
   a. *Egocentric:* enjoys being with peers, but it will take until age 7–8 before he can appreciate another's point of view.
   b. *Innovative* in activities.
   c. *Affection:* an egocentric reaction for approval and attention.
   d. *Assertive:* improving memory and language skills are used to direct his activities and to aid him to influence others.
   e. *Aggression:* a mode of behavior that continues through observing adult role models; a means of getting rid of unrelieved pressures.
   f. *Cooperation:* continues to bargain appropriate behavior for approval and attention.
   g. *Fear:* an expected reaction to his world of fantasy and to his increase in physical daring.
   h. *Shyness:* a lack of the feelings of competency and independence.
   i. *Passivity:* overcontrol by adults can make the child fearful to act on his own; a lack of developed built-in behavioral controls can prevent him from attempting activity.
   j. So much is to be accomplished in these 3 short years that occasional reversals to earlier behavior patterns can be expected.
3. High-risk factors
   a. Fearfulness.
   b. Anger.
   c. Inactivity.
   d. Withdrawal.
4. Child-rearing practices
   a. 3–4 years
      (1) Short periods of peer companionship under adult supervision. Needs sufficient time by himself to develop pleasure from initiating and accomplishing activities.
      (2) Open spaces and large equipment for play.
      (3) Safe boundaries and consistent limits on behavior.
      (4) A primary adult listener, confidant, and giver of attention and approval.
   b. 4–5 years
      (1) More time with peers, but with continued supervision.
      (2) Variety of activities and experiences.
      (3) Learning to use language rather than aggressive acts to get his own way.
      (4) Opportunities to take responsibility for his behavior.
      (5) A primary adult listener, confidant, and giver of attention and approval.

c. 5–6 years
   (1) Opportunity to use increased skills for independent planning and carrying out of activities.
   (2) Plan peer interaction and participation in simple group games.
   (3) Improve interaction by asking child to repeat ideas given by others.
   (4) Child still needs primary adult for attention and support.

C. Intellectual development—Piaget. These years continue the child's egocentric way of seeing the world. Learning intuitively through self-activity, having little concern for reality, and using his increasing memory and language, he keeps reconstructing his world to fit his needs. By 6 years of age, the influence of peers and his own experiences are forcing him to take a more realistic view of the world around him.

1. Expectations
   a. 3–4 years
      (1) Intuitive learning through freewheeling activities.
         (a) "Pretending"; trying on role activities of others.
         (b) Investigating and manipulating everything that can be reached.
         (c) Watching activities of others.
         (d) Magical world: limited experience gives incorrect explanations of events.
      (2) Memory continues storing up events and their outcomes.
   b. 4–5 years
      (1) Intuitive learning continues through the initiative to attempt new and creative ways to do things.
      (2) Magical world is giving way to reality as past experiences are used to predict the correct outcome.
      (3) Logical reasoning is still a long way off.
   c. 5–6 years
      (1) Beginning to learn through language.
      (2) Can maintain a single line of thought.
      (3) Listens to others, but with little exchange of ideas.
      (4) Integrating past experiences to form a more reliable version reality.
   d. High-risk factors
      (1) Passive and cautious in activities.
      (2) Magical thinking still dominating activity at age 5.
      (3) Impulsive, quarrelsome behavior at age 5.
      (4) No primary adult to provide support and affection.
   e. Child-rearing practices
      (1) Safe areas where high-level energy can be expended.
      (2) Variety of activities with the opportunity for some association with children slightly older.
      (3) Play equipment: for large-muscle activity, for perceptual learning; materials and opportunity for dramatic play.

(4) Discussion of activities; time for someone to listen to child.
(5) A primary adult to provide support and affection.

2. Language
   a. 3–4 years
      (1) Makes declarative statements about his own wants and feelings.
      (2) Thinks out loud; cannot be expected to keep a secret.
      (3) Conversations consist of each child talking only for himself, not attending to or responding to ideas of others.
      (4) Body language supplements these limited language skills.
   b. 4–5 years. A quarrelsome period of learning to interact with peers; quarrels force child to express his ideas and to listen to the ideas of others.
   c. By 5 years
      (1) Listening skills improving, but not until 7–8 years can he listen to others well enough to have an exchange of ideas.
      (2) Improving ability to use words in place of action; needs role model of people doing this and help in developing this skill.
   d. High-risk factors
      (1) Impulsive behavior; unable to use language as a controller of action.
      (2) Too quiet; retreating into silence in confrontations.
      (3) Continued baby talk and poor fluency.
   e. Child-rearing practices
      (1) Avoid correcting errors; child will make own corrections.
      (2) Absolutely no attention to stuttering; increased concern by child will add to problem.
      (3) Provide good speech and language role models.
      (4) Provide a patient listener to hear child express his feelings and ideas.
3. School readiness
   a. Able to manage away from home.
   b. Able to accept behavior control expectations.
   c. Able to interact with adults other than parents.
   d. Language skills sufficient to express his ideas.
   e. Listening skills sufficient to attend to directions of others.
   f. Sufficient self-esteem to be able to carry on independent activity.
4. Television watching
   a. Passive activity; replaces important learning from self-initiated activity.
   b. Child is fascinated by color, sound, and motion; energy put into watching, not taking in story.
   c. Child is unable to distinguish between fantasy and reality.
   d. By age 5, child relates to characters as role models; aggressive behavior seen as appropriate behavior.
   e. Usurps family conversations and interaction.
5. Television control

a. Make a family activity by discussing what programs are to be selected, each member having a limited choice.
b. Discuss programs in the family group.
c. Watch as many programs as possible with child. Pay attention to snacks eaten during TV watching; often they are "junk foods," which are high in calories and fat and low in nutrients.
d. Set up play equipment near the TV as an alternative to watching.
e. Set up definite times for TV watching and definite times when TV is turned off.

D. Social development

1. Expectations. Sequential development in becoming a member of society; by the time the child enters first grade, the following expectations must be met so that he is freed of his egocentric needs and can reach out to learn and enjoy the companionship of others.

a. 3–4 years
(1) Managing away from home; sufficient ability to control behavior.
(2) Observant of what is going on around him; peer relations consist of watching each other but playing independently.
(3) Instigating his own activities.
(4) Turning to adults for help and support.

b. 4–5 years
(1) Easily accepts the expected appropriate behavior.
(2) Peer relations are often quarrelsome, since child attempts to argue for his own way.
(3) Eager to please primary caretaker and remorseful if caught doing wrong.

c. 5–6 years
(1) Able to join peers in simple interactive games.
(2) Dogmatic; changes rules as needed to benefit himself.
(3) Internalizing behavioral patterns; standards of family and peer group accepted.
(4) Sufficient self-esteem for independent activities without constant demanding of attention.

2. Sexual identity

a. From 3 to 5 years, usually indiscriminate as to which sex he is with; will take on role of either sex in dramatic play.
b. By age 6, prefers the company of own sex; this preference continues until adolescence.
c. Social expectations of each sex are internalized.
(1) Boys are more combative and daring.
(2) Girls use words as weapons and coyness and guile to get their own way.
d. Modification of sex-typing patterns:
(1) Boys: gentleness and nonpunitive punishment.
(2) Girls: develop feelings of competence and industry by devising more challenging physical activities and intellectual projects.

3. High-risk factors

a. Parents with low self-esteem have difficulty enforcing consistent behavioral standards.
b. Inadequate environment for active, curious child.
c. Few opportunities to be with other children; little supervision if with other children.
d. No primary caring adult.

4. Child-rearing practices
   a. Promoting acceptable behavior by
      (1) Safe environment with sufficient space and equipment for constructive activities.
      (2) Daily schedule consistent; expected behavior defined and maintained.
      (3) Understanding child's ability to comply with demands put on him.
      (4) Spending some time with older children; imitating is easiest way for child to learn.
      (5) Positive reinforcers, such as hugs and kisses; approval needed for each small step; be aware of things he is doing right.
      (6) Remembering that logic and reasoning are not part of his skills yet.
   b. Discipline
      (1) Expect child to control his behavior for attention and approval.
      (2) Give positive reinforcers for any and all appropriate behaviors.
      (3) Harmful behavior to himself and others must be stopped but must not be the only way for the child to get attention.
      (4) Frequent aggressive and uncontrolled behavior needs investigation into the child's role models, unrelieved pressures, and physical problems.
      (5) Punitive punishment feeds into anger and violence.

E. Safety

1. Accidents happen most frequently
   a. When usual routine changes (holidays, vacations, illness in family).
   b. Following stressful events (either for caretakers or for child).
   c. When caretakers are tired or ill.
   d. Late in the afternoon.
2. Accident prevention
   a. Child is beginning to understand the consequences of actions.
   b. Responsibilities given as child demonstrates reliability.
   c. Magical thinking makes child think he can do the impossible.
   d. Family rules established and discussed.
      (1) Responsibilities outlined for each family member.
      (2) Fire drills practiced and meeting place established.
      (3) Emergency plans established and rehearsed.
      (4) Telephone numbers posted and practiced.
3. Investigate frequent injuries as possible child neglect or abuse.
4. Instructions to baby-sitters

OVERVIEW

6-YEAR WELL CHILD VISIT

I. Parents

A. Observing carefully the child's ability to:

1. Cope with his long day away at school.
2. Maintain appropriate behavior and his independence with new peer group.
3. Communicate with him and listen to his daily experiences (still difficult for him to express ideas and feelings).

II. Child

A. Physical

1. Slow growth rate for both sexes.
   a. Enjoying food and accepting a well-balanced diet. Family emphasis on physical fitness enjoyed.
   b. Sleep 10–12 hours. Nightmares should be occurring less frequently.
   c. Speech. Articulation of all sounds.
   d. Loosing teeth in same order as eruption.

B. Emotional

1. Initiates own activities but has difficulty following activities of others. He is still attempting to control his own world and expects things to be done his way.

C. Intellectual

1. No longer interested in his magical world but now thinks concretely or how things are and how they work.

D. Social

1. Experimenting with ways to interact successfully with teachers and peers.
2. Prefers associating with own sex.
3. Cultural and ethnic patterns of others difficult to understand.

III. High Risk Factors

A. Poor school adjustment or inappropriate school

B. Frequent illness or using illness as a way to escape these new developmental tasks.

C. No primary caretaker to "listen" to him.

IV. See Guidelines for specific factors of physical examination.

NOTES

NOTES

6-YEAR WELL CHILD VISIT

I. **Developmental process.**

The attitudes of competence, self-worth, and initiative that the 6-year-old has developed provide the impetus to separate more completely from his family and home. Both he and his family enjoy their increasing independence. Attending school and associating with teachers and peers provide the child with the new challenge to develop his own capabilities and self-confidence within his enlarging world.

- A. Parents
  1. Understand the importance of the change from a home- and family-centered child to a teacher- and peer group-centered child.
  2. Have consistent expectations of appropriate behavior.
  3. Continue to provide a safe, supportive environment.
- B. Child
  1. Maintains appropriate behavior.
  2. Busy and happy with projects at school and with peers.
  3. Continues to turn to family for support.

II. **Family status**

- A. Parental concerns and problems. Ability to identify problems and to cope.
- B. Illnesses in family since last visit.
- C. Parental assessment of child's development.
- D. Family interaction and support for each other.
  1. Organization of responsibilities for each member.
  2. Review and updating of emergency planning.
  3. Meetings for group decisions, problem solving, and sharing of experiences.

III. **Health habits**

- A. Nutrition and diet history
  1. Adequate diet offered.
  2. Intake of food during school hours; snacks.
  3. Child learning the basics of nutrition.
  4. Ethnic eating patterns evaluated.
  5. Continued involvement in shopping and preparation of foods.
- B. Sleep
  1. Restful 10 hours with fewer disturbances from nightmares.
  2. Falls asleep easily unless overtired or overstimulated.
  3. Beginning to realize when he needs rest and sleep.
- C. Elimination
  1. Managing independently.
  2. Family routine allows for regular time of bowel movements.
  3. Problems or discomforts discussed with caretaker.
  4. Enuresis: see Enuresis in Part II.
  5. Encopresis: refer to physician.

IV. Growth and development

A. Physical

1. Growth following established pattern.
   a. Participating in activities to develop endurance and large muscles, such as climbing, swimming, running.
   b. Developing muscle coordination with games of rhythm and music and with large ball games.
   c. Activity program needed that is designed to develop individual skills.
   d. Family emphasis on the importance of physical fitness.
   e. Careful supervision to de-emphasize competitive games until child is physically and emotionally ready.
2. Teeth
   a. Losing teeth in the same order as eruption.
   b. Child taking responsibility of daily care.
   c. Dental care available.

B. Speech development

1. Articulating all sounds by 6–7 years.
2. Correctly using verb tenses, plurals, and pronouns.
3. Vocabulary increasing, and most words used appropriately.

C. Emotional development—Erikson: initiative vs. guilt. The child demonstrates that he feels competent to manage his daily routine, can be a leader of his peers, and can accept and return the affection of his primary caretakers.

1. Is enthusiastic about daily happenings but cautious about routine changes and new experiences.
2. Enjoys companionship of peers but continues to want to do things his way.
3. Continues to turn to caretaker for affection and approval.
4. If these attitudes are not present, further assessment is needed.

D. Intellectual development—Piaget: from intuitive learning to concrete thinking. Child continues through sufficient experiences to distinguish fact from fantasy. This world of reality is established through increased memory of and ability to symbolize these experiences.

1. Learning
   a. Enjoys school, learning of facts; rather than "what does that do?" he asks "how does it work?"
   b. Turning to stories of actual adventures; no longer interested in fairy tales.
   c. Can define ways to both solve a problem and understand its consequences.
2. Language
   a. Enjoys words, riddles, puns.
   b. Experiments with sounds—chants, songs, poems.
   c. Exchanges factual information, but has trouble expressing ideas and feelings.

E. Social development. The continuing task is to learn to interact successfully with those in the child's enlarging world of school and community.

1. Inconsistent behavior in trying to find successful interactive patterns.
2. Has frequent changes in friendships.
3. Depends on his rules for expected ways of acting for himself and playmates.
4. Turns to adults for guides to cultural and moral behavior; is now internalizing the behavioral patterns of his culture.

F. High-risk factors
   1. Family
      a. Needs not being met.
      b. Inappropriate and inconsistent expectations of child.
   2. Child
      a. Inappropriate behavior patterns continue.
         (1) Lack of behavior control.
         (2) Not showing guilt when doing wrong.
         (3) No appropriate role models.
      b. Developmental lags (specifically neurologic and speech).
      c. Inability to relate appropriately with siblings, peers, and adults.
      d. Poor adjustment to school.

V. Physical examination

A. Appearance
   1. Body proportion.
   2. Muscle development.

B. Behavior
   1. Makes eye contact.
   2. Cooperative.
   3. Interested in visit.
   4. Able to contribute to history taking.

C. Growth
   1. Continues on established pattern.
   2. Investigate if more than 2 standard deviations in height or weight.

D. Specific factors to note while doing routine physical examination
   1. Skin. Check for excessive bruises, burns.
   2. Eyes. Equal tracking.
   3. Ears. Mobility of tympanic membrane.
   4. Teeth. Losing teeth in order of appearance; check occlusion; check for cavities.
   5. Throat. Tonsils—size, color, pitting.
   6. Heart. Sinus arrhythmia.
   7. Abdomen. Muscle tone, hernia.
   8. Genitalia. Irritation, discharge, phimosis.
   9. Musculoskeletal. Muscle development, strength, tone; check back for scoliosis.
   10. Neurologic. Coordination—gait, skip, hop; fine motor—draws triangle horizontal, vertical.

OVERVIEW

ANTICIPATORY GUIDANCE FOR THE PERIOD OF 6–9 YEARS

I. **Parents**

A. Appreciate their role to establish family standards and mores.

B. Discuss with child their expectations and devise plans toward cooperation in maintaining these expectations.

C. Plan sufficient time to be with child to "listen" and talk about his experiences.

D. Provide opportunities for successful experiences at school and with his peers.

II. **Child**

A. Physical

1. Slower growth pattern for both sexes but agility and coordination improving.
2. Early maturing girls can begin hormonal changes by 9. Evident by developing chubbiness.
3. Diet. Learning to take responsibility of eating a balanced diet.
4. Elimination. Boys have more evidence of encopresis and enuresis. Important to elicit this information and refer to M.D.
5. Safety. Accident-prone behavior needs evaluation.

B. Emotional

1. A period where successful experiences are important to continue his growth toward self-esteem and self-confidence. Without these a feeling of inferiority can take over his attitude towards himself and his ability.
2. See Guidelines for outline of characteristics of child's temperament.

C. Intellectual

1. The developing ability to think realistically helps him to manage himself and his affairs effectively.
2. See Guidelines for school and learning expectations for each age group.

D. Social

1. During these years the child turns from needing only a few friends to expecting to become a member of a group or gang. Community activities such as Scouts, church group, and sports can help to find appropriate groups.
2. See Guidelines for age-appropriate expectations.

III. **High Risk**

A. Poor school adjustment and not working up to capacity.

B. Using aggressive behavior to gain attention.

C. Accident prone or frequent illnesses.

D. Depending on TV or computer games for entertainment rather than enjoying companionship of others.

IV. **Safety and Accident Prevention**

A. See Guidelines for accident prevention.

NOTES

ANTICIPATORY GUIDANCE FOR THE PERIOD OF 6–9 YEARS

I. **Expectations of this period.**

Like the other age periods, the years 6–9 are not a single steplike unit. Contrasting a 6-year-old and a 9-year-old shows what a big step this is. The 6-year-old still retains many characteristics of earlier periods, including struggling to find a way to establish himself with his peers and turning back to his family for overt shows of affection. In contrast, the 9-year-old is a firm member of the gang, accepting its rituals and rules and taking his disappointments and hurts stoically. This period, the first that can be recalled chronologically, includes years of freedom, fun, and fond memories. By 9 years, the child

- A. Is separating from the family and making independent decisions.
- B. Is able to relate successfully to peers and adults other than his parents.
- C. Enjoys school and is eager to learn.
- D. Instigates projects; has perseverance and derives pleasure from completing tasks.
- E. Turns to his family for support and approval.
- F. Is guided in his behavior by the rules of his family and peers.

II. **Family status**

- A. Basic needs being met; self-direction in coping with problems.
- B. Parents
  1. Pride and enjoyment in child.
  2. Fostering independence and new experiences.
  3. Time for listening, discussions, and support.
  4. Giving responsibility as child demonstrates he can accept it.
  5. Acting as a moral guide and role model of love and affection.
  6. Spending time to see that family rules are adhered to.
- C. Child
  1. Moves away from a close association with the family to his own peer group.
  2. Accepts household responsibilities and schedules.
  3. Returns to family for support and belonging.
  4. Begins challenging family values with the values of peers and school; moral judgment limited by inability to appreciate views of others.
  5. Learning to accept consequences of his actions.

III. **Health patterns.**

The following areas are to be identified and discussed with the child at each of the well child visits.

- A. Nutrition
  1. Learning nutritional standards such as basic four food groups; knows nutritious foods vs. "junk foods."
  2. Participating in meal planning and shopping.
  3. Keeping chart for adequate calories and nutrition as needed.
- B. Elimination
  1. Responsibility for regular schedule.

2. Boys have more frequent problems with constipation and soiling than girls—refer to physician if a continuing problem.
3. Enuresis: see Enuresis in Part II.

C. Sleep
1. Individual pattern (8–10 hours).
2. Older child to stay up later than younger child; this gives parents time with each child and gives the children a feeling of individuality.
3. Able to awaken on time in the morning.

D. Exercise
1. High energy level and muscular development require adequate opportunity for exercise.
2. Supervised sports program in and after school.
3. Free play periods—safe environments, necessary limits.
4. TV watching limited.

E. Responsibility for own health
1. Adequate role models.
2. Realization of the pleasure and advantage of good health and the disadvantage of illness.
   a. Knowledge and willingness to obtain health care.
   b. Social and emotional problems identified—parents or school personnel used as resource.

F. Safety
1. Realistic thinking promotes more cautiousness.
2. Accident-prone children: investigate causes.
   a. Awkwardness.
   b. Daredevil behavior to get attention from peers.
   c. Unstable environment causing inattention and high level of frustration.

IV. Growth and development

A. Physical
1. Growth rate continues at a slow pace for both sexes.
   a. Chubbiness at 8–9 years does not mean future obesity; following puberty there is usually a return to the previous pattern.
   b. Muscle growth equal for both sexes; amount of exercise now determines muscle strength.
2. Teeth—"age of the loose tooth."
   a. Teeth replaced in the same order as eruption of deciduous teeth.
   b. Dental care: discuss fluoride treatments with dentist if no fluoride in drinking water.
3. Eyes. By 7 years, visual acuity of 20/20–20/30.
4. Speech
   a. Articulation: refer to speech therapist if problems with enunciation, slurring, or fluency continue.
   b. More complex sentences used (5–7 words).
   c. Rapid increase of vocabulary.

d. Careless enunciation can be improved by whistling, repeating jingles and tongue twisters, and singing; listening to tape of his own voice also is helpful.

5. Development of secondary sex characteristics. Organ enlargement begins 2–4 years before puberty.

a. Girls: growth spurt at 9–14 years; breast enlargement at 8–13 years; menses at 10–16 years.

b. Boys: growth spurt at 10 1/2–13 1/2 years; enlarged testes at 9 1/2–13 1/2 years.

6. Child-rearing practices

a. School athletic program: Title IX specifies equal time and money for girls and boys.

b. 6–7 years

(1) Child is learning to interact and to play according to rules, but he finds it difficult to be a loser.

(2) Physical coordination makes possible simple games such as kickball; eye/hand coordination and depth perception are not sufficient for much success at more skilled games.

(3) Muscle strength and development progressing rapidly; equipment needed to enhance this.

(4) Endurance greatly improved, but signs of fatigue need to be identified.

c. 8–9 years

(1) Sportsmanship is now a gang standard.

(2) Child can interact well enough to enjoy team sports.

(3) Girls need sufficient opportunities to develop muscle strength and have team participation.

B. Emotional development—Erikson: industry vs. inferiority. Building on the previously developed attitudes of self-confidence, competence, and independence, the child attempts new projects. Completing these projects fosters pleasure and satisfaction in doing and succeeding. These same skills apply to participating in school and making new friends successfully. Without opportunities for these successes, feelings of inferiority develop.

1. Temperament

a. *Egocentric thinking:* continues until age 7–8, when child can include his peer group in his world.

b. *Affection:* turning from family to teacher and peer group for affection and approval.

c. *Spontaneous and enthusiastic:* enjoys his new outside world.

d. *Assertive:* attempts to persuade others to do things his way; demands his share, his turn, and his belongings.

e. *Self-concept:* sees himself as different from others and begins to perceive his own abilities.

f. *Self-identity:* moving away from family; becoming dependent on gang's assessment.

g. *Self-esteem:* approval or disapproval of those important to him reflects how he sees himself.

h. *Sexual identity:* interacts best with own sex (both adults and peers); taking on society's role expectations.

i. *Frustrations:* learning to cope with disappointments; learning to have more realistic expectations.

2. *High-risk factors.* Attitudes of defiance, rebellion, aggression, and overpassivity need a careful and intense workup; treatment now is more likely to be successful than in the future.
3. Child-rearing practices
   a. Independence of parents and child: important to have specific times together for planning, companionship, and support.
   b. Carefully watch child's success and failure in school and with friends; promote open communication so that understanding of problems is possible.
   c. Provide opportunities for successful experiences.
      (1) Appropriate school experience for child's ability.
      (2) Playmates available of same size, age, and interests; playing with older or younger child causes him either to be bossed or to do the bossing with no possibility of reciprocal interaction.
   d. Affection and approval
      (1) Child is now keen enough to know when approval is not deserved; demands honest opinions and gives honest opinions.
      (2) Child needs help expressing affection and love; compassionate role model needed.
   e. Seek help if
      (1) Child continues to be unsuccessful in school or in making friends.
      (2) Child is unable to control acting out or is predominantly passive in his behavior.
      (3) Communication between parents and child is poor.

C. Intellectual development—Piaget. During this age period, the child progresses from learning through intuition to learning through concrete experiences. The difference between fantasy and reality is being sorted out and replaced by facts and order, systematic thinking, organizing, and classifying. Problems need to be tested in actuality; hypotheses are not yet comprehended.

1. Expectations
   a. 6–7 years
      (1) Still learning intuitively, but with good memory and building up of experiences, will soon become a realist.
      (2) Ready for learning.
      (3) Can still be unrealistic in his explanations of events.
      (4) Can remember letters and numbers.
      (5) Expends much energy in learning to manage away from home and to interact with teacher and peers—this can cause learning difficulties if this becomes an overriding concern.
   b. 7–8 years
      (1) Learning concretely; logical reasoning improving.
      (2) Able to sit still longer.
      (3) Lengthening attention span and improving listening skills.
   c. 8–9 years

(1) Looks for cause and effect (scientist).
(2) Comprehends reading material more easily.
(3) Time and place: past becomes important; interest in far-off places.
(4) Basic writing, spelling, reading skills accomplished.

d. Identify intellectual behavior by the following:
(1) Successfully adapts to new situations.
(2) Changes thinking to new requirements.
(3) Manages himself and his affairs effectively.
(4) Has an acute sense of humor.
(5) Is goal-directed.

e. High-risk factors
(1) Difficult and unhappy adjustment away from home.
(2) Inappropriate schooling for child's abilities.

f. Child-rearing practices
(1) Sincere, consistent interest in child's schoolwork.
(2) Participation in school organizations by parents.
(3) Defined, realistic expectations of child, following teacher conference and own judgment.
(4) Consistent insistence on child's appropriate behaviors.
(5) "What's the hurry?": if either social or academic problems arise, this is the best time to give the child a chance to catch up. Watch
(a) If boy, whether one of the youngest and smallest in the class.
(b) If girl, whether one of the youngest in the class, with a maternal history of late pubertal maturation; by sixth to seventh grade, still a little girl while classmates are becoming young ladies; socially a misfit at a crucial time of development.

2. Language

a. Vocabulary development important for expression of an increasing range of feelings and experiences.

b. Expressing ideas and feelings; used as a coping and problem-solving mechanism.

c. Child-rearing practices
(1) Vocabulary development
(a) Encourage word games, crossword puzzles, word tests of synonyms and antonyms, dictionary use.
(b) Provide new experiences and find specific new words from these experiences.
(c) Encourage reading: read to child until his reading skills are sufficient for him to take over; library visits.
(d) TV: learning from pictures and voices; can cause difficulty in shifting to letters.
(2) Help in developing communication skills
(a) Expressing feelings; finding precise vocabulary.
(b) Stating problems; defining problem areas.

(c) Developing "think tank" solutions.

(d) Predicting outcome of each solution.

(e) Appropriate listener available.

(3) Bilingual home

(a) Most children handle bilingualism successfully.

(b) If problems, child should develop proficiency in one language, then return to the second.

(4) Listening skills

(a) For awareness of speech, encourage memorizing and reciting, repeating digit lists (backward and forward), learning nonsense verse.

(b) Music: have child learn to play an instrument and read music.

(c) Encourage child to repeat statements of others before giving an answer.

(d) Constant high background noise discourages efforts to listen.

(e) Approving adult with whom to talk.

(5) Writing skills

(a) By 6 years: has muscle control for printing large letters.

(b) By 7–8 years: writes simple, short sentences; one idea or fact, few adjectives or adverbs.

(c) By 9 years: can write compositions of 200 words.

(d) Spelling: connecting sound to written form demands attention to detail, a difficult task for a child with other concerns.

D. Social development

1. Expectations

a. 6–7 years

(1) Successfully managing a whole day at school; taking the bus; eating away from home, bathroom independence; now able to sit still, listen, answer questions, and most particularly, aware of what others are doing.

(2) Interaction with teacher established.

(3) Still controls behavior for attention and approval.

(4) Makes friends with a few classmates.

b. 7–8 years

(1) Enjoys school; eager to learn.

(2) Reliable, and accepts behavioral expectations.

(3) Makes friends but changes affections frequently.

(4) Groups have loose ties, easily change members.

(5) Rules not absolute, change to serve own purpose.

c. 8–9 years

(1) An exceptional period of good health, good academic skills, good friends, and few concerns.

(2) Peer groups: a behavioral phenomenon that appears to develop in all societies.

(a) Rules and rituals are rigid, form boundaries of behavior.

(b) Leadership given to those who are largest (in boys' group) and the best talkers (in girls' groups) and who have the ability to understand the feelings of other gang members.

(c) Satisfy urge for companionship and approval.

(d) Give opportunity to practice comparing gang mores with standards of the family.

(e) Perpetuates segregation; continued sex discrimination, even beyond this age group (fraternities, lodges, service clubs); usually part of a neighborhood group, which perpetuates ethnic affiliations.

(f) Organized peer groups such as scouts, church groups, etc. continue society's cultural patterns.

2. High-risk factors

a. Inability to form friendships.

(1) Becomes a loner or makes extra demands on teacher for approval by being especially helpful, etc. (teacher's pet).

(2) Uses pets as center of affection (most common in girls who have difficulty maintaining friendships).

(3) Uses unacceptable behavior to get attention from peers—role as class clown, daredevil, thief, etc.

(4) Label received from gang can continue throughout school years—fatty, clown, teacher's pet.

b. Peer group with unacceptable behavioral standards.

(1) Appreciate that peers are necessary for approval and affection.

(2) Criticism and maligning of friends demand that child defend those on whom he depends for his own self-esteem.

c. Overwhelmed by pressure of school and peers; acting out or passive behavior.

d. Divorce particularly shattering.

(1) Awareness of others and the feelings of others.

(2) Fear of abandonment.

3. Child-rearing practices

a. Expectation that family mores and standards will be upheld.

b. Review developmental tasks accomplished, and identify those unmet.

c. Provide loving, approving adult with time to talk with and listen to child.

d. Provide child advocate for developing a plan to remove unattainable pressure on child, and find a way to have child operate in an environment in which he can succeed.

e. Environmental and family inadequacies necessitate referral of family to social service agencies and/or parent education classes.

4. Sexual identity

a. 6–7 years. Beginning to prefer playmates of own sex.

b. 7–8 years

(1) Prefers company of own sex, to whom child relates more easily.

(2) Boys aspire to maleness, girls to femininity.

(3) Parents and teachers of child's sex used as role models.

c. 8–9 years

(1) Curiosity and interest in the other sex.

(a) Secretive whisperings about sex; telling of off-color stories; experimenting and inspection of each other; searching in dictionary for words.

(b) Appropriate time for information and vocabulary to be supplied before emotions become mixed with facts.

(2) Sex roles more clearly defined and adhered to.

(a) Boys more aggressive and set higher vocational goals than girls.

(b) Girls less aggressive and less motivated for success than boys; new role of women is slow to change these deep cultural patterns.

(3) Parents' attitudes and actions are models for love and affection.

E. Safety

1. Statistics—frequency and type of accidents (age 5–14 years)

Mortality Rates	**Boys (per 100,000)**	**Girls (per 100,000)**
Motor vehicles	13.3%	7.8%
Pedestrian	5.2%	3.3%
Drowning	5.6%	1.3%
Fires and flames	1.9%	1.5%
Falls	0.5%	0.2%

2. Education

a. Responsibilities given as child proves reliable.

b. Awareness of incidence of accidents.

c. Discussions and prevention planning.

d. Emergency plans established and rehearsed.

3. Accident-prone children

a. Accidents follow stressful events.

b. Accidents more frequent when aggressive behavior is reactive pattern.

c. Accidents used as a means of getting attention.

OVERVIEW

9- TO 11-YEAR WELL CHILD VISIT

I. As chronological age does not now determine the preadolescent child's physical and psychological stage of development, the information in these guidelines needs to be individualized for each child. Please refer to guidelines for overall picture of these years.

II. **Family**

A. The onset of this transitional period depends on the child's own genetic, physical, and environmental history. Both the parents' and child's understanding of the child's individual growth pattern can make this a successful and happy period. As children of the same age may be in a different developmental level, peers and gangs will find they are shifting their interests and loyalties.

III. **Parents**

A. Maintaining family and moral standards.

B. Providing opportunity for health care and counseling as needed.

C. Providing appropriate schooling, recreational, and community activities.

D. Giving them opportunities to make independent decisions as they demonstrate the ability to be responsible and accept the consequences of their activities.

E. Provide consistent and caring "listener."

IV. **Child. Understanding and accepting his individual pattern of development.**

A. Physical

1. See Guidelines for physical changes and development of secondary sex characteristics.
2. Taking responsibility for good health habits.
3. Use Guidelines for parameters of physical changes.
4. Safety. Awareness of incidents of accidents and prevention planned.

B. Emotional

1. A period of confusion and indecision. Through trial and error he is working toward developing his confidence and self esteem to become an independent, reliable member of society. This can make for a very self-conscious, indecisive, stubborn, argumentative preadolescent.
2. Continues to need family to provide acceptance and feeling of self-worth.

C. Intellectual

1. A transitional period progressing from concrete thinking to abstract thinking, giving him the ability to express his ideas and feelings better and to begin to accept ideas of others. However, because he does not have the experience to realize practical limitations, he can become impractical in his expectations of others and critical of those around him.

D. Social

1. Peers, teachers, and other adults outside the family give him the opportunity to observe other cultures and values. His behavior is still directed by the need to be accepted by those important to him. An understanding adult is important for him to turn to for support to maintain his expected behavior.

V. **High Risk**

A. Not using language to express feelings. Resorting to aggressive behavior.

B. Inappropriate environment of school and peers.

C. Frequent illnesses or accidents.

VI. **See Guidelines for specific factors of Physical Examination.**

NOTES

9- TO 11-YEAR WELL CHILD VISIT

I. **Developmental process.**

The third cycle of growth comprises the physical and psychosocial steps from childhood to adulthood. It is divided into two periods: a transitional stage, including the years of approximately 9–11, and adolescence, from 12–17. Individuals enter and exit these stages according to their own genetic, environmental, and physical status. The preadolescent period has been defined as one of "mismatch," since one's peers are the same chronological age, but their physical development, interests, and abilities can be at different stages.

A. Parents
   1. Understand this natural process of growth and change.
   2. Establish and maintain home, school, and social guidelines and standards.
   3. Provide a safe, supportive environment.

B. Child
   1. Appreciates the importance of this growing process.
   2. Maintains school and family responsibilities and standards.
   3. Developing ability to assess peer group values relative to own values.

II. **Family status**

A. Parental concerns and problems. Ability to identify problems and to cope; single parents, divorce, remarriage, step-parents, step-siblings.

B. Parents' and child's assessment of development.

C. Family interaction and support for each other.

D. Review and updating of emergency planning.

III. **Health habits—as maintained by child**

A. Nutrition
   1. Understanding basic nutritional requirements during this rapid growth period.
   2. Taking responsibility for and obtaining adequate diet.
   3. Participating in food shopping and preparation.

B. Sleep
   1. Maintaining adequate schedule of sleep and rest to meet needs.
   2. Able to discuss sleep disturbances if present.

C. Hygiene
   1. Takes pride in good grooming.
   2. Understands and copes with body changes, i.e., increased perspiration, menstruation, acne, weight increase.
   3. Able to discuss problems and concerns.

IV. **Growth and development**

A. Physical
   1. Parameters of second period of rapid growth, lasting 2–4 years:
      a. Onset: girls, 9–13 years; boys, 11–14 years.
      b. Height: girls, 9 cm/yr; boys, 11 cm/yr.
      c. Weight: girls, 5 kg/yr; boys, 6 kg/yr.
   2. Body changes

a. Extremities grow faster than trunk and head.
b. Facial proportions change, nose and chin enlarge first.
c. Figure changes: girl's pelvis enlarges; boy's shoulders enlarge.
d. Subcutaneous fat increases.
e. Skin: increased function of sweat glands and increased activity of sebaceous glands.

3. Secondary sex characteristics
   a. Girls—age range at onset
      (1) Breast enlargement: 8–13 years.
      (2) Axillary hair: 11–13 years.
      (3) Pubic hair: 10–12 years.
      (4) Menarche: 10–16 years.
   a. Boys—age range at onset
      (1) Genitalia enlargement: 9–13 years.
      (2) Axillary hair: 12–14 years.
      (3) Facial hair: 11–14 years.
      (4) Pubic hair: 12–15 years.

B. Emotional development—Erikson. The task of the age of pubescence (prepuberty) is to begin the process of developing a self-identity that is independent of both family and peers. The first steps inherent in this process are the following:
   1. An increase in self-awareness, self-consciousness, and self-appraisal.
   2. Becoming preoccupied with how one measures up to peers.
   3. No longer accepting only parental evaluation, but beginning to use the values of peers as criteria with which to judge own values.
   4. Continuing to need family to provide acceptance and a feeling of self-worth.

C. Intellectual development—Piaget. This stage marks the progression from concrete thinking to formal operation; the ability to conceptualize and hypothesize; the beginning of abstract thinking.
   1. The excitement of thinking through possibilities leads to argumentativeness.
   2. The joy of putting across ideas and listening to ideas (of peers) leads to a constant need for gabfests, long telephone conversations, and writing of songs and verse.
   3. Learning is rapid and efficient if school provides a challenging program.

D. Social development
   1. School. The wide range of physical, emotional, and intellectual growth of students makes age grouping unsatisfactory; individual programming of school classes and extracurricular activities is essential.
   2. Community activities (scouts, church, sports)
      a. Provides contact with a wider group than child's own clique.
      b. Provides projects that help child to reach beyond his own self-interests.
   3. Sexual maturity
      a. Boys becoming more masculine, girls becoming more feminine.

b. Interest in each other continues to increase.
c. New self-consciousness makes physical appearance to the opposite sex an overriding concern.
d. Behavioral patterns less established than in the past, since society's expectations and adult role models have been changing.
e. Factual information needed on the reproductive process, the female body, the male body, terminology, birth control, and venereal disease.

4. Antisocial behavior
   a. Drugs. Knowledge of classification and street names, availability, effects, physical and emotional problems with use.
   b. Sexual experimenting. Evaluate:
      (1) Dependence on peer group for acceptance and attention.
      (2) Role models from television, movies, friends, relatives.
      (3) Ability to conceptualize the consequences of behavior.
      (4) Need for consistent, caring adult.
   c. Destructive acts toward society. Evaluate:
      (1) Impulsive behavior.
      (2) Inability to delay gratification.
      (3) Inability to give and accept affection.
      (4) Lack of a consistent, caring adult.
5. Developing sense of community
   a. Cooperation with others—family, school, peers.
   b. Leadership qualities and self-actualizing activities.
   c. Consistent, caring adults with whom to relate.

E. High-risk factors
   1. Family
      a. Poorly defined parental role functions.
      b. Lack of clear and consistent expectations for preadolescent's behavior.
      c. Inability to allow preadolescent to participate in decision-making process.
   2. Preadolescent
      a. Inability to gain peer acceptance.
      b. Participation in socially unacceptable behavior.
      c. No caring adult for support and open communication.

V. Physical examination

A. Growth. Continuing on established pattern; deviations reflected by growth spurt (see Appendix B, Physical Growth NCHS Percentiles).

B. Appearance and behavior
   1. Overall hygiene, appropriateness of dress.
   2. Posture.
   3. Coordination.
   4. Self-assurance.
   5. Communication skills.
   6. Interest in health care.
   7. Eye contact.

C. Specific factors to note while doing routine physical examination
   1. Skin. Enlargement of pores.
   2. Hair. Becoming oily.
   3. Dental occlusion; need for orthodontia.
   4. Decrease in lymph tissue (dependent on maturational level).
   5. Heart. Heart rate slower, particularly in athletes; normal blood pressure slowly rises.
   6. Breasts. Breast budding; gynecomastia in males.
   7. Genitalia
      a. Boys
         (1) Pubic hair at first sparse and straight.
         (2) Enlargement of testes
      b. Girls
         (1) Pubic hair sparse and straight along labial border.
         (2) Labia enlarged.
         (3) Vaginal discharge.
   8. Musculoskeletal. Increased muscle mass, strength, and tone; check back for scoliosis; check for leg length discrepancy.

D. Parent-child interaction
   1. Parent
      a. Allows child to have health maintenance visit alone, but is made aware of any problems and care plans.
      b. Expresses health care concerns with provider and child.
      c. Discusses emerging sexual development openly with child.
   2. Child
      a. Discusses concerns with parent and provider.
      b. Open communication with parent—trusting, supportive relationship.

VI. Assessment

A. Physical
B. Developmental
C. Emotional
D. Environmental

VII. Plan

A. Immunizations. Complete schedule as needed.
B. Screening. Hematocrit; urinalysis; blood pressure check; hearing and eye tests.
C. Problem list (devised with child); SOAP for each.
D. Appropriate timing for office, home, and/or telephone visits; continue individual scheduling.

OVERVIEW

ANTICIPATORY GUIDANCE FOR THE PERIOD OF 9–11 YEARS

I. **Expectations for this period**

   A. Family, school, and community provide opportunities for each child to continue on his own path to maturity.

   B. The child has understanding and acceptance of his own pattern of growth.

II. **Health**

   A. Child taking responsibility for maintaining good health habits and coping with physical changes.

   B. Individual sport activities appropriate to developmental stage.

   C. Health care available.

III. **Emotional**

   A. Moving toward having sufficient self-esteem to make appropriate decisions.

   B. Able to predict and willing to accept the consequences of these decisions.

IV. **Intellectual**

   A. Continuing to move forward from concrete thinking to hypothesize or think abstractly, leading to indecision, being impractical, and critical of others.

   B. Language becomes an important tool in this development.

   C. Lack of language skills can lead to continued use of aggressive act.

V. **Social**

   A. Family and school behavioral standards needed.

   B. Sexual identify established. Appropriate time for self education.

   C. Peer group. See Guidelines.

VI. **Safety**

   A. Accident prevention important.

   B. Accident proneness needs further evaluation.

NOTES

ANTICIPATORY GUIDANCE FOR THE PERIOD OF 9–11 YEARS

Review the previous anticipatory guidelines to help identify child's accomplished or unaccomplished developmental tasks.

I. **Expectations of this period.**
This is a transitional period and a time of new challenge. The strengths and weaknesses that are brought to these preadolescent years will influence the success of the passage from childhood to adulthood. Especially important during the preadolescent years are the understanding and guidance of the family, school, and community organizations to ensure the optimal opportunities for each child to continue his own individual path to maturity.

- **A.** Knowledge of the sequence of the physical changes of preadolescence so that the individual pattern of growth can be predicted.
- **B.** Understanding of the development from concrete to abstract thinking, so that the preadolescent's ability to assume responsibilities and independent activities, to think through planned activities, and to predict outcomes can be assessed.
- **C.** Opportunities provided for the preadolescent to have successful accomplishments and thereby develop an understanding of his own capabilities and continue to develop an attitude of self-esteem and self-worth.
- **D.** Availability of a consistent, caring adult to insist that standards of behavior be upheld and to act as an appropriate role model, a source of encouragement, and a patient listener.

II. **Family status**

- **A.** Basic needs being met; referrals as needed.
- **B.** Parents
  1. Adequate understanding of the use of communication skills and problem-solving techniques.
  2. Appreciation of changing family dynamics and need for developing opportunities for independent decision-making by child.
- **C.** Preadolescent
  1. Ability to establish close relationships outside the family group.
  2. Maintaining school and home responsibilities and behavioral standards.
  3. Keen interest in outside activities such as sports, church, or community groups.
  4. Continues to return to family for support.

III. **Health patterns**

- **A.** Nutrition. Status of growth cycle and level of activity determine the nutritional requirements.
  1. The fastest growing period is the year before puberty; chubbiness before and during this year may lead to extreme dieting, which may interfere with optimal growth.
  2. Preadolescent assuming responsibility for knowledge of nutritional standards, adequate intake, and appropriate eating habits.
- **B.** Health maintenance
  1. Knowledge provided for appropriate care of skin, hair, body odor, and menses.

2. Extreme self-consciousness respected; appropriate fitness and grooming classes available.
3. Exercise
   a. Team sports and competition favor those who mature early.
   b. Individual sports activities are needed for late maturers so that they also may continue to develop and appreciate their capabilities.
4. Health supervision and counseling available.
5. Sickness treated and evaluated; attitude toward illnesses assessed.
6. Health care available.
7. Proneness to accidents evaluated for underlying causes and referrals made as needed.

IV. Growth and development

A. Physical
   1. Growth pattern evaluated by the Tanner scale.
   2. Awkwardness expected because of large muscle growth before refinement of fine motor muscles.
   3. Teeth. Dental care available; orthodontia as needed.
   4. Speech
      a. Enjoyment of and interest in words, rhymes, puzzles.
      b. Increasing vocabulary to handle expanding knowledge and expression of ideas and emotions.
      c. Problems in speech, articulation, or syntax need referrals.

B. Emotional development—Erikson: identity vs. role confusion. The first task is to move from the security of family and friends and develop a positive self-identity. Another task is to develop the ability to make independent decisions and to understand and assume their consequences. Thus, the development of the child's own self-esteem and integrity continues.
   1. The first steps of these tasks need careful attention so that the taking on of independent activities can be geared to both the physical and the intellectual stage of development.
   2. High-risk factors
      a. Regressive patterns of overdependence on family, shyness, passivity, or aggression.
      b. Use of illness as a means of not taking on new challenges.
      c. Use of food, either too much or not enough, as a means of gaining attention and satisfaction.
      d. Lack of opportunities for taking on new responsibilities.
      e. Inability to make and maintain friends; becoming a loner.

C. Intellectual development—Piaget. This is a period of transition from concrete thinking to formal (abstract) thinking. During this process, horizons are broadened to include such learning as calculus and appreciation of the images in poetry. However, because the preadolescent does not have the experience to realize the practical limitations of life, he can be indecisive, accepting of impractical ideas, and lacking understanding of others.
   1. Opportunities provided for taking on new responsibilities with careful supervision.
   2. Readings and experiences broaden the understanding of others.

3. Academic programs stimulate independent work.
4. Discussion groups help child formulate and express ideas and listen to and counter the ideas of others.
5. High-risk factors
   a. Unsuccessful in maintaining scholastic expectations.
   b. Inappropriate classes for developmental stage.
   c. Assuming responsibilities beyond his ability to understand and assume the consequences of these actions.
6. Language now becomes the most important tool in understanding and accepting the new experiences of this transitional period.
   a. Aggressive acts replaced by use of communication skills and problem-solving techniques.
   b. Peer groups and "best friend" used to try out new ideas.
   c. Broad reading programs introduce cultural heritages.
   d. A consistent, caring adult listens to problems and new ideas and provides alternative approaches.
   e. High-risk factors
      (1) Too much time watching TV and computer play: inhibits discussions with peers and family; limits vocabulary development.
      (2) Not using language to express feelings and ideas; still resorting to aggression to take control.
      (3) No consistent listener to provide a sounding board for feelings and ideas.

D. Social development. It is important for the preadolescent to turn to peer groups, school, and community groups to observe the cultures, mores, and values of others; evaluating these in relation to family patterns and establishing one's own standards take an extended period of trial and error with reinforcement of appropriate behavior by a significant adult.
   a. Guidelines established by the family for behavioral standards, curfews, and extracurricular activities.
   b. Guidelines indicate parents' interest and concern and provide the security of behavioral limits.
2. Sexual identity
   a. Dependent on stage of growth development with respect to awareness of and interest in the opposite sex.
   b. Girls' maturing earlier than boys makes chronological age activities difficult, as in sports, clubs, discussion groups.
   c. Now is the appropriate time for necessary information and vocabulary about sex to be supplied, before emotions become mixed with facts.
3. Peer group
   a. Positive developmental process
      (1) Facilitates learning about interpersonal relationships.
      (2) Source of support, guidance, and esteem.
      (3) Role model for appearance and behavior.
      (4) Leads to awareness of social class, prestige, and power of belonging to "right" group.
      (5) Pressure to perform provides opportunity for testing out own values and evaluating them against values of others.

b. Parental role
   (1) Continue expecting conformance to family behavioral limits, values, and standards.
   (2) Understand importance of peer group to preadolescent.
   (3) Reserve evaluation of peer group until concrete evidence available.
   (4) Remember that preadolescent considers criticism of group a personal attack.
   (5) When intervention necessary, explain parental responsibility to protect him—genuine concern can be appreciated by preadolescent and used as a means of extracting himself from an unhappy situation.

4. High-risk factors
   a. Antisocial behavior.
   b. Poor school performance.
5. Child-rearing practices
   a. A time to investigate and evaluate carefully the forces that are causing the preadolescent to reject this next step toward becoming a responsible member of society.
   b. Appropriate intervention and referrals.

E. Safety
   1. Statistics—frequency and type of accidents (age 5–14 years)

Mortality Rates	Boys (per 100,000)	Girls (per 100,000)
Motor vehicles	13.3%	7.8%
Pedestrian	5.2%	3.3%
Drowning	5.6%	1.3%
Fires and flames	1.9%	1.5%
Falls	0.5%	0.2%

   2. Education
      a. Responsibilities given as child proves reliable.
      b. Awareness of incidence of accidents.
      c. Discussions and prevention planning.
      d. Emergency plans established and rehearsed.
   3. Accident-prone children
      a. Accidents follow stressful events.
      b. Accidents more frequent when aggressive behavior is reactive pattern.
      c. Accidents used as a means of getting attention.

V. Suggested readings for preadolescents and parents

A. Calerone, M., and Ramey, J. *Talking with Your Child About Sex.* New York, Ballantine Books, Inc., 1983.

B. Johnson, E.W. *Love and Sex in Plain Language,* 3rd ed. Philadelphia: J.B. Lippincott, 1988.

C. Faber. *How to Talk so Kids Will Listen.* New York: Avon, 1982.

D. Rosenberg. *Growing Up Feeling Good.* New York: Penguin Books, 1989.

E. Elkind, D. *Your Hurried Child.* Reading, MA: Addison-Wesley, 1992.

F. Johnson & Rosenfeld. *Divorced Kids.* New York: Fawcett Crest, 1990.

OVERVIEW

12- TO 17-YEAR WELL CHILD VISIT

I. During these years the increasing stability of both physical and psychological development can be expected. These guidelines can be used to identify the essential parameters of this development.

A. Family

1. Assessment of adolescents' growth toward maturity with successes and concerns identified. Problem-solving session planned and referrals made as needed.

B. Adolescent

1. Physical

a. Changes can be predicted and a more realistic thought process can help the adolescent understand and appreciate his own uniqueness.

b. Concerns and problems identified and referrals made as needed.

c. Accepting responsibility for good health habits and safety practices for himself and others.

2. Emotional

a. Developing a more self-directed and assured behavior pattern.

b. Establishing the confidence to rely on his own self-esteem and competence.

c. Becoming more discriminating in making friends and group involvement.

3. Intellectual

a. Able to think more realistically about his own capabilities and values.

b. Becoming more tolerant of others.

c. Feels comfortable in his society and taking on the role of a responsible member of society.

4. Social

a. Becoming less dependent on peer group for his self-confidence.

b. Establishing own standards of behavior and values.

c. Accepting own values and self-awareness of sexual role.

II. **High Risk Factors**

A. Indications of substance abuse.

1. Changes in behavioral habits.

2. Changes in emotional stability.

3. Withdrawing from friends and family activities.

B. Indication of risk of suicide.

1. Talking about this is a serious call for help.

2. Careful evaluation and intervention indicated.

III. See Guidelines for specific factors of physical examination.

NOTES

12- TO 17-YEAR WELL CHILD VISIT

I. Developmental process.

The adolescent is now settling into a more stable growth and behavioral pattern. The individuality of this process can be identified, and strengths and problems can be assessed. Physical changes can be predicted, and the emergence of a more realistic thought process helps the adolescent understand and appreciate his own uniqueness.

A. Parents
   1. Providing opportunities for the adolescent to make independent decisions.
   2. Assessing with the adolescent the appropriateness of these decisions.
   3. Allowing increased independence when teenager is able to make appropriate and realistic decisions and bear the consequences of his activities.

B. Adolescent
   1. Understanding physical changes, and taking responsibility for health maintenance.
   2. Successful accomplishments at home, at school, and in extracurricular activities.
   3. Accepting his sexuality and the cultural standards of society.

II. Family status

A. Basic needs being met; referrals as needed.

B. Parents
   1. Assessment of adolescent's development.
   2. Concerns identified.
   3. Family communication skills and problem-solving techniques assessed.
   4. Problem-solving session including both parent and adolescent planned; referrals as needed.

C. Adolescent
   1. Understanding and acceptance of the individuality of his development.
   2. Concerns and problems identified.
   3. Ability to relate to and cooperate with parents or another significant adult.
   4. Problem-solving sessions planned; referrals as needed.

III. Health habits

A. Health maintenance
   1. Attitude toward and appreciation of health maintenance.
   2. Knowledge of requirements for good health.
   3. Availability of health supervision and crisis care.
   4. Accident prevention:
      a. Driver education.
      b. Swimming and lifesaving proficiency.
      c. Knowledge of sports injuries; appropriate equipment, supervision, physical fitness needed for particular activity.
      d. First aid course and emergency planning available.
      e. Proneness to accidents evaluated for underlying causes.

5. Prevention of infectious diseases:
    a. Knowledge of communicability, symptoms, course of disease, complications, and sequelae.
    b. Most common infectious diseases of adolescents: mononucleosis, upper respiratory infections, herpes, hepatitis, gonorrhea.
6. Information for those who are sexually active:
    a. Knowledge of endocrine and reproductive systems.
    b. Birth control information.
    c. Symptoms of physical problems and infections.
    d. Pregnancy testing and abortion counseling.

B. Nutrition
1. Knowledge of nutritional requirements.
2. Nutritional assessment for poor weight gain, slow muscle tissue growth, obesity, and intense physical activity:
    a. Twenty-four-hour recall or diary of food intake.
    b. Eating habits: more than three meals per day to spread metabolic load for better absorption.
    c. Evaluate intake of protein, milk products, fruits, vegetables, grains.
        (1) Protein: 2 servings/day; high percentage of fish, poultry, dried beans, peas, nuts.
        (2) Milk products: 2 servings/day, including cheese and ice cream.
        (3) Fruits and vegetables: 4 servings/day, including potatoes.
        (4) Cereal and grains: 4 servings/day.
        (5) Fluids: increased amount to compensate for increase of sweat glands; avoid caffeine and soda drinks.
    d. Athletes and those who need to gain weight: increase the size of servings of high-value foods (e.g., whole-grain bread, cereal, potatoes, cheese, nuts).
3. Refer to nutritionist as needed.

C. Sleep
1. Established pattern of work and sleep.
2. Ability to maintain daily schedule.
3. Willingness to discuss problems.

D. Elimination
1. Established schedule.
2. Understanding and knowledge to cope with problems.
3. Symptoms of urinary tract infections known.
4. Willing to ask for help as needed.

E. Menstruation
1. Regularity of periods.
2. Premenstrual symptoms.
3. Menstrual discomforts.
4. Able to maintain daily schedule.
5. Willing to ask for information and help.

F. Nocturnal emission
   1. Understanding of normal physical development.
   2. Willing to ask for information and help.
G. Masturbation
   1. Infrequent experimenting is normal.
   2. If a frequent and obsessive practice, intervention and referral needed.

IV. Growth and development

A. Physical
   1. Slower rate of growth in height and weight; return to percentiles of preadolescent pattern.
   2. Facial features and adult stature obtained by 18 years for females and 20 years for males.
   3. Muscle strength and size now influenced by sex hormones as well as by nutrition and exercise.
   4. Endurance dependent on lung capacity, heart size, and muscle strength, as well as on sex hormones and physical fitness.
   5. Speech
      a. Voice changes in resonance and strength in both sexes—more pronounced in males.
      b. Problems in articulation, pitch, and rhythm need investigation.
B. Emotional development—Erikson: self-identity vs. role confusion. These years see the development of a more self-directed and assured behavioral pattern. As in all steps to maturity, optimal growth is more easily reached when opportunities are available to try out and experiment with new roles in an understanding and safe environment.
   1. More even-tempered and cooperative.
   2. Self-directed in planning educational and vocational goals.
   3. More discriminating in making friends and group involvement.
C. Intellectual development—Piaget. Concrete thinking to formal operation; the ability to conceptualize and hypothesize.
   1. Continues to be excited about presenting ideas and countering ideas of others; debating and rap groups help organize and define ideas and force one to listen to ideas of others.
   2. Able to think realistically about vocational goals.
   3. Accepts own capabilities and appreciates own values.
D. Social development
   1. Continues to work through establishing his own standards of behavior and values.
   2. Becoming less dependent on peer groups for social stature and behavior pattern.
   3. Increase in tolerance and appreciation of others.
   4. Sexual maturity
      a. Adjusting to body changes and functions.
      b. Accepting societal standards for sexual identity.
      c. Developing own values for and self-awareness of sexual role.

5. Antisocial behavior
    a. Developing better judgment toward and control of drug use, smoking, alcohol, and sexual behavior.
    b. Able to respond to school and community counseling groups.
6. Destructive acts toward society
    a. Impulsive behavior.
    b. Need to gain attention from peer group.
    c. Inability to delay gratification.
    d. Inability to give and accept affection.
    e. No consistent, caring adult.
7. Developing sense of community
    a. Cooperation with others—family, school, peers.
    b. Leadership qualities and self-actualizing activities.
    c. Consistent, caring adults with whom to relate.

E. High-risk factors

1. Family, school, community
    a. Not providing an understanding and safe environment.
    b. Punitive measures of behavior control attempted in place of open communication, problem-solving techniques, and defined behavioral standards.
    c. Unrealistic expectations of adolescent's ability to control and take responsibility for his actions.
2. Adolescent
    a. Physical problems not under medical supervision.
    b. Not accepting of physical appearance and capabilities.
    c. Not taking on the role of a self-directed, caring individual.
3. Indication of substance abuse and risk of suicide
    a. Changes in behavior patterns of sleep, eating, friendship, and school performance.
    b. Changes in personality: boredom, agitation, bursts of anger, apathy, evasiveness, carelessness.
    c. Increasing attitudes of discouragement and disgust with the affairs of the world.
    d. Difficulty in accepting disappointment and failure.
    e. No supportive companion to share and evaluate new perceptions of his role for himself and his obligations to society.
    f. Suicidal calls for help.
        (1) Talking about ways of committing suicide.
        (2) Giving away prize possessions.
        (3) Previous attempts.
        (4) Withdrawal from friends and family.

V. Physical examination

A. Growth. Height and weight percentiles return to preadolescent pattern.

B. Appearance and behavior

1. Grooming and hygiene.

2. Posture.
3. Coordination.
4. Self-assurance.
5. Communication.
6. Interest in health care.
7. Eye contact.

C. Specific factors to note while doing routine physical examination
1. Hair. Oily; body hair appears on chest and face in males, axilla in both sexes.
2. Skin. Acne on face, back, and chest; large pores in skin.
3. Lymph. Decrease in lymph tissue.
4. Teeth. Caries; dental hygiene; need for orthodontia.
5. Heart. Decrease in heart rate; increase in blood pressure.
6. Lungs. Decrease in respiratory rate.
7. Breasts. Breasts developing; gynecomastia in males.
8. Genitalia
   a. Males
      (1) Pubic hair: increase in amount to adult distribution; becomes coarse and curly.
      (2) Penile enlargement continuing.
      (3) Enlargement of testes.
   b. Females
      (1) Pubic hair: increase in amount to adult distribution; becomes coarse and curly.
      (2) Labia mature.
      (3) Vaginal discharge.
9. Musculoskeletal. Increased muscle mass, strength, and tone; check back for scoliosis; check for leg length discrepancy.

D. Parent-adolescent interaction
1. Parent
   a. Expecting adolescent to take responsibility for health care.
   b. Made aware of health problems and care plan.
   c. Follow-up visits and financial responsibility planned.
2. Adolescent
   a. Turns to parents for support and comfort.
   b. Discusses health care plans with parents.

VI. Assessment

A. Physical
B. Developmental
C. Emotional
D. Environmental

VII. Plan

A. Immunizations. Complete schedule as needed.
B. Screening. Hematocrit; urinalysis; blood pressure check; hearing and eye tests.

C. Problem list (devised with adolescent); SOAP for each.

D. Appropriate timing for office, home, and/or telephone visits; continue individual scheduling.

OVERVIEW

ANTICIPATORY GUIDANCE FOR THE PERIOD OF 12–17 YEARS

I. **Expectations**

A. Parents and adolescents appreciate the strengths needed to become an independent, responsible, and caring member of society.

B. The family, school, and community provide opportunities for development of these strengths.

C. Adolescent developing pride in his capabilities and accepting responsibility of his actions.

II. **Family**

A. Better able to accept change in family structure such as divorce and remarriage—step-siblings.

III. **Health**

A. Period of rapid growth so adequate nutrition essential.

B. Responsibility for health maintenance accepted.

IV. **Emotional**

A. Evaluation of positive attitudes towards himself and others.

B. Negative attitudes indicate need for referral.

V. **Intellectual**

A. Continuing ability to think abstractly leads to more accurate and tolerant assessment of himself and others.

VI. **Social**

A. At home, in school, and in community is now a responsible, caring member.

NOTES

ANTICIPATORY GUIDANCE FOR THE ADOLESCENT YEARS

Expectations of this period. In these fascinating and challenging years, both the parents and the adolescent come to understand and appreciate the strengths and individuality that are needed to become an independent, responsible member of society.

I. Adolescent

A. Accepting and developing pride in one's capabilities and working toward vocational goals.

B. Establishing independent values that provide a framework to assess appropriate behavior.

C. Having role models of caring, responsible members of society.

II. Family status

A. Basic needs being met; self-direction in coping with problems.

B. Parents

1. Have positive attitudes toward the changing emotional ties between parents and adolescent.
2. Provide time to listen (not argue), and encourage the adolescent to verbalize new ideas and feelings.
3. Provide a role model for maintaining family mores and cultural values.

C. Step-parents

1. Shift in family relationship demands that parents be role models of mature, caring people.
2. Understanding and appreciation of each adolescent's individuality.
3. Poor adjustment can lead to behavioral and school problems for the adolescent and jealousy and abuse by the parent.

D. Adolescent

1. Single-parent homes
   a. Has extra responsibility.
   b. Feels left out of some activities.
   c. Misses attention of other parent.
   d. Can be embarrassed by having only one parent.
2. Divorce of parents
   a. Better able to think through and understand the problems.
   b. Relieved by the cessation of family discord.
   c. Can feel despair and abandonment.
3. Remarriage of a parent
   a. Can appreciate and be happy for the parents.
   b. Glad to be relieved of some of the responsibility he has been carrying.
   c. Jealousy and resentment can be present if parent has been dependent on adolescent for his emotional satisfaction.

E. Step-siblings

1. Important that each child be seen as an individual.
2. Parents establishing a caring relationship with each child.

3. Parents providing opportunities for open communication.
4. Children given opportunity to take part in and develop outside interests.

F. Siblings
   1. Different developmental stages cause different needs and expectations.
   2. Important to provide privacy and respect for each person's possessions.
   3. Expect a united front if one sibling is hurt or maligned.

III. Health patterns

A. Nutrition. Period of rapid physical growth, so special attention to adequate nutrition is essential.
   1. Considerations. Ethnic food habits, past growth pattern, nutritional history, familial diseases such as high blood pressure, heart attacks, diabetes, obesity.
   2. Nutritional requirements
      a. Boys: 45 kcal/kg, or 25 cal/lb.
      b. Girls: 38 kcal/kg, or 20 cal/lb.
   3. Problems to be evaluated
      a. Inadequate food available.
      b. Obesity.
      c. Anorexia nervosa/bulimia.
      d. Poor eating habits.

B. Health maintenance—responsibility assumed by adolescent.
   1. Established patterns of grooming, elimination, and sleep.
   2. Physical fitness and pride in maintaining good health.
   3. Accepting responsibility of sexual identity.
   4. Seeking help when problems arise.

C. Exercise
   1. Variability of growth pattern makes individualized program necessary.
   2. Endurance and muscle strength improving, but type of activity geared to stage of development.
   3. Girls: equal opportunities and equal money allotted for their activities (Title IX)—school programs evaluated.
   4. Evaluate growth progress by frequent measurement of height, weight, muscle mass, and energy level.

D. Safety—accident prevention
   1. Able to accept the reality that accidents can happen to him.
   2. Impulsive and aggressive behavior a reactive pattern to stressful events.
   3. Ability to identify and assume responsibilities.
   4. Controls activities for the benefit of others.

IV. Growth and development

A. Physical
   1. Individual growth pattern can now be recognized.
   2. Information on the order of expected body changes can be provided to the adolescent—see Tanner scale.
   3. Self-concern and rapid body changes can cause overconcern with health problems.

a. Parents and health professionals appreciate reality of problem to adolescent.
b. Care plan devised with parent, adolescent, and professional.
c. Identify adolescent's use of illness as a way of avoiding emotional or social concerns—plan intervention and referrals.

B. Emotional development—Erikson. The preadolescent developmental task of beginning to establish an identity as an independent, self-sufficient, caring person continues during the next years. Assess by the following:
1. A positive developmental process
a. Showing confidence in his own judgment and accepting the consequences of his actions.
b. Appraising his abilities and working toward vocational goals.
c. Decreased self-consciousness and increased understanding of others.
2. A negative developmental process
a. Lack of self-esteem and confidence in his potential abilities.
b. Frequent illnesses, accidents, and periods of depression.
c. Continued use of self-destructive behavioral patterns, such as drugs, promiscuity, cheating, stealing.

C. Intellectual development—Piaget. The process of the development from concrete thinking to formal operation continues at an individual pace.
1. The first steps are identified by the ability to think abstractly.
a. Conceptualizes and theorizes about ideas that include several variables—seen by parents as having difficulty making decisions and being slow to start projects.
b. Theorizes from own perspective; unable to incorporate ideas of others—seen by parents as being stubborn, uncooperative, and argumentative.
c. Idealistic in problem solving, since expectations are unrealistic—seen as "disgust" with "stupidity" of adult world.
2. Final steps toward formal operation:
a. Makes decisions on basis of more accurate appraisal of options, so can become independent of societal and peer pressure.
b. Incorporates ideas of others, so can become more tolerant of both peers and adults.
c. Experience leads to less idealism about the ease of solving problems.
d. Feels comfortable in society and takes on the role of a responsible member of society.

D. Social
1. Beyond their academic purpose, schools are a safe environment that can be used as a common meeting ground.
a. In the school environment the adolescent intellectually and emotionally can do the following:
(1) Appreciate other cultures and mores.
(2) Observe a wide range of socioeconomic strata, with their privileges and inequalities.
(3) React to the importance placed on academic performance and the pressures of testing and scoring.

(4) Try out and develop interpersonal relation skills.

b. The school provides opportunities for the adolescent to develop abilities, find pride in accomplishments, and obtain leadership skills.

c. The adolescent needs teachers and administrators who will maintain standards by which actions and abilities can be fairly judged.

2. The community

   a. Provides the adolescent with an opportunity to observe and take part in projects that serve other segments of society.

   b. Maintains sufficient recreational activities to provide wholesome outlets for adolescents' energy and need to be together.

   c. Demonstrates interest, concern, and pride in its adolescent population.

3. The family continues its important role of

   a. Providing a safe and wholesome environment.

   b. Offering help and encouragement when problems occur.

   c. Respecting the adolescent's ideas and opinions.

   d. Giving open, honest answers and suggestions when asked.

   e. Demonstrating the roles of caring, responsible citizens.

V. Suggesting readings for adolescents and parents

A. Bell, R. et al. *Changing Bodies, Changing Lives.* New York: Random House, 1986.

B. Coles, R. *The Moral Life of Children.* Boston: Houghton Mifflin, 1986.

C. Gordon, S., and Saydor. *Personal Issues in Human Sexuality.* Rockleigh, N.J.: Allyn & Bacon, 1989.

D. Elkind, D. *All Grown up and No Place to Go.* Bradbury Press, Inc., 1984.

E. Clarke. *Self-Esteem—A Family Affair.* New York: Harper.

COMMON CHILD-REARING CONCERNS: TEMPER TANTRUMS

Temper tantrums are a developmental stage in learning to cope with frustration and gain self-control. In *The Process of Human Development,* Spitz defines five sequential stages in the development of self-control (Schuster & Ashburn; see Section V: Suggested readings). These are:

1. Passive acceptance: protest, bewilderment, and noncompliance.
2. Physical aggression: biting, hitting, throwing objects, running, stamping feet.
3. Verbal aggression: using the word "no," name calling, making demands, using expletives.
4. Socially acceptable behavior: bargaining, accepting alternative means or goals.
5. Cooperation: compromising one's wishes and maintaining self-control.

According to Schuster, these stages may overlap, but they "resolve quickly in normally developing children."

I. Manifestations of frustration

A. Infant

1. Uncontrolled crying can be caused by the baby's inability to stop once he has started.
2. This behavior requires quiet soothing and rocking to let the baby know there is comfort for him.
3. If such crying spells occur frequently, further physical and environmental factors need investigating.

B. Toddler

1. Still completely ego-centered; his needs and wishes come first.
2. Does not tolerate fatigue, hunger, pain, and overstimulation well.
3. His schedule, physical condition, nutrition, and family patterns of behavior should be investigated.
4. Best to head off temper tantrums by carefully noting precipitating events and trying to avoid these.
5. Having to make choices can be frustrating to a toddler. A definite schedule and decisive tone of voice ("Now it is time to eat," "Now it is time for bed," etc.) can help the toddler accept the rules and standards of his world.

C. Preschool child

1. Verbal aggression is best ignored.
2. Adults are excellent role models—parents should express frustration in positive ways, such as by singing, laughing, reciting poetry, and stating clearly why they are upset.
3. A 4-year-old realizes he can get attention by using forbidden words.
   a. If the child is getting enough attention and having success in his daily routine, this language will soon pass.
   b. Playing word games with the child and listening to his stories seem to be the best ways to handle this problem.
4. Preschoolers are learning socially acceptable ways of handling frustration.
   a. Language skills should now be sufficient for the child to state his wishes and needs.

b. Child is becoming an expert in bargaining.

5. A 4-year-old is usually still working on these skills and may still occasionally lose control and have a temper tantrum. It is important for the adults in his world to help him develop positive ways of handling frustration.
6. By age 5 years, the child has become an expert in bargaining. Girls learn this skill earlier than boys; boys need more supervision and male role models to help them control their behavior through words rather than aggression.
7. Learning self-control enhances self-esteem; punishment control will only lessen the child's feeling of being able to control himself.

D. School-age child

1. If uncontrolled outbursts of frustrations still persist at this age, referral to appropriate professionals is imperative.
2. School, family, and environmental pressures must be evaluated before new skills in behavior control can be established.
3. Frequent outbursts at this age may be a precursor of delinquency.
4. A child's ability to control his behavior is seen in his success with peers and teachers, in school, and at home.
5. The school-age child has come a long way since toddlerhood; with his caretakers providing good examples and guidance, he has learned to stand up for what he thinks is right and yet is willing to cooperate and bargain when that is appropriate.

II. Caretaker responsibilities

A. To appreciate that they are role models for their child with respect to behavior patterns for coping with anger and frustration.

B. To demonstrate the processes of bargaining, accommodation, compromise, and cooperation.

C. To review the successes or problems the child is encountering with each developmental task.

D. To understand the child's individual temperament and let a fiery tempered child know that he will need to work harder than others to build up his behavior control.

E. To respect the child's need to protect his own self-esteem and his growing need for independence.

F. To identify precipitating events that lead to loss of self control and head them off.

G. To create a family environment in which all members are expected to respect and help one another.

H. To help children develop positive ways of expressing anger and frustration so that they experience the satisfaction of learning to be in control of their behavior.

1. Set up time-out periods or a "thinking bench" to be used when the child's behavior is unreasonable.
2. Watch for and praise successful attempts at self-control.
3. Help the child develop a vocabulary to express feelings, and talk about one's own feelings so that the child will learn how adults handle their frustrations.
4. Learn songs and poems to use to relieve anger and frustration.

5. Provide the child with plenty of opportunity for physical exercise.
6. Have available a caring adult with whom the child can share his concerns.
7. Understand that their own emotional states may be reflected in the child's behavior.

III. Tips for handling temper tantrums

A. Infant. Hold closely, rock, play music, sing.

B. Toddler. Pick up, hold under arm of caretaker (child may be frightened by his loss of control), keep calm, sing; do not reason or explain.

C. Preschooler. Don't allow the child to hurt himself or others, hold under your arm if necessary. Walk out of the room if possible, and don't try to reason or explain. Don't take the episode too seriously; respond with a casual statement, such as "Oops, see if you can't hold on to your temper," or "Now that you are 4, you don't need to do that anymore; tell me why you are angry." Praise the child for getting his behavior under control. Do not use threats or punishments.

D. In public. Remove from scene, walk with the child outside until he calms down. Take him home if possible. Help him practice how to act in public and set limits he knows about before going out. Carefully study his world to make sure such episodes are not his only way of getting attention.

E. Refer to limit-setting protocol

IV. High-risk factors

A. Children who are too quiet, too good, and too shy; their behavior may be controlled by low self-esteem or fear of punishment.

B. Sudden burst of destructive acts toward himself or others may occur, as the child has not learned a positive way to cope with his frustrations.

C. Early identification and family interaction needs further investigation and/or referral for these destructive behaviors.

V. Suggested reading

A. Schuster, C., and Ashburn, S. *The Process of Human Development,* 3rd ed. Philadelphia: J.B. Lippincott, 1992.

COMMON CHILD-REARING CONCERNS: TOILET TRAINING

Toilet training is a developmental task of toddlerhood. Success will help the toddler continue to develop awareness of his own ability for self-control and self-esteem. There appears to be a critical period at about 18 to 24 months of age when the child becomes aware of his body functions; attempts at training too early or too late may influence long-range behavior.

I. Indications of readiness

A. Physical maturation of muscles and nerves to allow for voluntary sphincter control. Given that myelination takes place in a cephalocaudal direction, the ability to walk well indicates that myelination has taken place in the trunk of the body and that sphincter control is now possible.

B. Body awareness. Toddler shows discomfort in soiled diapers, can locate pain, and is developing some coordination.

C. Toddler can follow simple directions and use language to make his wishes known.

D. Toddler can anticipate and postpone events in his daily schedule.

E. Toddler is not under any new stresses.

F. Toddler has primary caretakers to look to for approval and attention.

II. Technique

A. Pretraining when the above indicators are present.

1. Have child observe others using bathroom.
2. Talk about it as an expected accomplishment; comment with appropriate word when child is observed having bowel movement (BM) so that he becomes aware that this will get attention.
3. Have potty chair or insert ring for toilet seat available.
4. Use training pants occasionally.
5. Toddler shows awareness of plan by bringing to caretaker's attention that he is having a BM; this is the beginning of gaining the child's cooperation and may take more time and effort than seems necessary.
6. It is important to remember that this is only one of the many tasks the toddler is attempting to master at this age and to understand his frequent lapses.

B. Bowel control

1. First make sure toddler is becoming aware of the connection between the potty chair and the BM.
2. If child's bowel movements are regular, use the potty chair at those times.
3. If no regularity is apparent, watch for signal from child and then take him to the bathroom. This is where patience and perseverance by the caretakers are rewarded.
4. Leave child on potty chair for only a short time; long sitting sessions may lead him to rebel. Be aware that he may be afraid of the toilet seat.
5. Do not distract child with books or toys; he is there for one reason.
6. Treat success as a normal expectation. Overenthusiasm may cause child to use toileting as a way to get attention; positive feedback should be given for other daily activities.

7. If training unsuccessful, reevaluate maturation indicators and repeat pre-training techniques. It seems to take more time and effort to train boys than girls, particularly if they are larger than average.

C. Daytime bladder control

1. Follows BM control, since voiding signal is less intense.
2. Small bladder size makes control more difficult.
3. Watch for increasingly long periods of dryness as this signifies an increase in bladder size.
4. Put child on potty chair before and after meals, naps, and playtime; treat as usual part of daily schedule.
5. Dress child in clothing that is easy to remove.
6. Boys may prefer to sit backward on toilet seat.
7. Treat success casually.

D. Nightime bladder control

1. Follows daytime control; may not be accomplished until after the age of 3 years.
2. Bladder must have capacity of 8 oz before child will be dry all night.
3. Getting child up at night may be helpful in the short term but is not a good long-term solution to nighttime voiding.
4. Put child on toilet or potty chair as soon as he is awake, whether dry or not, to develop routine.
5. Outside pressure makes child feel inadequate and discouraged with his ability to please those important to him.
6. In a happy, healthy child, bladder control is a natural process.

E. Success

1. Depends on toddler's physical maturation.
2. Depends on parents' positive attitudes and patience in following through and helping child.

F. Problems. See Enuresis in Part II.

COMMON CHILD-REARING CONCERNS: LIMIT SETTING*

Discipline can best be defined as training that helps a child develop self-concept and character. Parents are often hesitant to set firm and consistent limits on their child because they are afraid of damaging his "psyche" or fear that their child won't love them or feel loved by them if they are stern. To the contrary, being allowed to act in a way he knows should not be tolerated causes a child anxiety and makes him feel insecure. A child feels that his parents do not love him if they do not make an effort to help him develop inner controls.

The ultimate goal for any child is parental approval; a child will do his best to live up to parental expectations. For example, if a mother conveys the impression that she does not expect her toddler to go to bed without a struggle, a struggle will surely ensue. Furthermore, if parental expectations are that a child will "pass" in school, he probably will, though if the same parents were to expect "A's," the child would probably strive to achieve them. Parental disapproval helps the child develop a conscience; he knows that, with a naughty deed, he has not "measured up."

Health care providers involved in routine physical concerns must be careful not to neglect the issue of discipline. This is especially important as the child develops initiative and autonomy. The following points can be discussed with parents. It is generally helpful to raise the issue before the need arises and to reinforce significant areas when the parents have a specific concern.

I. Principles of limit setting

A. United front.
   1. Parents must be in accord.
   2. Parents must agree on what limits will be.
   3. Parents must agree on penalties for infractions.

B. Consistency.
   1. Rules must be consistently enforced.
   2. Expectations must be consistent.
   3. The child should not be allowed to perform unacceptable behaviors at some times and be punished for similar behaviors other times.

C. Limits must be clearly delineated.
   1. Parental expectations must be defined.
   2. Rules and regulations must be clear.

D. Behavioral expectations must be in relation to the developmental and intellectual level of the child.
   1. A 12-month-old cannot be relied on not to touch something because mom or dad said "no."
   2. A 2-year-old does not understand what can happen to him if he goes in the street or gets into a car with a stranger.
   3. A school-aged child can be expected to understand that he must go home after school before playing with his friends.

*This section written by Elizabeth Dunn.

4. Expectations must be clear to the child; he will strive to achieve them.

E. "Bumping point"

1. Every parent has a point up to which he can be pushed and beyond which he cannot, and every child quickly learns his parent's "bumping point" and uses it to his own advantage.

F. Unemotional approach

1. Children repeat behaviors that they know get a parental response, whether positive or negative.
2. A toddler learning to walk takes another step when Mom and Dad laugh and applaud.
3. The perfect entertainment for a school-aged child on a boring, rainy day is to tease his sister and watch Mom hop!
4. Overreacting under stress and in anger leads to irrational threats and perhaps violence.

G. The deed is "bad," not the child.

1. Attack the deed, not the child; this preserves the child's respect for himself and for his parent.
2. "Breaking windows, throwing stones, etc., are naughty things to do."
3. Child needs to know, however, that he is responsible for his actions.

H. Immediacy of action.

1. For most effective learning, especially with a toddler or preschool child, the consequences of inappropriate behavior should not be delayed.
2. With older children and adolescents, a "conference" with Mom and Dad may be more appropriate; in this case the consequence is delayed.
3. Do not threaten with "wait till your father gets home." This threat can cause an enormous amount of anxiety for a child and makes it appear not only that Dad is the "bad guy" but also that Mom does not care enough to set limits. Alternatively, for a child whose father comes home from work and then usually spends his time in front of the TV, a secondary gain may be involved in the form of attention, albeit negative attention.

I. "Punishment" must fit the "crime."

1. There should be a logical connection between the two; banning after-school play for two weeks for an infraction unrelated to such activity is usually not only inappropriate but also unhealthy.
2. Punishment should not exceed the child's tolerance.
3. Punishment should not negate educational aims.
4. Coming in half an hour after curfew does not warrant restricting an adolescent for one or two months; instead, make the curfew half an hour earlier next time and give the child one of the parent's tasks the next day because "Dad is so tired from waiting and worrying."
5. As the child gets older, parental disapproval is often the only punishment needed; guilt at letting his parents down is often punishment enough.

J. Punishment should educate.

1. Punishment is done for and with children, not to them.
2. Spanking
   a. Produces an external rather than an internal motive for controlling the impulse and therefore does not help develop child's conscience.

b. Cancels the crime.
c. Relieves sense of guilt too readily.
d. Parental anger often escalates with spanking, resulting in injury.

3. Isolation
   a. Appropriate length of time, e.g., "until you can act like a young lady," is preferable to isolating for a specified length of time once child is old enough to understand what behaviors are expected.
4. Sit on chair. Tell child timer is set for 3 minutes, not "sit there until I tell you that you can get up."
5. Restrictions on privileges
   a. For bike rule infraction, take bike away.
   b. TV restrictions work well for most children.
   c. It is best not to restrict learning experiences such as Boy Scout camping.
   d. Withhold positive rewards such as social or verbal approval.
   e. Never offer a reward that cannot be fulfilled.

K. Treat child with respect.
   1. This teaches him to respect in turn.
   2. Allow him to share in decision-making process.
   3. Child models behaviors he sees in parents; be the kind of person you expect your child to be.
   4. Earliest approach to limit setting is based on baby's ability to learn.

L. Threats are useless.
   1. Any self-respecting child will try to see whether parents will follow through; threats are an invitation for unwanted behaviors.
   2. Threats are often made in a moment of anger and may be unreasonable.

M. An ounce of prevention is worth a pound of cure and is certainly easier on parents.
   1. Clearly define limits.
   2. Remove temptation.
   3. Do not pick on insignificant things.
   4. Do not threaten with punishment that you cannot or are unwilling to carry out.
   5. Distract your child if he looks as though he is getting in trouble.
   6. When your child is losing control, pick him up and remove him.
   7. If you know that your child has misbehaved, do not ask him whether he has done the misdeed; confront him with it and thereby avoid tempting him to lie.

COMMON CHILD-REARING CONCERNS: SIBLING RIVALRY*

Sibling rivalry occurs when children feel displaced, frustrated, angry, and unloved. It is normal for an older child to feel jealous at the arrival of a new baby. Competition and feelings of envy can also occur among older siblings; fighting between brothers and sisters is common. However, if such behavior is allowed to continue, it can persist into adolescence and even adulthood.

Often the arrival of a second child occurs when the first child is at the developmentally stressed age of 2 years. All children show signs of regression after the birth of a sibling; it is best to allow this regression to take place without interference. If the parents continue to reinforce positive behavior, the older child will gradually begin to feel as important and loved as his younger sibling, and the relationship between the two will become stronger and more supportive.

Parents are responsible for establishing a positive, supportive environment in which competition among siblings is reduced and replaced by a caring, concerned, affectionate relationship. This takes place over a long period of time. Parents must be fair and consistent in teaching children both by example and by good management of negative behavior.

One successful method used to change negative behavior is "time out." This is a proved method in which the fighting children are separated and sent to separate rooms. All the fighting children are treated equally, with no favoritism. Parents must verbally praise and encourage positive play, rewarding good behavior and discouraging name-calling, baiting, and arguments.

Feelings of jealousy naturally occur at the birth of siblings. If this event does not interfere with the time spent with the older child or affect the love and affection shown, these feelings eventually dissipate.

The age of the child is an important factor in sibling rivalry. The younger the older child, the greater will be the degree of rivalry. Children age 5 years or older are fairly secure and therefore less intensely jealous of a new baby. Anticipatory guidance is advisable; parents should set the stage well in advance of the birth. A few simple practices may help decrease the jealousy between the first child and the new baby:

1. Take the older child to the prenatal exam to hear the baby's heartbeat.
2. Allow the child to feel the baby move in Mom's tummy.
3. When talking about the new baby, use terms such as "our baby" and describe what babies do, e.g., wear diapers, coo, smile, etc.
4. Borrow a small baby or visit a friend with a newborn to acquaint the child with babies.
5. Have a special time each day, called "our time," to be spent reading or playing with just the older child.
6. Read books together (many are available at the library) about "arrival of new baby."
7. Supply the older child with a doll, a "baby" of his own.
8. Establish the older child in his new bed or room long before the baby is due.

After the baby arrives:

1. Allow the child to visit you in the hospital each day.
2. Phone the child daily from the hospital.
3. Bring a special gift to the child when you come home with the baby.

---

*This section written by Rose Boynton.

4. Allow the child to assist in baby care by bringing you diapers, etc.
5. Spend some time each day exclusively with each child.

Parents must be fair about the attention they give each child. If a child matures in a loving, sharing, charitable environment, he will have the self-esteem he needs to grow into a well-rounded, strong adult who likes and enjoys his siblings.

I. Sibling interaction

A. Siblings interact independently of other family relationships; relationships with parents and extended family members may be more or less intense, or more or less caring.

B. Birth order influences the development of the sibling bond. Since all the children in family both initiate behaviors and react to others' behaviors, this development continues into and through adulthood.

C. Families provide a social arena in which children learn to explore language, observe behavior (both negative and positive), and learn to assess their influence on other people. Therefore, children's personalities outside the family and their ability to deal socially with others are first established with family members.

1. Children without siblings are more critical of themselves and often find peer relationships more uncomfortable and difficult to sustain than do children with siblings. "Only" children relate to older people and adults much more successfully than to other children their own age. Single children are perfectionists, expecting perfect behavior from others as well as from themselves. "Only children often quietly wish they could move in, take over, and'do it right,'" (Leman, K. *The Birth Order Book.* See Section V: References).
2. First-born children are often confident, conscientious, organized children who grow up to be hard-driving, successful adults. A lot of pressure is exerted on the oldest child, who receives more attention and more discipline and has more expectations made of him. He is the pathfinder and the one all the other children in the family look up to.
3. Middle children learn social skills early in life. They learn how to negotiate and that it is futile constantly to compare themselves with others. They are forced to form their own identities, usually by adolescence, and grow up to be people-oriented adults.
4. Last-born children are often pleasant, cheerful, outgoing, and uncomplicated. They can be impatient, spoiled, and clownish. Last-borns live in the shadow of the children born before them. They are often "put down" and not taken seriously. Often they get attention by clowning, making jokes, or behaving badly in school, but they secretly wish to be very successful.

D. Gender influences the interaction between siblings. Rivalry is likely to be most intense in a two-child family with two boys; however, if such brothers are born close together, there is less chance for the older one to establish clear superiority. In a two-child family with two girls, the rivalry is likely to be much less serious; the father is usually the key family figure, and the girls compete for his attention. In a two-child family with a girl and a boy, rivalry is much less serious, the difference in expectations of the two sexes having been made clear since birth.

E. Sibling rivalry is an important consideration in the age spacing of children in families. The children closest in age often share experiences and friends and therefore form a stronger bond than do siblings born 8 or 9 years apart. Siblings born close together become more reciprocal in their relationship and are more intimate and intensely involved with each other than are siblings born years apart.

II. Parents can influence sibling rivalry

A. Set a good example; be supportive of all the children in the family, and reinforce positive behavior within the family.

B. Teach the children to be loyal to each other regardless of the anger they feel toward each other; allow competition between them to be verbalized and to be resolved openly and swiftly.

C. Verbalize the frustration the angry child is feeling; always show concern and compassion for the child.

D. Try to teach the children constructive ways of expressing feelings of rivalry rather than punishing them for negative rivalrous behaviors.

E. Expect the children to be accountable for their words and actions, and thereby teach them coping skills.

F. Be consistent; the discipline should fit the "crime."

G. Separate the children for a period of time if they are constantly fighting (time out).

H. Treat the children with respect, and show confidence in their ability to get along.

III. Sibling rivalry in step-families.

Sibling rivalry among children in step-families is a difficult problem. The family system is complex owing to the large number of persons involved, and often the parents are preoccupied with their own new marriage.

A. Special attention should be focused on cementing a step-parent-step-child bond; allow time to build a caring relationship.

B. Parents should remember children in step-families are often angry and sad at the loss of their original families.

C. Children should be taught that "sharing" is a key component to success, and the advantages of sharing within the family should be pointed out to them.

D. Step-families must clearly and consciously work out the rules of the family, and the children should be included in this process.

E. Adolescents find the new family structure in step-families difficult; often they withdraw from both parents and become closer to their own siblings.

IV. Siblings of handicapped children

A. Sibling relationships between handicapped and nonhandicapped children are more complex; special problems arise owing to the intense nature of the relationship.

1. Siblings of a handicapped child
   - a. Resent the attention and time given to the handicapped child.
   - b. Fear catching the handicapped condition.
   - c. Feel angry toward the disabled child because they feel ignored and unappreciated by the parents.
   - d. Feel upset by the unfairness of the family situation; long for a "normal" family.
   - e. Feel embarrassed by the handicapped sibling.
   - f. Feel guilty about their own hostility toward their sibling.

g. Feel confused about their role in caring for their sibling.
h. Feel afraid that outsiders won't accept the handicapped child.

2. Parents of a handicapped child
    a. Communicate with the handicapped child; be truthful with him about the degree of his handicap and nonsecretive in approaching the problems of working with him.
    b. Treat all the children individually, reinforcing their positive characteristics.
    c. Schedule quality time to be spent with the nondisabled children.
    d. Strive to attain a normal home life by providing a comfortable home environment that welcomes the participation of other children in family activities.
    e. Establish or join a support group in which each family member obtains a balanced perspective on his role within the family and can compare his experiences with those of others.

V. Suggested readings

A. Farber, A., and Mazlish, E. *Siblings Without Rivalry: How to Help Your Children Live Together so You Can Live Too.* Ontario: Penguin Books, 1987.

B. Leman, K. *The Birth Order Book.* New York: Dell, 1985.

C. Lofas, J., and Sova, D. B. *Step-Parenting: A Guide to the Joys, Frustrations and Fears of Step-Parenting.* New York: Zebra Books, 1986.

D. Powell, T. H., and Ahrenhold-Olgie, P. *Brothers and Sisters: A Special Part of Exceptional Families.* Baltimore: Paul H. Brookes, 1985.

BIBLIOGRAPHY

American Academy of Pediatrics. *Caring for Your Baby and Young Child.* New York: Bantam Books, 1991.

Brazelton, T. *Infants and Mothers: Differences in Development.* New York: Dell, 1986.

Dreikurs, R., and Soltz, V. *Children: The Challenge.* New York: Hawthorn, 1987.

Dreikurs, R. Discipline *Without Fear.* New York: Hawthorn, 1974.

Eastman, P., with Barrm, J. *Your Child is Smarter Than You Think.* New York: William Morrow, 1985.

Erikson, Erik. *Childhood in Society.* New York: W.W. Norton, 1991.

Fraiberg, S. H. *The Magic Years.* New York: Scribner's, 1984.

Gibson, J. T. *Discipline: A Positive Learning Approach.* Lexington, MA: Lewis Publ., 1983.

Johnson, T. R., Moore, W. M., and Jeffries, J. E. (Eds.). *Children Are Different: Developmental Physiology,* 2nd ed. Columbus, Ohio: Ross Laboratories, 1978.

Kagan, J., and Coles, R. *The Twelve to Sixteen Year Old.* New York: W.W. Norton & Co., Inc.

Normans, J., and Harris, M. *The Private Life of the American Teenager.* New York: Rawson, Wade, 1981.

Pillitteri, A. *Maternal and Child Health Nursing.* Philadelphia: J.B. Lippincott, 1992.

Schowalter, J. E., and Anyan, W. R. *The Family Handbook of Adolescence.* New York: Knopf, 1981.

Schuster, C., and Ashburn, S. *The Process of Human Development,* 3rd ed. Philadelphia: J.B. Lippincott, 1992.

Singer, D., and Revenson, I. *How a Child Thinks: A Piaget Primer.* New York: New American Library, 1978.

Stone, L. J., and Church, J. *Childhood and Adolescence,* 3rd ed. New York: Random House, 1984.

Valadian, I., and Porter, D. *Physical Growth and Development from Conception to Maturity.* Boston: Little, Brown, 1977.

White, B. L. *The First Three Years of Life.* Englewood Cliffs, NJ: Prentice-Hall, 1984.

II

Management of Common Pediatric Problems

Elizabeth S. Dunn

Part II covers common pediatric health problems within the scope of practice for a nurse practitioner and others responsible for the delivery of primary health care. It is developed according to the SOAP format, an outline form that includes Subjective data, Objective data, Assessment, and Plan.

The subjective data include the information with which the child and/or parent presents or the provider expects to elicit in a history of the presenting illness.

The objective data include the information that would be obtained from the physical examination of the child as well as from laboratory tests.

In the assessment, the differential diagnoses for each management problem are listed and include relevant information to assist the provider in making an accurate diagnosis.

The plan consists of various treatment modalities used in managing the case. The plan is comprised of specific pharmaceutical treatment as well as symptomatic treatment.

Additionally, for each protocol there is an extensive education section which includes pertinent information for parents. It incorporates physical care, psychosocial issues, medication information, and general information about the presenting problem.

The etiology, incidence, communicability, and incubation period have been included for each protocol where applicable. Similarly, indications for follow-up, complications, and indications for consultation and/or referral are a part of every protocol.

Prior to initiating a treatment plan for any management problem, several factors must be recognized and assessed. First, a high anxiety level may interfere with the parent's or child's ability to hear and remember the recommended plan; the provider should recognize this anxiety and deal with it. Second, the ability to follow through with recommendations should be assessed; for example, a parent already stressed by the daily care of several small children may find the additional tasks involved in coping with a sick child overwhelming. Third, given that compliance is enhanced by knowledge, it is essential to evaluate the parent's or child's understanding of the disease and treatment. The provider must be aware of potential barriers to compliance, such as ethnic or religious customs or restrictions, and address them as necessary. Fourth, with regard to pharmaceuticals, it is necessary to ascertain whether the family can afford the prescribed medication, how they intend to measure the dosage, whether they understand the route of administration, whether they can give it at proper intervals, and whether they know the importance of continuing the medication for the duration prescribed.

Protocols are included for some of the most common childhood problems. Space has been left at the end of each protocol for changes and additions since specific practices and geographic locations may necessitate minor revisions. For most effective use, each protocol should be carefully reviewed by the health care team and amended, if necessary, for their particular health center. Once reviewed and amended by the nurse practitioner and collaborating physician, they can be used as guidelines for practice as required for nurses practicing in an expanded role.

Indications for use and dosages for drugs are from current literature. However, since medicine is a constantly changing science, recommendations for management and standards for use of drugs are subject to frequent change. For that reason, current recommendations should be reviewed on a regular basis.

AIDS, anorexia, and bulimia have been included in this section. Although they are not necessarily problems which should be managed in the primary health care setting, the health care provider is responsible for the diagnosis and referral of these contemporary issues. The above are presented with pertinent background information, presenting signs and symptoms, indicators for diagnosis, and referral sources. Space has been left for the health care provider to list local resources at the end of each of these protocols.

In addition, Child Abuse and Suicide Prevention, authored by Rose Boynton, are included in this section. They contain pertinent background information, indicators for diagnosis, and management techniques.

ACNE

An inflammatory eruption involving the pilosebaceous follicles characterized by comedones (open and closed), pustules, and/or cysts.

I. Etiology

Pilosebaceous follicle activity is stimulated by increased androgen levels during puberty. Desquamation of the follicular wall occurs, creating a number of cells that, combined with sebum, result in a plug obstructing the lumen of the follicle. *Corynebacterium acnes* enzymes hydrolyze these trapped sebaceous lipids, causing distention and rupture of the sebaceous ducts. An inflammatory reaction occurs in the dermis with the release of the keratin, bacteria, and sebum.

II. Incidence

Affects 30–85% of adolescents. Generally disappears by the early 20s in males, somewhat later in females. Severe disease affects males 10 times more frequently than females.

III. Subjective data

Vary according to the degree of severity.

A. Complaints include
   1. "Bumps," blackheads, whiteheads, pimples, cysts, scarring.
   2. Pain on application of pressure.
   3. Premenstrual flare.
B. Location. Face, chest, back, buttocks.
C. Pertinent subjective data to obtain
   1. Does patient see acne as a problem and want treatment for it?
   2. Does acne flare with stress or emotional upheaval?
   3. Does acne flare premenstrually?
   4. Do seasonal changes affect acne (e.g., improve in summer or worsen with high humidity)?
   5. Is acne worse in response to certain foods? What are they?
   6. What treatment has been used in the past?
   7. What was the response to previous treatment?
   8. Has female patient been on birth control pills?
   9. Are there any associated endocrine factors?
      a. Are menses regular?
      b. Does patient complain of hirsutism?
   10. Does patient use cosmetics or creams on skin?
      1. Determine type—oil based or water based.
   11. Is patient exposed to heavy grease and oil?

Note: Often the patient will not complain of any symptoms because of embarrassment. It is the responsibility of the nurse practitioner to raise the issue.

IV. Objective data

A. Inspect the entire body. Lesions may be found on the face, earlobes, scalp, chest, back, buttocks; they generally recur in the same areas.
B. Lesions
   1. Mild acne

a. Closed comedones (whiteheads).

b. Open comedones (blackheads).

c. Occasional pustules.

2. Moderate acne

a. Comedones—open and closed.

b. Papules.

c. Pustules.

3. Severe acne

a. Comedones—open and closed.

b. Erythematous papules.

c. Pustules.

d. Cysts.

C. Scarring may be present in any stage.

D. Hair is often very oily.

V. Assessment

A. Diagnosis is easily made by the appearance of the different lesions present on the skin.

B. Assess degree of involvement—both physical and emotional—to determine the best therapeutic plan.

VI. Plan

A. Mild acne

1. Exposure to sunlight. Start with brief periods (15–20 minutes), extending the time daily by 5 minutes. Too much sun exposure can exacerbate acne.

2. Topical agents.

a. Benzoyl peroxide—a potent antimicrobial agent as well as an exfoliant, a sebostatic, and comedolytic agent.

(1) Use one of the following:

(a) Desquam-X (clear aqueous gel).

(b) Benzagel (clear alcohol gel).

(c) PanOxyl (clear alcohol gel).

(d) Persa-Gel (clear acetone gel).

(2) Begin with 5% used once daily. (With fair or sensitive skin, use every other day and increase frequency accordingly.)

(3) Follow-up telephone call in 2 weeks. If no sensitivity, gradually increase application to twice daily.

or

a. Retin-A 0.05% cream—a comedolytic agent.

(1) Use once daily.

or

b. T-Stat pads (an antimicrobial agent).

(2) Use once daily.

3. Recheck in the office in 1 month. Continue regimen if condition responds to treatment. If there is no response to treatment and no sensitivity to the medication:

a. Increase strength of benzoyl peroxide preparations to 10% used once daily. Increase frequency to twice daily after 2 weeks if no sensitivity.

   b. Increase strength of Retin-A to 0.1% cream or 0.025% gel used once daily. Increase frequency to twice daily after 2 weeks if no sensitivity.
   c. During early treatment, an increase in inflammatory lesions is common. Improvement may take as long as 2 months.
4. Further follow-up should be individualized according to the patient's needs and the degree of response to therapy.

B. Moderate acne
1. Benzoyl peroxide gel and/or
2. Retin-A Cream
3. Hot soaks to pustules 5–6 times a day.
4. Tetracycline 250 mg qid, or 500 mg bid.
5. Recheck in 4 weeks.
   a. With no improvement:
      (1) Increase tetracycline to 1.5 gm/day for 2 weeks, then 2 gm/day for 2 weeks.
      (2) Increase strength of keratolytic gel to 10% or increase Retin-A to 0.1% cream or 0.025% gel.
   b. With marked improvement, decrease tetracycline to 250 mg bid.
6. Recheck again in 4 weeks.
   a. With no improvement:
      (1) Continue tetracycline at 2 gm/day.
      (2) Use keratolytic gel at bedtime, Retin-A in the morning.
   b. With improvement:
      (1) Decrease tetracycline to 250 mg qid, or discontinue if already decreased to bid.
      (2) Continue with topical medication.
7. Continue individualized follow-up:
   a. Every 4–8 weeks while on tetracycline.
   b. Every 3–6 months while on topical medication.

C. Severe or inflammatory acne
1. Topical medication as above.
2. Hot soaks to inflamed lesions 5–6 times a day.
3. Tetracycline 250 mg qid.
4. Recheck in 4 weeks. With no improvement, increase tetracycline as above.
5. Refer to dermatologist if no improvement on this regime.

D. Note
1. Limit refills on tetracycline to ensure follow-up visits.
2. Sulfur can be comedogenic.
3. Keratolytic gels penetrate better than creams or solutions.
4. When discussing acne, do not hesitate to touch the area so child does not feel he is "dirty." Tell child that blackheads are not dirt but oxidized melanin.
5. Psychological scarring may occur.
6. Appropriate therapy should be instituted if patient perceives acne as a problem.

VII. Education

A. Acne is chronic. It cannot be cured, but it can be controlled.

B. Explain etiology (for psychological support).

C. When local treatment is instituted, acne may appear worse before it improves.

D. For mild and moderate acne, the aim is to dry and desquamate the skin. Expect some dryness, peeling, and faint erythema of the skin.

E. Topical medication.

1. If marked erythema and pruritus develop in response to topical medication, discontinue use temporarily and then resume with less frequent application.
2. Apply 20—30 minutes after gentle washing.
3. Apply lightly to affected area. Do not rub in vigorously.
4. Expect a feeling of warmth and slight stinging with application.

F. Hygiene.

1. Avoid abrasive agents, e.g., over-the-counter scrubs.
2. Shampoo frequently; no special shampoo is necessary.
3. Change pillowcase daily.
4. Do not pick or squeeze lesions—this will retard healing and cause scarring.
5. Use facecloth and hot water for soaks. Try to soak for 10–20 minutes 5–6 times a day.
6. Wash face gently three times daily with mild soap; excess scrubbing can exacerbate acne.
7. "Facials" may exacerbate acne.
8. Use only water-based cosmetics.
   a. Oil-free is not necessarily water-based.
   b. Use loose powder and blush.
9. Acne medications can be applied under cosmetics and sunscreens.
10. Avoid oily sunscreens. Sundown and PreSun are generally acceptable.

G. Avoid foods that seem to make acne worse.

H. Overexposure to sunlight can have adverse effects, alone or in combination with Retin-A and tetracycline. It may be necessary to discontinue these medications in the summer.

I. High humidity and heavy sweating exacerbate acne, as does exposure to heavy oils and grease.

J. Tetracycline.

1. While on medication, restrict exposure to sunlight.
2. Do not take if there is any question of pregnancy.
3. Take 1 hour before or 2 hours after a meal.
4. If unable to take four times a day because of schedule, take 500 mg every 12 hours. Nurse practitioner should acknowledge that it may be a problem for an adolescent to have an empty stomach 4 times a day.
5. Patient must take the *full* dose for at least 1 month for effective treatment.
6. Moniliasis may occur in females.

K. Discuss preparations available over the counter. Explain to adolescent (and parent, if applicable) that it is more cost-effective to follow the treatment regimen than to try all the latest acne products for the dramatic cures that advertisements promise.

L. Birth control pill may need to be changed to one that does not contain norgestrel, norethindrone, or norethindrone acetate.

M. T-Stat should be applied with the disposable applicator pads. Drying and peeling can be controlled by reducing the frequency of application.

VIII. Follow-up

Acne is chronic. Treatment should be continued until the process subsides spontaneously. Return visits need to be individualized according to the severity of the acne and the emotional needs of the adolescent. Once control has been achieved, however, the frequency of follow-up can be decreased. The patient may need to remain on a 250- to 500-mg daily maintenance dose of tetracycline for several months, in which event 6- to 12-week return visits should continue. If patient is on topical medications alone, after acne is controlled the frequency of application can be adjusted by the patient, and telephone follow-up may sufficient.

IX. Complications

A. Psychological problems.

B. Secondary bacterial infection.

C. Scarring.

X. Consultation/referral

A. Moderate acne. Consult for treatment. if no improvement noted after treatment with tetracycline for 2 months, consult before continuing treatment plan.

B. Severe or inflammatory acne. Consult for treatment. Refer if no improvement noted after treatment with tetracycline for 1 month. May require more aggressive therapy such as treatment with accutane.

NOTES

AIDS (ACQUIRED IMMUNE DEFICIENCY SYNDROME)

A severe, debilitating disease that destroys the immune system. It is characterized by increased vulnerability to bacterial, protozoan, fungal, and other viral infections as well as by malignancies. These opportunistic infections eventually cause death.

I. Etiology

A. RNA cytopathic human retrovirus, human immunodeficiency virus, type 1 (HIV-1).

B. The virus infects the CD4+ lymphocyte. When stimulated by an antigen, the infected CD4 cell replicates the HIV instead of itself. The new HIV then infects other T cells. With its CD4+ lymphocytes depleted, the immune system is impaired by severely diminished antibody production. Overwhelming infections then occur when organisms, some of which do not generally cause disease, invade the body.

II. Communicability

HIV is a low-contagion virus and is not spread by casual contact. There have been no documented instances of transmission to family members other than by sexual contact. It is not transmitted by fomites, by hugging, social kissing, or shaking hands, or through swimming pools or hot tubs. There are no known cases of AIDS transmission by insects.

HIV is transmitted by blood, blood products, semen, transplacental infection, vaginal secretions, and possibly breast milk.

There is a higher incidence of transmission from infected men to women than from infected women to men.

Humans are the only known reservoir of HIV.

HIV cannot reproduce outside a living cell.

III. High-risk persons

A. Homosexuals. Approximately 70% of AIDS victims are homosexual or bisexual.

B. Bisexuals.

C. Heterosexuals. Risk increases in relation to number of sexual encounters.

D. Prostitutes.

E. Intravenous-drug users. Approximately 20% of AIDS patients use IV drugs, most commonly heroin and cocaine.

F. Hemophiliacs.

G. Persons who received transfused blood products before March 1985.

H. Persons of Haitian ethnic background comprise 3.6% of individuals infected in the Unites States. Most of these persons are not involved in high risk behaviors.

I. Infants or children of high-risk persons. Approximately 1,800 HIV-infected infants are born annually in the United States.

J. Sexual contacts of high-risk persons.

IV. Incubation period

A. Six months to 5 years or more.

B. Antibodies develop in 2 weeks to 4 months (average, 6 weeks). If an exposed person shows no antibodies after 4 months, he has not been infected.

C. AIDS symptoms appear on an average of 18 months after infection. (Dormant periods have been estimated to be 1.9 years for children up to age 4 at time of infection to 8.23 years for persons aged 5–59 years at time of infection.)

V. Incidence

A. AIDS

1. AIDS was first reported in the United States in mid-1981.
2. Twenty thousand cases had been reported in the United States by spring of 1986.
3. By August 1987, 40,532 cases had been reported.
4. By 1991, over 160,000 cases had been reported to the CDC.
5. As of January 1, 1993, total cases reported were:
   a. United States—242,146
      (1) Males—214,315
      (2) Females—27,831
   b. World—1,500,000
6. One percent of cases of AIDS are adolescents.
7. Twenty percent of cases of AIDS are 20 to 29 years old, representing infection as teens.

B. ARC—AIDS-related complex

1. Caused by the AIDS virus; patient tests positive for HIV and demonstrates symptoms of immunodeficiency.
2. An estimated 100,000–200,000 persons infected with the AIDS virus will get ARC.

C. Infection by AIDS virus

1. Estimates vary; between 1 and 1 1/2 million persons in the United States have been infected by the AIDS virus.
2. Current worldwide cumulative counts of infected persons are:
   a. 10 to 12 million adults
   b. one million children
3. Those persons infected with the HTLV-III virus
   a. Have no visible signs of illness.
   b. May not be aware that they harbor the virus.
   c. Can transmit the virus throughout their lifetime.
   d. Will not necessarily get AIDS.
   e. May get ARC, with symptoms taking as long as 9 years to appear.

D. Less than 2% of people with AIDS are children.

1. 1982—16 cases.
2. 1983—35 cases.
3. 1984—48 cases.
4. 1985—132 cases.
5. 1986—410 cases.
6. January 1993—4,051 cases.

E. Health care workers (6.8 million in US).

1. Documented cases of occupational transmission through September 1992: 32.

2. Cases with possible occupational transmission through September 1992: 69.

VI. Mortality

(Statistics may be inaccurate due to underreporting or under diagnosis.)

A. Sixty-six percent of persons with AIDS have died.

B. One hundred percent of infected persons are expected to die from AIDS.

C. Centers for Disease Control statistics indicate that as of January 1993, 160,372 people have died from AIDS.

D. Seventy percent of persons with AIDS die within 2 years of diagnosis.

E. Eighty percent of children with AIDS have died within the first 2 years of diagnosis.

F. In 1987, AIDS was the 15th leading cause of all deaths in the United States.

G. In 1989, AIDS was the second leading cause of death in males ages 25 to 44.

H. In 1991, AIDS was estimated to be the fifth leading cause of death in females ages 25 to 44.

VII. Diagnostic indicators

A. AIDS

1. Positive history of risk factors.
   a. Haitian ethnic background.
   b. Sexual partners of:
      (1) Intravenous drug users.
      (2) Bisexuals and homosexuals.
      (3) Prostitutes.
   c. Mother with immunologic abnormalities.
2. Low birth weight.
3. Failure to thrive or poor growth rate; unexplained weight loss of greater than 10 lb.
4. Hepatosplenomegaly.
5. Diffuse lymphadenopathy.
6. Recurring fever and/or night sweats.
7. Recurrent severe viral or fungal infections.
8. Episodic or chronic diarrhea.
9. Persistent cough; shortness of breath.
10. Persistence of an infection in spite of appropriate treatment.
11. Infections in diffuse sites rather than a single site.
12. Candidiasis.
13. Chronic interstitial pneumonitis.
14. Increased bruising; unexplained bleeding.
15. *Giardia* or other opportunistic infections.
16. *Pneumocystis carinii* pneumonia.
17. Kaposi's sarcoma (most common cancer seen with AIDS); pink or purple blotches on or under the skin and inside the mouth, nose, eyelids, or rectum.
18. Positive HIV antibody test.

B. Congenital AIDS

1. Pediatric AIDS is predominantly perinatally acquired (80% of cases).
2. Fetal transmission both transplacentally and during delivery is 25 to 30% in the United States. If infected during pregnancy, the risk of transmission to the fetus is 27% as opposed to a 16% risk if infected prior to pregnancy.
3. Positive history of risk factors.
4. Prematurity.
5. Low birth weight (small for gestational age).
6. Failure to thrive.
7. Respiratory infections.
8. Dysmorphic features.
   a. Microcephaly.
   b. Hypertelorism.
   c. Prominent forehead.
   d. Flat nasal bridge.
9. Positive HIV antibody test after 4 months of age.

C. ARC
1. Clinical symptoms less severe than those of AIDS.
   a. Anorexia.
   b. Weight loss.
   c. Fever.
   d. Night sweats.
   e. Rashes.
   f. Diarrhea.
   g. Fatigue.
   h. Generalized lymphadenopathy.
   i. Oral candidiasis.
   j. Decreased resistance to infection.
2. Positive ELISA and Western blot tests.

VIII. Differential diagnosis—Congenital immunodeficiency disorders

A. X-linked agammaglobulinemia. B-cell deficiency characterized by recurrent bacterial sinopulmonary infections, diarrhea, and otitis media.

B. Wiskott-Aldrich syndrome (chronic granulomatous disease). T-cell deficiency characterized by severe eczema, thrombocytopenia with platelets of reduced size and function, and recurrent infection with encapsulated bacteria.

C. Ataxia-telangiectasia. T-cell deficiency characterized by telangiectasias, ataxia, recurrent sinopulmonary infection, malignancy, and dysarthric speech.

D. DiGeorge anomolad. T-cell deficiency characterized by hypertelorism and ear anomalies; abnormalities of the aortic arch and neonatal tetany candidiasis are common.

E. Severe combined immunodeficiency. T- and B-cell deficiency characterized by low immunoglobulin levels and by absent antibody responses with recurrent or chronic bacterial, fungal, viral, and protozoan infections.

IX. Plan

A. Order blood test for HIV after appropriate counseling and signing of informed consent. Schedule return visit to inform patient of results of HIV testing.

B. Blood test should include: CBC, differential, platelets, LFT's, BUN, TP albumin, serology for syphilis, hepatitis B screen.

C. Chest X-ray.

D. Urinalysis.

E. TB test.

F. Pap test, vaginal cultures, endocervical tests for GC, *Chlamydia.*

G. Urethral test for GC, *Chlamydia.*

H. Referrals should also include:

1. Local AIDS service groups.
2. Social workers (for planning of physical and financial assistance).
3. Mental health personnel.

I. List local referral sources here. (See Appendix G for national and state organizations, and state boards of health telephone numbers.)

J. There is no known cure for AIDS. Opportunistic infections can be treated with appropriate therapy, although they may not respond. Over 200 investigational drugs have been tried, but none has effectively halted or reversed the immunodeficiency.

1. Zidovudine (AZT): Prolongs quality and duration of life by delaying progression of immunodeficiency and onset of symptoms.
2. Zalcitabine (HIVID): Approved for use in combination with AZT for adult patients with advanced infection.
3. Dideoxyinosine (ddI): Used for treatment in adults and children who cannot tolerate zidovudine or in whom AZT treatment has failed.

K. Routine monitoring of clinical status: Growth, nutrition, development, associated infections.

L. Prophylaxis for PCP as indicated. (Trimethoprim-sulfamethoxazole)

M. Aggressive treatment of HIV-associated infections.

X. Education

A. General public

1. Education is the best method of controlling the spread of AIDS. Prevention relies on both education and behavior change.
2. Intravenous drug abuse is the most important factor in maternal spread.

3. Sexual promiscuity increases one's chances of contracting AIDS; sexual partners should be chosen with care.
4. Couples who have had a mutually monogamous relationship for at least 6 years will not contract AIDS through sexual intercourse unless one or both partners has illicitly used intravenous drugs.
5. Use latex condoms for sexual intercourse (vaginal or rectal); they afford some protection as does nonoxynol-9 either on a condom or intravaginally.
6. Do not have sex with prostitutes or intravenous drug abusers.
7. Avoid sexual activities that could cause tears in the vaginal or rectal lining or injury to the penis.
8. Avoid oral contact with vagina, penis, or rectum.
9. Rectal intercourse is particularly dangerous, since the rectal mucosa tears easily and provides direct access to the circulatory system by HIV.
10. Genital ulcers, i.e. herpes, facilitate transmission of the virus.
11. Transmission occurs less easily from women to men than from men to women.
12. A pregnant woman infected with the AIDS virus is more apt to develop AIDS or ARC than a nonpregnant woman with the AIDS virus. An infected pregnant woman can also transmit the virus to the fetus.
13. Since a number of reports have implicated breast-feeding as a mode of transmission, HIV-infected mothers should avoid breast-feeding.
14. Do not share syringes, needles, or other implements used for injecting drugs.
15. Do not donate blood if you have a history of homosexual activity or illicit drug use.
16. Donating blood poses no threat to the donor.
17. Do not have tattoo done.
18. The virus can be transmitted by acupuncture if the instruments are not properly sterilized.
19. Ear piercing should be done only under aseptic conditions in a physician's office.
20. Do not share toothbrushes, razors, or any other personal effects that can be contaminated by body fluids.

B. Health care workers

1. Intact skin is an effective barrier against HIV; health care workers with exudative dermatitis or lesions should not provide direct patient care.
2. Hands should be washed carefully and thoroughly before and after patient contact and after any contact with body fluids.
3. Gloves should be used for any contact with body fluids (blood, vomitus, feces, urine); the gloves should be discarded and the hands washed after contact.
4. Gloves should be worn by all dental health personnel.
5. Body spills should be disinfected with bleach (1 part bleach to 10 parts water); this solution should be prepared daily.
6. Use chlorine bleach in laundry for items soiled with blood, urine, feces, or vomitus.
7. Health care workers should be careful to avoid accidental puncture by lancets, needles, and other sharp objects.

8. All used needles, lancets, and other sharp objects should be disposed of in puncture-proof containers.
9. Disposable diapers, dressings, syringes, gloves, etc., should be placed in plastic bags, which should be tied securely.
10. Disposable ambu-bags should be used for mouth-to-mouth resuscitation.
11. Use masks for direct, sustained contact with patients who are coughing.
12. Protective eye wear (i.e., goggles) should be worn if splattering of body fluids is anticipated.
13. Gowns are necessary only if soiling of clothing with body fluids is anticipated.
14. Continuing education programs concerning infection control procedures should be ongoing in every health care facility.

C. Children

1. Children with AIDS and members of their families should not receive live virus vaccines.
2. Children with AIDS who have cutaneous eruptions or draining lesions that cannot be covered should not attend school or day care.
3. Children with AIDS who have bloody diarrhea or have inappropriate behaviors, such as biting of an unusual frequency which would result in transfer of blood from the biter, should not attend school or day care.
4. Children with AIDS should not attend school or day care during outbreaks of chicken pox or other communicable diseases. Advise home tutoring when child with AIDS is at risk of getting infections from other children.
5. For all children, a comprehensive sex education curriculum should be instituted at the earliest age possible.

D. Adolescents

The high incidence of AIDS in the 20–29 age group (20% of cases of AIDS) is clearly indicative of infection in the adolescent years. Comprehensive substance abuse and HIV prevention education must be provided to adolescents by parents, schools, and health care providers.

1. Twenty percent of all people with AIDS (adults ages 20–29) were probably infected in teenage years.
2. As of January 1, 1993, there were 912 cases of AIDS in teenagers.
3. 51.5% of adolescents females report having intercourse between 15 and 19 years of age.
4. 25.6% of 15 year old females have had intercourse.
5. Adolescents who have intercourse at younger ages are more likely to have multiple partners.
6. Adolescents are less apt to use condoms after drinking or using drugs.
7. Use of crack cocaine is associated with high levels of risk-taking and sexual activity.
8. By age 21, 25% of teens have been infected with a STD.
9. Homelessness, poverty, and abuse may increase exposure to HIV.

NOTES

ALLERGIC RESPONSE TO HYMENOPTERA

A local or systemic reaction to the sting of an insect, generally a bee, wasp, or hornet.

I. Etiology

Hypersensitivity is an IgE-mediated response. Generally an initial exposure is followed by reexposure, and the rechallenge elicits the reaction.

- **A.** Hymenoptera
  - **1.** Bee family. Bees and honey bees.
  - **2.** Wasp family. Yellow jackets, wasps, and hornets.
- **B.** Ant family. Fire ants of southeastern United States (attack en masse).

II. Incidence

- **A.** 90% of children experience a normal reaction of less than 2 inches in diameter and less than 24 hours in duration.
- **B.** 10% of children will have a large local reaction greater than 2 inches in diameter and lasting up to seven days.
- **C.** Anaphylaxis occurs in 0.4 to 0.8% of the general population.
- **D.** Approximately 50 deaths from stings occur in the United States every year.

III. Subjective data

- **A.** History of bite or sting
- **B.** Local reaction
  - **1.** Swelling and redness at site of sting.
  - **2.** Intense local pain.
- **C.** Systemic reaction. May be a combination of the following:
  - **1.** Anxiety initially.
  - **2.** Nausea.
  - **3.** Itching.
  - **4.** Sneezing, coughing.
  - **5.** Hives or frank angioedema, with various parts of skin swollen.
  - **6.** Swelling of lips and throat.
  - **7.** Difficulty swallowing.
  - **8.** Difficulty breathing.
  - **9.** Stridor.
  - **10.** Respiratory compromise with ultimate collapse.
  - **11.** Vertigo.

IV. Objective data

- **A.** Local reaction
  - **1.** Local wheal and flare reaction with central punctum.
  - **2.** Edema around sting site.
  - **3.** Normal reaction
    - **a.** Swelling less than 2 inches in diameter.
    - **b.** Duration less than 24 hours.
  - **4.** Large local reaction

a. Swelling greater than 2 inches in diameter.
b. Duration 1–7 days.

B. Systemic reaction—signs of anaphylaxis
1. Anxiety.
2. Urticaria.
3. Dysphagia.
4. Laryngeal edema.
5. Bronchospasm.
6. Dyspnea.
7. Cyanosis.
8. Drop in blood pressure and pulse.

V. Assessment

A. Hymenoptera sting by history (honey bee if the stinger is left intact)

B. Differential diagnosis of anaphylaxis
1. Vasopressor syncope—self-limited. No pulmonary involvement, rarely occurs when child is prone, blood pressure and pulse do not drop, child rouses after breathing amyl nitrite.
2. Cardiac failure.
3. Anxiety attack.
4. Penicillin allergy.
5. Obstruction in laryngotracheobronchial tree.
6. Aspiration of foreign body.

VI. Plan

A. Normal local reaction
1. Remove stinger.
2. Topical application of ice.
3. Benadryl, 5 mg/kg/day in 4 divided doses.
4. Calamine lotion.

B. Large local reaction or multiple stings
1. Local measures as above.
2. Prednisone, 1mg/kg/day for 5 days may be helpful.

C. Systemic reaction
1. Apply tourniquet proximal to sting.
2. Remove stinger; shave off stinger of honey bee (has reverse serrations).
3. Administer epinephrine 1:1000, 0.01 ml/kg sc (maximum 0.3 ml); rub injection site to speed absorption. Repeat in 15–30 minutes.

Kilos	Pounds	Dosage (ml)
10	22	0.1
15	33	0.15
20	44	0.2
25	55	0.25
30 & over	66	0.3

4. Transport patient immediately to emergency room.

5. Refer patient to allergist for testing and possible immunotherapy.
6. Order Anakit or EpiPen.

VII. Education

A. Do not wear perfumes, hairspray, aftershave, etc. when outside.
B. Wear neutral colors; flowery prints are apt to attract bees.
C. Do not walk barefoot outside. Yellow jackets, the most aggressive hymenoptera, nest in the ground.
D. Avoid flower beds, playgrounds, picnic areas, and trash or garbage disposal areas.
E. Do not run or engage in physical activity after a sting.
F. The honey bee stinger has reverse serrations and leaves its stinger in the skin, the venom sac attached to it. The venom sac continues to eject venom and will empty out completely if compressed. Do not squeeze it; instead, shave the stinger off.
G. Seventy percent of deaths due to hymenoptera are caused by airway edema or respiratory compromise.
H. Eighty-five percent of children who go into anaphylactic shock do so within the first 15–30 minutes of exposure.
I. Anaphylaxis has occurred as late as 6 hours following exposure, but this is highly unusual.
J. Steroids do not help against the initial insult but will help against a delayed recurrence after the initial treatment.
K. Skin testing for allergy may yield a false-negative result if done too soon after treatment for a sting; wait 3–4 weeks after a sting before doing such testing.
L. Immunotherapy reduces risk of life-threatening complications from 60% to less than 5%.
M. Anakit contains 2 chewable antihistamines, 2 vials of epinephrine, and a syringe.
N. EpiPen spring-loaded syringe contains epinephrine in a premeasured dose (pediatric or adult size). Epinephrine is administered when the pen is pressed against the skin of the thigh.
O. Child should wear a MEDIC ALERT bracelet.

VIII. Follow-up

Contact after discharge from hospital to ensure that parent and/or child has made appointment with allergist for testing.

IX. Complications

A. Anaphylaxis following rechallenge.
B. Delayed systemic reaction.

X. Consultation/referral

A. Refer to allergist any patient who has had an immediate systemic reaction.
B. Consult with allergist on any patient who has had a large local reaction.

NOTES

ALLERGIC RHINITIS AND CONJUNCTIVITIS

An allergic response characterized by chronic, thin, watery nasal discharge with or without concurrent conjunctival discharge, inflammation, and pruritus.

I. Etiology

IgE-mediated immunologic reaction to common inhaled allergens (pollens, molds, dust, animal dander). Seasonal allergic rhinitis is generally caused by non-flowering,wind-pollinated plants. Perennial allergic rhinitis is caused by animal dander, dust, and molds. The mediators cause increased permeability of the mucosa and produce vasodilation, mucosal edema, mucous secretions, stimulation of the itch receptors, and a reduction in the sneezing threshold. Foods are not a common cause of allergic rhinitis.

II. Incidence

Allergic rhinitis is the most common atopic disease. It is usually seen after 3–4 years of age and affects approximately 10% of the population.

III. Subjective data

A. Nasal stuffiness—varies from mild to chronic obstruction.

B. Rhinorrhea—bilateral, thin, watery discharge.

C. Paroxysms of sneezing.

D. Itching of nose, eyes, palate, pharynx.

E. Conjunctival discharge and inflammation.

F. Mouth breathing.

G. Snoring.

H. Fatigue, irritability, anorexia may be present during season of offending allergen.

I. Allergic salute—rubbing the tip of the nose upward with the palm of the hand.

J. Pertinent subjective data to obtain

1. History of associated allergic symptoms—asthma, urticaria, contact dermatitis, eczema, food or drug allergies.
2. Family history of allergy.
3. Does child always seem to have a cold, or does it occur at specific times of the year (perennial versus seasonal)?
4. Are symptoms worst in any particular season?
5. Do parents or child notice that symptoms are worse after exposure to specific allergens, such as animals, wool, feathers, going into attic or cellar, etc.?
6. Are symptoms worse when child is indoors or outside?
7. What do parents and/or child think causes symptoms?
8. Can child clear nose by blowing?
9. What makes child feel better?
10. How much do symptoms bother child and family?

IV. Objective data

A. Allergic shiners—bluish cast under eyes.

B. Allergic crease—transverse nasal crease at junction of lower and middle thirds of nose.

C. Clear mucoid nasal discharge.

D. Pale edematous nasal mucosa.

E. Nasal turbinates swollen and may appear bluish.

F. Nasal phonation.

G. Mouth breathing.

H. Conjunctivae may be inflamed. "Cobblestoning" of upper lids may be present.

I. Tearing.

J. Edema of lids.

K. Laboratory test. Nasal smear positive for eosinophilia.

V. Assessment

A. Diagnosis. Differentiate between the following:

1. Seasonal allergic rhinitis occurs seasonally as a result of exposure to airborne pollens—generally tree pollens in late winter and early spring, grass pollens in spring and early summer, and weeds in late summer and early fall.
2. Perennial allergic rhinitis occurs all year but is usually worse in winter due to increased exposure to house dusts from heating systems, pets, wool clothing, and other allergens.

B. Differential diagnosis

1. Infectious rhinitis or recurrent colds: by detailed history.
2. Foreign body: unilateral purulent nasal discharge with foul odor.
3. Vasomotor rhinitis: symptoms precipitated by exposure to temperature changes or specific irritants (smoke, air pollutants, strong perfume, chemicals). Symptoms appear suddenly and disappear suddenly.
4. Rhinitis medicamentosus: by history of chronic use of nose drops.
5. Acute or chronic sinusitis: nasal mucosa is usually inflamed and edematous, discharge is generally mucopurulent, may have low grade fever.
6. Cystic fibrosis: consult if nasal polyps are present.

VI. Plan

Involve child in treatment plan as much as developmental level allows.

A. Pharmacologic therapy

1. Antihistamines for seasonal rhinitis

   Ages 6–12 years

   a. Benadryl, 5 mg/kg/day.

   b. Tavist syrup, 0.5 mg/5ml—1 tsp every 12 hours.

   Ages 12 and over

   c. Tavist D—one tablet every 12 hours.

   d. Seldane, 60 mg—one tablet every 24 hours.

   e. Hismanal, 10 mg—one tablet every 12 hours.

2. Decongestant-antihistamine combination.

   a. Pseudoephedrine (Actifed, Sudafed).

   b. Phenylephrine (Dimetapp).

3. Nasalcrom (cromolyn sodium nasal solution)—one spray in each nostril 3–4 times a day.

4. Acular 0.5% (ketoralac tromethamine) ophthalmic solution.
    a. 1–2 drops in each eye 4–6 times a day.
    b. For maximum effect, use at regular intervals as directed.

B. Avoidance.

Identify and avoid offending allergens (see Environmental Control for the Atopic Child, p. 257).

1. Seasonal allergic rhinitis: ragweed, trees, grasses, molds.
2. Perennial: house dust, feathers, animal dander, wool clothing or rugs, mold.

C. Desensitization. Referral indicated if

1. Symptoms are severe and cannot be controlled with symptomatic therapy.
2. Recurrent serous otitis occurs with resultant hearing loss.
3. Symptoms become progressively worse or asthma develops.
4. Allergen avoidance is impossible.

VII. Education

A. Advise parents that this is a chronic problem, although symptoms sometimes decrease with age and then disappear. Exacerbation of symptoms may occur, particularly as child approaches puberty.

B. Discuss indications for hyposensitization.

1. Inability to suppress symptoms with conservative treatment.
2. Inability to avoid allergens.
3. Severe symptoms affecting child's normal life-style—school, sleep, play.
4. Thirty to 50% of children with allergic rhinitis who are not treated develop asthma.

C. Discuss specific allergen control (see Environmental Control for the Atopic Child).

D. Advise child and parents of possible hearing loss due to serous otitis.

E. Notify school of child with hearing loss.

F. Side effects of antihistamines.

1. Sedation—often resolves with continued use.
2. Excitation, nervousness, tachycardia, palpitations.
3. Dryness of mouth.
4. Constipation.

G. Antihistamines relieve nasal congestion, itching, sneezing, rhinorrhea. Continuous therapy is more efficacious than sporadic use.

H. Hismanal and Seldane are less apt to cause sedation.

I. Cromolyn nasal solution

1. Inhibits release of histamines.
2. Generally takes 2–4 weeks for full effect.
3. Antihistamines and/or decongestants can be used concomitantly during initial phase of treatment and can be discontinued once Cromolyn becomes effective in controlling symptoms.
4. Treatment with Nasalcrom should be started prior to expected exposure to allergens and in seasonal allergic rhinitis, continued until pollen season is over.

J. Child should not wear soft contact lenses when using Acular.

K. Acular may cause transient stinging or burning.

L. Child with allergic rhinitis is more prone to upper respiratory and ear infections.

M. Child cannot clear nose by blowing it.

N. Child may not be able to chew with his mouth closed.

O. Epistaxis may be a problem because of nose picking and rubbing. Control nosebleed by compressing lower third of nose (external pressure over Kiesselbach's triangle) between fingers for 10 minutes.

VIII. Follow-up

A. Return visit or telephone follow-up in 2 weeks for reevaluation. Contact sooner if adverse reaction to medication occurs.

B. If no response to medication, increase dosage to control symptoms. Reevaluate in 2 weeks. Change type of antihistamine if indicated.

C. If symptoms under control, continue medication until suspected allergen no longer a threat. Medication may then be used as needed to control symptoms.

D. Return visit at any time that child or parent feels symptoms are worse or medication has ceased to control symptoms.

IX. Complications

A. Bacterial infection.

B. Recurrent serous otitis media.

C. Malocclusion.

D. Psychosocial problems.

X. Consultation/referral

A. Symptoms have not abated after a trial period of 4 weeks on antihistamines.

B. Parent or child sees symptoms as a major problem and requests skin testing.

C. Recurrent serous otitis affecting hearing or school progress.

NOTES

ANOREXIA NERVOSA

A symptom complex of nonorganic cause resulting in extreme weight loss in the preadolescent or adolescent.

I. Etiology

Anorexia nervosa is generally hypothesized to be due to reactivation at puberty of the separation-individuation issue—the adolescent's attempt to maintain or initiate a sense of autonomy and separateness from the mother. Starvation gives the adolescent a sense of identity and control over what is happening to her body.

II. Incidence

A. Affects approximately 3–4% of the adolescent population.

B. Ninety to 95% of anorexics are female, with the onset occurring between ages 13 and 20 in 85%.

C. Found in the middle and upper classes and commonly among members of the same family.

D. Generally seen in perfectionists or "model children" with poor self-images. They are high-achievers academically and are frequently engaged in strenuous physical activity such as varsity sports or vigorous exercise programs. Parents are often overprotective, controlling, and demanding. Children feel unable to live up to parental expectations despite strict adherence to these expectations.

E. Eighty percent of anorexics respond to therapy in terms of body weight, although other psychosocial problems may be prolonged. Amenorrhea persists in 13–50% even after weight returns to normal or is stabilized at 85–90% of ideal weight.

F. Mortality from physiological complications or suicide is 5–18%.

III. Subjective data

A. Weight loss.

B. Amenorrhea—absence of three consecutive menstrual periods.

C. Constipation.

D. Abdominal pain.

E. Cold intolerance.

F. Fatigue.

G. Insomnia.

H. Depression, loneliness.

I. Pertinent subjective data to obtain

1. Preoccupation with food and dieting.
    - **a.** History of dieting.
    - **b.** Denial of hunger.
    - **c.** Patient finds food revolting but spends time preparing gourmet meals for others.
    - **d.** History of food rituals.
2. Morbid fear of gaining weight.
3. Weight history—highest and lowest weights achieved.
4. Vomiting after meals.
5. Poor body-image; patient complains of being fat, when in reality, she is not.

6. Excessive exercising.
7. Laxatives, diuretics, or other medications used to control weight.
8. Recent family or social stress.
9. History of unpleasant sexual encounter; patient may be using starvation to try to halt development of secondary sex characteristics.
10. History of sexual activity; condition may be unconscious attempt to abort a pregnancy.

Note: Anorexia nervosa may be identified in its early stages by a conscientious health care provider eliciting a history during a routine health maintenance visit. Any combination of the above should create a high index of suspicion. (See Appendix, *Are You Dying to be Thin?)*

IV. Objective data

A. Weight loss—20% or more of body weight.
B. Emaciation—patient appears gaunt, skeletal.
C. Bradycardia.
D. Hypotension.
E. Hypothermia.
F. Skin: dry and flaky, lanugo hair, loss of subcutaneous fat, yellow.
G. Hair loss: scalp and genital.
H. Extremities: edema, cyanosis, mottling, cold.
I. Compulsive mannerisms (e.g., hand washing).
J. Apathy, listlessness.
K. Occasionally, scratches on palate from self-induced vomiting.
L. Laboratory findings
   1. Usually normal until later stages of malnutrition.
   2. With malnutrition.
      a. Leukopenia.
      b. Lymphocytosis.
      c. Low sedimentation rate.
      d. Low fibrinogen levels.
      e. Low serum lactic dehydrogenase estrogens.
      f. Low T3.
      g. Electrolyte imbalance.
   3. Cranial MRI to rule out hypothalmic tumor if neuro symptoms present and in all males (cerebral atrophy often seen).

V. Assessment

A. Diagnosis is made by evaluation of the subjective and objective data. Primary among these are the adolescent's intense or morbid fear of being fat, a poor or distorted body image, and a loss of 20% or more of body weight (patient weighs less than 75% of mean weight for age).
B. Differential diagnosis
   1. Inflammatory bowel disease.
   2. Endocrine disorders.
   3. Psychiatric illnesses (e.g., schizophrenia, or depressive disorder).
   4. Pregnancy (starving to abort pregnancy).

VI. Plan

A. Outpatient treatment
   1. Refer to psychotherapist.
   2. Refer to nutritionist.
   3. Weekly visit to check weight and urine (water loading will be detected by specific gravity).
   4. Refer family for counseling and/or parents group.
   5. Clearly identify parameters for admission:
      a. Unstable vital signs.
      b. Abnormal blood work.
      c. Failure to make progress as an outpatient in 4 weeks (less than one pound a week weight gain).
      d. Refusal to eat.
      e. Suicidal ideation.

B. Hospitalization indicated with severe malnutrition. Or for failure to make progress as an outpatient over a 4-week trial. Treatment includes the following:
   1. Family therapy.
   2. Behavior modification.
      a. Operant conditioning with positive reinforcers.
      b. Negative reinforcers.
   3. Pharmacotherapy.
      a. Amitriptyline.
      b. Cyproheptadine.

VII. Education

A. Counseling may need to be continued for as long as 2–3 years.

B. A consistent approach by all caretakers and family is necessary.

C. Aversion to food decreases as self-image improves.

D. Emphasis should be on weight gain, not eating.

E. Recommended weight gain is about 3 lb/week. Too rapid weight gain may cause adolescent to begin dieting again.

F. Weekly weights preferable to daily weights.

G. Child may drink copious amounts of water or conceal weights on body prior to weigh-in.

H. Bathroom use may need to be monitored for prevention of self-induced vomiting after meals.

I. Laxative use may continue if not closely monitored.

J. Anorexics who are cured generally stabilize at 85–90% of normal weight.

K. Television use should be monitored. Cultural influences such as television promote a preoccupation with food. In addition, television and fashion magazines are dedicated to a "thin is in" image—an ideal figure that few can hope to achieve.

VIII. Follow-up.

Contact patient and/or family following referral to ascertain that appointments have been made and kept as well as to provide support.

IX. Resources

A. National Association of Anorexia Nervosa and Associated Disorders, Box

271, Highland Park, IL 60035.

B. Anorexia Bulimia Care Inc., Box 213, Lincoln Center, MA 01773. (617) 259-9767

C. National Anorexic Aid Society, 1925 E. Dublin-Granville Road, Columbus, Ohio 43229. (614)436-1112

X. List local referral sources

NOTES

APHTHOUS STOMATITIS

Recurrent small, painful ulcers on the oral mucosa, commonly known as "canker sores."

I. Etiology

Unknown. Emotional and physical factors often precede eruptions and have been implicated in the etiology, but no definite proof is available. Herpes simplex is *not* the cause.

II. Incidence

Most commonly seen between the ages of 10 and 40. The estimated prevalence is about 20% of the general population.

III. Subjective data

- **A.** History of tingling or burning sensation preceding eruption for up to 24 hours.
- **B.** Complaint of canker sores or recurrent painful oral lesions.
- **C.** Pertinent subjective data to obtain. Do lesions occur after a specific triggering factor such as the following?
  1. Trauma.
  2. Ingestion of certain foods—chocolate, tomatoes, nuts.
  3. Ingestion of drugs.
  4. Stress—emotional or physical.

IV. Objective data

- **A.** Lesions.
  1. Single or multiple.
  2. Small: 1–10 mm.
  3. Oval, shallow.
  4. Light yellow or gray.
  5. Erythematous border.
- **B.** Distribution: buccal or labial mucosa, lateral tongue, pharynx.
- **C.** Rarely any systemic symptoms or adenopathy.

V. Assessment

- **A.** Diagnosis is made by the characteristic appearance of the lesion, its recurrent nature, and the absence of systemic symptoms.
- **B.** Differential diagnosis
  1. Herpes simplex: lesions are on the skin, most commonly at the mucocutaneous junction.
  2. Herpangina: elevated temperature, sore throat, vesicular eruptions on an erythematous base on the anterior pillars. No lesions found on gingival or buccal mucosa.

VI. Plan

- **A.** Kenalog in Orabase applied to lesion 3 times daily.
- **B.** Topical anesthetics for pain.
  1. Dyclone, 0.5% topical solution: apply directly to lesion every 1–2 hours.
     or
  2. Chloraseptic Mouthwash every 2 hours (for children over 6 years of age).

3. Xylocaine Viscous Solution: Over 12 years of age: 1 tbsp (15 ml or 300 mg) swished around mouth every 4 hours (dosage is 4.5 mg/kg). For children 5–12: 3/4–1 tsp every 4 hours.

C. Tetracycline mouthrinse (250 mg/5 ml)—four times a day for children over 8 years of age.

or

D. Tetracycline compresses 4–6 times a day for 5–7 days for children over 8 years of age.

E. Oral hygiene: rinse mouth gently with warm water.

VII. Education

A. With recurrent lesions, use Kenalog in Orabase as soon as tingling or burning is felt. This may be useful in aborting aphthae or shortening duration of ulcers.

B. Topical anesthetics.
   1. Dry lesion before using topical anesthetic.
   2. Apply to lesion only; do not use on surrounding skin.
   3. Topical anesthetics provide pain relief for about 1 hour; do not overuse. Do not eat within 1 hour after using.
   4. Do not use more than 120 ml (approximately 8 tbsp of Xylocaine Viscous) in 24 hours for children over 12. Maximum 40 ml for children ages 5–12.

C. Tetracycline compresses abort lesions, shorten healing, and prevent secondary infection.
   1. Dissolve 250 mg tetracycline in 30 ml water. Apply for 20–30 minutes.
   2. Do not eat or drink for 1/2 hour following treatment.

D. Identify triggering factor if possible; avoid specific foods or drugs felt to be precipitating factors.

E. Use soft toothbrush if trauma seems to precipitate lesions.

F. Encourage liquids.

G. A bland diet is helpful; avoid salty or acidic foods.

H. Recurrences are common.

I. Lesions heal in 1–2 weeks.

J. Lesions are not the same as cold sores.

VIII. Follow-up

A. Telephone follow-up in 24 hours if child is not taking liquids well.

B. Routine follow-up visit is not indicated.

IX. Complications

Dehydration in a small child with several lesions (see Appendix D, Clinical Signs of Dehydration).

X. Consultation/referral

A. Infants.

B. Any signs or symptoms of dehydration.

C. Child with very large or many lesions.

NOTES

ASTHMA

A disease of the lungs characterized by partially reversible airway obstruction, airway inflammation, and airway hyperresponsiveness. The usual manifestations are wheezing, cough, and dyspnea although any of the three can be the sole presenting complaint. It is the most common chronic disease and the most serious atopic disease in children.

I. Etiology

Hyperreactivity of the tracheobronchial tree to chemical mediators.

A. Allergens
   1. Environmental inhalants such as dust molds, animal dander, pollens.
   2. Food allergens such as nuts, fish, cow's milk, egg whites, and chocolate provoke asthma in about 10% of children.
   3. Anaphylactic reaction.

B. Infection. Upper and lower viral respiratory tract infections. Viral infections are more common ln younger children, particularly those in day care who may easily have more than 12 infections a year. In the younger age group, viral infections are the primary cause of asthmatic attacks.

C. Exertion. Exercise induced asthma.

D. Rapid temperature changes. Cold air, humidity.

E. Air pollutants. Smog, smoke, paint fumes, aerosols.

F. Emotional upsets. Fear, anxiety, anger.

G. Gastroesophageal reflux.

II. Incidence

Prevalence of asthma has been increasing. An estimated 5.2% of children under 18 years of age are affected. Prior to puberty, twice as many males are affected as females. At puberty, the incidence becomes about equal.

III. Subjective data

A. Onset may be abrupt or insidious.

B. Generally preceded by several days of nasal symptoms (sneezing, rhinorrhea).

C. Allergic salute—rubbing the tip of the nose upward with the palm of the hand.

D. Dry, hacking cough.

E. Tightness of chest.

F. Wheezing.

G. Dyspnea.

H. Anxiety, restlessness.

I. Rapid heart rate.

J. Pertinent subjective data to obtain
   1. History of upper respiratory tract infections, particularly in infants.
   2. History of allergic rhinitis or atopic dermatitis.
   3. Family history of atopic disease (e.g., allergic rhinitis, bronchial asthma).
   4. History of incitant factors that may have initiated current attack.
   5. Review of environment (e.g., pets, heating system).
   6. History of bronchospasm occurring after vigorous exerclse .
   7. History of recurrent pneumonia or bronchitis.

K. Clues to diagnosis in nonacute phase.
   1. Symptoms.
      a. Cough. Exercise-induced asthma may be manifested as a cough with no wheezing.
      b. Wheezing—episodic. Acute wheezing may indicate aspiration of a foreign body.
      c. Shortness of breath.
      d. Tightness of chest.
      e. Excessive mucous production.
   2. Pattern of seemingly isolated symptoms.
      a. Episodic or continuous.
      b. Seasonal.
      c. Frequency.
      d. Timing—i.e., after exercise, consider exercise-induced asthma; during night, consider gastroesophageal reflux.
   3. Factors precipitating symptoms.
      a. Exposure to common triggers—allergens, viral infections, exertion, pollutants, emotional upheavals.

L. History negative for symptoms that would indicate other chronic diseases (e.g., cystic fibrosis, cardiac disease).
   1. Wheezing associated with feeding.
   2. Failure to thrive.
   3. Sudden onset of cough or choking.
   4. Digital clubbing.

IV. Objective data

A. Rales; sibilant or sonorous throughout lung fields.

B. High pitched rhonchi.

C. Prolonged expiratory phase; exhales with difficulty.

D. Bilateral expiratory wheezes. Sometimes expiratory wheezes as well which reflects exacerbation of the process. Patient with severe respiratory distress may not have enough air exchange to generate wheezing.

E. In infants, inspiratory and expiratory wheezes with tracheal rales.

F. Hyperresonance to percussion.

G. Tachypnea.

H. Child sits upright with shoulders forward to use accessory muscles of respiration.

I. Fever, if concurrent infection.

J. History of atopic disease.

K. In infants, intercostal and suprasternal retractions.

L. Flaring of alae nasi.

M. Altered mental status; indicative of impairment of gas exchange.

N. Exam may be negative in a child with mild or moderate asthma who presents between episodes except for signs of allergic rhinitis(see p. 194).

O. Exam negative for clinical features suggestive of other diseases: failure to thrive, digital clubbing, cardiac murmur, unilateral signs.

P. Laboratory findings/diagnostic procedures

1. In acute attacks, laboratory studies are not generally indicated; diagnosis is generally clinical, depending on history and physical examination.
2. X-ray studies are not generally indicated except to rule out a foreign body or infectious process.
3. For recurrent episodes or mild asthma, skin testing and cytology provide the most valuable data.
4. Pulmonary function tests
   a. Spirometry. A 10% improvement in the forced expiratory volume in one second or a 25% increase in the mean forced expiratory flow at 25–75% of the vital capacity after inhaling a bronchodilator indicates reversible airway obstruction is present. (Simple spirometry can be done in the primary care physicians office.)
   b. Bronchial challenge tests. Refer to pulmonologist for testing and evaluation.
5. CBC is generally not indicated for diagnosis but, if done, eosinophilia would be indicative of allergies. Blood gasses should be done with a severe episode.

V. Assessment

A. Acute asthmatic attack—diagnosis in an acute asthmatic attack is clinical, dependant on history and physical examination.

B. Asthma

1. The diagnosis is generally made by history of symptoms and pattern of occurrence, physical exam, and, if indicated, PFTs.
2. The severity can then be classified clinically or with PFTs. Clinical classifications:
   a. Mild asthma Less than two attacks a week. Few symptoms between attacks. No significant lifestyle disruptions. Peak expiratory flow rate (PEFR) greater than 80% of normal.
   b. Moderate asthma More than two attacks a week. Symptoms between attacks. May have nocturnal symptoms 2–3 times a week. Disruption of lifestyle. Exercise tolerance decreased. PEFR 60–80% of normal.
   c. Severe asthma
      (1) Daily wheezing with frequent, often severe exacerbations.
      (2) Low-grade coughing and wheezing almost constantly.
      (3) Poor exercise tolerance.
      (4) Nocturnal symptoms almost nightly.
      (5) School/work attendance affected.
      (6) PEFR less than 60% of normal.

C. Differential diagnosis

1. Infectious bronchitis. Characterized by elevated temperature, poor response to epinephrine, negative family and/or patient history of atopy.
2. Foreign body in bronchus. Especially common in young children with negative history of atopy and unilateral wheezing. Confirm with bronchoscopy if history, physical examination, and x-ray studies are not conclusive.
3. Bronchiolitis. Most common in infants under 6 months, although it can occur in children up to 2 years of age. Temperature is variable; infant pre-

sents with paroxysmal cough, dyspnea, tachypnea, shallow respirations, marked hyperresonance, and markedly diminished breath sounds. A challenge with epinephrine usually does not cause improvement. Strongly suspect asthma if child has a second episode of bronchiolitis.

4. Pertussis. Rule out by history of exposure.
5. Cystic fibrosis. Rule out by previous history and, if indicated by history and physical examination, a sweat test.
6. Laryngotracheobronchitis. Usually seen in children under 3 years; characterized by insidious onset, with history of upper respiratory tract infection; harsh, barking cough with severe inspiratory stridor; slightly elevated temperature.
7. Bronchopneumonia. Characterized by dyspnea and tachypnea; rales may be present; expiratory wheezes are generally not present; in advanced, consolidative phase, decreased breath sounds.

VI. Plan

A. Acute severe attack

1. Immediate treatment
   a. Albuterol (nebulized) 5mg/ml

      Dosage—0.10–0.15 mg/kg (up to 5 mg)

      Frequency—every 20 minutes, up to 3 doses or

   b. Epinephrine hydrochloride 1:1000 sc

      Dosage—0.01 m/kg (up to 0.3 mg)

      Frequency—every 15–20 minutes, up to 3 doses

      Auscultate chest and heart after each dose. Do not repeat if pulse is over 180/minute.

      Refer stat if no response to epinephrine for probable status asthmaticus.

   c. Oxygen as needed
   d. Prednisone—if incomplete or poor response to bronchodilators. Dosage—1–2 mg/kg as a single dose continue with a tapering dose given once in the AM for 5–10 days or give 1–2 mg/kg/day in divided doses.

B. Long-term treatment. The goal of treatment is to control chronic symptoms, maintain normal activity levels, maintain normal or near-normal pulmonary function, and to prevent acute episodes. The frequency of exacerbations can be diminished by continuous therapy. Side effects of prescribed drugs diminish with long term administration.

1. Mild/episodic asthma
   a. Inhaled beta-agonist prn for wheezing
2. Moderate asthma
   a. Inhaled beta-agonist 3 to 4 times a day
   b. Inhaled cromolyn sodium—3 to 4 times a day *or*
   c. Inhaled corticosteroids—2 to 3 times a day If control not achieved, increase inhaled corticosteriod *or add:*
   d. Oral beta-agonist or
   e. Theophylline (particularly if nocturnal asthma)
3. Severe asthma
   a. Inhaled beta-agonist as needed
   b. Inhaled corticosteroid

c. Long acting bronchodilator (oral beta-agonist or theophylline)

d. Oral corticosteroid

4. Exercise-induced asthma

a. Inhaled beta-agonist—2 puffs prior to exercise. If control not achieved, *add:*

b. Inhaled cromolyn sodium—2 inhalations 5 to 10 minutes after albuterol inhalation prior to exercise or exposure to allergen.

5. Peak flow monitoring program with moderate or severe asthma.

6. Environmental control.

VII. Medications

A. Beta Agonists—Albuterol (Ventolin, Proventil), metaproterenol (Alupent)

1. Metered-dose inhaler—2 inhalations every 4–6 hours (1 inhalation every 4–6 hours under age 12)

2. Powder inhaler—1 capsule every 4–6 hours

3. Nebulizer solution

a. Albuterol—0.10–0.15 mg/kg every 4–6 hours, up to 5 mg.

b. Metaproterenol—0.3–0.5 mg/kg every 4–6 hours up to 15 mg.

4. Oral

a. Albuterol

Liquid—0.1 mg/kg every 4–6 hours for children ages 2–6 years of age. Maximum dose is 2 mg (one tsp.) 3 times a day.

Tablets—2 or 4 mg every 4–6 hours or sustained release, 4 mg every 12 hours

b. Metaproterenol

Liquid—0.3–0.5 mg/kg every 4–6 hours

Tablets—10 or 20 mg every 4–6 hours

B. Cromolyn Sodium (Intal)

1. Metered-dose inhaler—2 inhalations, 2–3 times a day

2. Powder inhaler—1 capsule, 2–3 times a day

3. Nebulizer solution—1 ampule, 2–3 times a day.

C. Theophylline—dosage is based on serum level and should achieve a serum concentration of 5–15 μg/ml

Begin with low dose and increase at 3 to 4 day intervals, depending on clinical response and serum concentration.

Children's dosage should not exceed 400–800 mg a day.

1. Liquids, extended release capsules, or tablets

a. 1–9 years: 16–22 mg/kg/day

b. 9–12 years: 16–20 mg/kg/day

c. 12–16 years: 16–18 mg/kg/day

D. Corticosteroids

1. Metered-dose inhaler (Beclovent, Vanceril)

a. 2 inhalations 4 times a day *or*

b. 4 inhalations every 12 hours

2. Oral—liquid (Pediapred) or tablets (Prednisone)—1–2 mg/kg/day

a. 1 year: 10 mg bid for 5–7 days

b. 1–3 years: 20 mg bid for 5–7 days
c. 3–13 years: 30 mg bid for 5–7 days
d. over 13 years: 40 mg bid for 5–7 days
e. chronic: 20–40 mg 1–3 times a day. When controlled for one month, taper by 5–10 mg every 2 weeks to lowest dose that keeps child symptom free.

E. Epinephrine hydrochloride 1:1000
1. 0.01 mg/kg
a. 10 kg: 0.1 ml
b. 15 kg: 0.15 ml
c. 20 kg: 0.20 ml
d. 25 kg: 0.25 ml
e. 30 kg: 0.30 ml maximum dose

VIII. Education

A. Do not give antihistamines during an acute attack; they dry respiratory secretions and may produce mucous plugs.
B. Try to keep child calm during acute attack; anxiety can increase bronchospasm.
C. Postural drainage: lie on bed with head hanging over the side.
D. Side effects of medications:
1. Epinephrine: tremor, tachycardia, anxiety, sweating.
2. Theophylline: gastric irritation, nausea, vomiting, diarrhea, headache. palpitations, restlessness, insomnia.
3. Albuterol: palpitations, tachycardia, tremor, nausea, dizziness, headache, insomnia, drying or irritation of oropharynx.
4. Intal: cough, wheezing, nasal congestion, dizziness, headache, nausea, rash, urticaria.

E. Theophylline:
1. Metabolism varies in individuals.
2. Metabolism may be decreased by drugs such as tagamet, Cipro, corticosteroids, causing an increase in serum concentrations.
3. Smoking may increase theophylline metabolism and decrease its effectiveness.

F. Cromolyn sodium:
1. Prevents and reduces inflammation.
2. Prevents allergen or exercise-induced bronchoconstriction.
3. Action is comparable to theophylline or inhaled corticosteroids.
4. Has no bronchodilating activity and is useful only for prophylaxis. It does not work for acute attacks.

G. Albuterol:
1. Produces bronchodilation with less cardiac stimulation than older sympathomimetics.
2. Provides the most rapid relief of acute asthmatic symptoms with fewest adverse side effects.
3. Improvement should be noted within 15 minutes of use.
4. Do not exceed recommended dosage; action may last up to 6 hours.

H. Tablets are less expensive than liquids or chewables.

I. Metered dose inhalers:
   1. Shake inhaler.
   2. Breathe out, expelling as much air from lungs as possible.
   3. Place mouthpiece in mouth, holding inhaler upright.
   4. While breathing deeply, depress top of metal canister, then remove from mouth.
   5. Hold breath as long as possible.
   6. If 2 inhalations are prescribed, wait 5 minutes and repeat steps 1–5
   7. Clean plastic case and cap in warm water after each use.

J. Aerosol-holding chambers—Aero chamber:
   1. Consider using inspirease or aerochamber with metered dose inhaler.
   2. Improves delivery for children who cannot inhale all of medication in one breath.
   3. Provides more efficient delivery to the lungs.
   4. Eliminates the need to synchronize the actuation and inhalation.

K. Peak flow meter (see tables in appendix):
   1. Used to detect airflow obstruction before child is symptomatic.
   2. Peak flow will have decreased by 25% or more before wheezing can be detected by auscultation.
   3. PEFR should be measured each morning prior to taking medication.
   4. Monitoring before and after medication in the morning and at bedtime yields the best information.
   5. Healthy children generally will have a PEFR 90% or above predicted value.
   6. Measurements below 80% of predicted value suggest obstruction that requires treatment.
   7. Measurements 50% or lower herald a severe attack.

L. Avoid offending allergens.

M. Environmental control. See protocol, p. 259.

N. Encourage child to participate in all activities that he is capable of.

O. There is no "cure" for asthma, but child should be symptom free with proper medication.

P. Without adequate treatment to control asthma, life-threatening pulmonary complications may develop.

Q. Parents and/or health care provider should maintain working relationship with the school.
   1. Ensure that school nurse has information on all of child's medications, including side effects. Request that she share this information with teachers.
   2. Identify allergen and irritant exposures in the classroom—e.g., animals, carpeting, chalk dust, plants.
   3. Periodic hearing impairment is common in allergic child. Suggest periodic audiometric evaluations and preferential seating if indicated.

IX. Follow-up

A. Call immediately if:
   1. Breathing difficulty worsens.
   2. Skin or lips turn blue.

3. Restlessness or sleeplessness occurs.
4. Cough or wheezing persists, or chest pain or fever develops.
5. There are side effects from medication (e.g., nausea, vomiting, irritability, palpitations.)

B. Measure theophylline level 2–3 days after initiating oral therapy and every 2–3 months while on medication.

C. Return visit is indicated for medication adjustment if asthma is not well controlled.

D. Routine follow-up every 6 months.

E. When asthma is stable or under control, measure PEFR in office.

X. Complications

A. Pulmonary infections (especially in children under 5 years).

B. Status asthmaticus.

C. Atelectasis.

D. Emphysema (after recurrent attacks).

E. Death (uncommon).

XI. Consultation/referral

A. Initial episode.

B. Acute attack not responsive to treatment.

C. Side effects from medication.

D. Persistent wheezing.

E. Secondary infection (bacterial, viral, or fungal).

F. For respiratory therapy.

G. For allergy testing if indicated.

NOTES

BULIMIA

An eating disorder that consists of recurrent episodes of binge eating and subsequent purging. Most patients are within a normal weight range but can have frequent fluctuations of weight of 10 lb or more due to alternating binges and fasts.

I. Etiology

Psychological and organic theories have both been proposed, but etiology is unknown.

II. Incidence

Occurs primarily in late adolescence or early adulthood and is seen primarily in females (90–95% of cases). An estimated 19% of college females and 5% of college males use purging as a method of weight control. However, not all cases of self-reported over-eating and occasional purging are true bulimia. A significant number of cases may be overdiagnosed on the basis of the simple criteria of binge eating and subsequent purging. According to Schotte and Stunkard, the prevalence of bulimia in a sampling of 994 university women was no greater than 1.3%.

III. Indications of bulimic behavior

A. Recurrent episodes of rapid consumption of high-calorie foods.

B. Binge eating done secretly, usually terminated by external factors (e.g., abdominal pain, sleep, visitor).

C. Abdominal pain following binge eating.

D. Purging by vomiting following binge eating; alternating binge eating and fasting.

E. Reasonably normal weight range with periodic fluctuations of about 10 lb.

F. Preoccupation with weight.

G. Attempts at weight loss through rigid dieting, vomiting, laxative and/or diuretic use, episodes of fasting.

H. Fear of losing control and not being able to stop eating.

I. Depression following binge eating.

J. Awareness of abnormal eating pattern.

K. Poor impulse control, also exhibited in other behavioral aberrations.

L. Excessive exercising.

M. Erosion of tooth enamel.

N. Amenorrhea may occur.

O. Electrolyte imbalance.

III. Subjective data

A. Sores in mouth.

B. Dental caries.

C. “Heartburn.”

D. Chest pains.

E. Bloody diarrhea (with laxative abuse).

F. Bruising.

G. Muscle cramps.

H. Fainting.

I. Menstrual irregularities.

IV. Objective data

A. Weight—normal or overweight.

B. Parotid gland hypertrophy.

C. Dental caries and enamel erosion (from contact with stomach acid).

D. Pyorrhea.

E. Callouses and abrasions on dorsum of hands (from contact with teeth from self-induced vomiting).

F. Abdominal distention.

G. Muscular weakness.

H. History positive for indications of bulimia. See Appendix K, (*Are You Dying to Be Thin?)*

VI. Assessment

A diagnosis of bulimia may be made if three of the following are present (according to Vaughan, et al.):

A. Consumption of high-calorie, easily digested food during a binge.

B. Inconspicuous eating during a binge.

C. Termination of eating episodes by abdominal pain, sleep, social interruption, or self-induced vomiting.

D. Repeated attempts to lose weight through severely restrictive diets, self-induced vomiting, or use of amphetamines, cathartics, or diuretics.

E. Frequent weight fluctuations of greater than 10 lb due to binges and fasts.

VII. Plan

A. Psychotherapy

1. To resolve underlying psychological issues.
2. To restore normal nutrition.
3. To increase self-esteem.
4. To help development of self-control.

B. Family therapy

C. Behavior modification

D. Drug therapy

1. Antidepressants.
    a. Phenelzine.
    b. Imipramine.
2. Anticonvulsants (phenytoin). Research has shown that binge eaters often have an EEG abnormality; anticonvulsants can sometimes control binge eating.

E. For the occasional "binger and purger" whose physical examination and laboratory tests (CBC, electrolytes, urinalysis) are within normal limits, office management can be attempted for a short time. The duration of office treatment must be individualized for each patient.

1. Counseling should concentrate on following issues:
    a. Body image.
    b. Normal weight for height.
    c. Nutrition.
    d. Dental.
    e. Excessive exercising.

f. Self-control.

g. Self-esteem.

2. Have child keep careful record of intake and of any episodes of binging and purging.

3. Recheck weekly.

a. Obtain weight.

b. Review dietary history.

c. Counseling.

4. Refer if episodes continue or if depression or despair is present.

VIII. Follow-up

Contact after referral for support and encouragement.

IX. Complications

A. Esophagitis.

B. Esophageal tears.

C. Gastric dilatation.

D. Hypokalemia.

E. Depression.

X. Resources

A. National Association of Anorexia Nervosa and Associated Disorders, Box 271, Highland Park, IL 60035.

B. Anorexia Bulimia Care Inc., Box 213, Lincoln Center, MA 01773. (617) 259-9769

VIII. List local referral sources

NOTES

CANDIDIASIS—DIAPER RASH

Diaper dermatitis characterized by inflammation with a well-defined, scaling border.

I. Etiology

Candida albicans is the usual causative agent.

II. Incidence

The most common form of cutaneous candidiasis is in the diaper area of infants. It is most prevalent in infants under 6 months of age.

III. Incubation period

Unknown.

IV. Subjective data

A. Bright red rash in diaper area.

B. Satellite lesions—outside border of rash.

C. Baby does not appear uncomfortable.

D. History of vaginal infection in mother.

V. Objective data

A. Diaper area

1. Beefy, red, shiny.
2. Sharply demarcated borders.
3. Satellite lesions—erythematous papules and/or pustules.

B. Inspect entire body; candidiasis may be found in intertriginous areas (e.g., neck, axilla, umbilicus).

C. Inspect mouth for oral candidiasis (thrush).

VI. Assessment

A. Diagnosis is made by a detailed history and/or the clinical picture.

B. Potassium hydroxide (KOH) fungal preparation reveals yeast cells and pseudohyphae.

C. Differential diagnosis.

1. Ammoniacal diaper rash.
2. Chronic mucocutaneous candidiasis reflecting an underlying immunodeficiency.

VII. Plan

A. Lotrimin (Clotrimazole) cream. Apply small amount twice daily.
or

B. Miconazole (Monistat Derm). Apply small amount bid.

C. Nystatin (Mycostatin) cream. Apply liberally twice daily.

D. Nystatin powder three times daily for use for concurrent candidiasis in moist intertriginous areas.

VIII. Education

A. Change diapers frequently.

B. Cleanse diaper area with tepid water at each diaper change.

C. Keep baby clean and dry, with special attention to warm, moist areas.

D. Careful hand-washing technique; candidiasis is transmitted by direct contact with secretions and excretions.

E. Check entire body for appearance of rash in intertriginous areas.

F. Medication.

1. Use medication sparingly.
2. Be alert for drug sensitivity—itching, irritation, maceration, secondary infection.
3. Do not use medication for other rashes.
4. Continue medication for at least 2 full days following disappearance of rash.

G. Do without diapers as often as possible; *C. albicans* thrives in warm, moist areas.

H. Do not use plastic pants.

I. Do not use cornstarch; it may be metabolized by microorganisms.

J. If mother is suspect for vaginal candidiasis, refer for diagnosis.

IX. Follow-up

A. Check mouth frequently; call immediately if white spots are present.

B. Call back in 3 days if no improvement.

C. Telephone call to report progress in 6–7 days.

X. Complications

Overuse of topical corticosteroids may result in striae or telangiectasia.

XI. Consultation/referral

A. Frequent recurrences: may require oral nystatin therapy to eliminate *C. albicans* in the intestine. May also reflect an underlying immunodeficiency.

B. Failure to respond to treatment after 1 week.

NOTES:

ACUTE CERVICAL ADENITIS

Inflammation of one or more cervical nodes. In children it is most commonly reactive hyperplasia in response to an infection of the ear, nose, mouth, or throat. Pharyngitis or tonsillitis is the most common primary infection. Cervical adenitis is characterized by a 3 cm (or more) enlargement with tenderness and erythema of involved node(s).

I. Etiology

- **A.** Group A beta-hemolytic streptococci: 75–80% of cases.
- **B.** Staphylococci: approximately 10% of cases.
- **C.** Viruses: rubella, measles, herpes simplex, and adenoviruses account for remainder of cases.

II. Incidence

Seen most frequently in preschool children. 70–80% of cases are seen in children 1 to 4 years of age.

III. Subjective data

- **A.** Painful swelling of the neck—may be of acute onset.
- **B.** Fever: variable; may be high.
- **C.** Complaint of malaise, anorexia, or vomiting common.
- **D.** Pertinent subjective data to obtain
  1. History of upper respiratory infection, sore throat.
  2. History of toothache, impetigo of face, or severe acne.
  3. History of exposure to streptococcal pharyngitis.
  4. History of exposure to animals or history of cat scratch.
  5. History of exposure to tuberculosis.
  6. Duration of swelling, temperature, and concurrent or preceding illness.

IV. Objective data

- **A.** Fever.
- **B.** Cervical nodes—generally unilateral.
  1. Enlarged—measure size of node. Usually 2.5 to 6 cm.
  2. Tender.
  3. Erythematous if infection is present for several days without treatment.
  4. Firm, but may become fluctuant.
- **C.** Examine the following:
  1. Ears for infection of canal or tympanic membrane.
  2. Nose for rhinitis, infection.
  3. Throat for erythema, exudate, petechiae.
  4. Face and scalp for impetigo or infected acne.
  5. Teeth: examine and percuss each tooth for evidence of infection.
  6. For lymphadenopathy in other areas.
- **D.** Laboratory tests
  1. Elevated white count—20,000/mm^3.
  2. Throat culture for streptococcal infection.

3. Heterophil antibody or Monospot test indicated with posterior cervical adenitis or generalized adenopathy.

V. Assessment

A. Consider streptococcal infection with history of acute onset, pain, elevated temperature, history of pharyngitis, petechiae of soft palate, and vomiting.

B. Consider staphylococcal or viral infection with a sustained high fever and no response to penicillin therapy.

C. Diagnosis is made by the history, clinical findings, and appropriate laboratory tests.

D. Differential diagnosis

1. Infectious mononucleosis: posterior cervical and generalized adenopathy; heterophil or Monospot positive.
2. Chronic adenitis: by history and presence of smaller, less tender node.
3. Cat-scratch fever: by history and evidence of trauma.
4. Tuberculosis: by tine or PPD test.
5. Leukemia: firm, nontender, more generalized involvement of glands characteristically in posterior triangle or supraclavicular areas; hepatosplenomegaly; peripheral blood changes.
6. Mumps: location of swelling (crosses the angle of the jaw) and no clear, palpable border; inflammation of Stensen's duct; leukopenia.

VI. Plan

A. Throat culture.

B. Tuberculin test.

C. Antibiotic therapy. Empirical therapy directed against staph aureus and group A strep.

1. Dicloxacillin: 25 mg/kg/day in 4 divided doses.
   or
2. Cloxacillin: 50 mg/kg/day in 4 divided doses.
   or
3. Keflex: 50 mg/kg/day in 2 divided doses.
   or
4. Erythromycin: 30–50mg/kg/day in 2 or 4 divided doses.

D. Antipyretics/analgesics

1. Tylenol (see Drug Index).
2. Motrin (see Drug Index).

E. Local measures: warm compresses to enlarged node for 10 minutes 5–6 times a day for symptomatic relief.

VII. Education

A. Call back immediately:

1. If child
   a. Seems worse.
   b. Has difficulty swallowing.
   c. Has difficulty breathing.
2. If node
   a. Enlarges.
   b. Becomes inflamed.

c. Drains.

d. Becomes fluctuant ("pointing" or looking like a pimple).

B. Encourage liquids; do not worry about solid food if child is anorexic.

C. Compresses: use wet facecloth or other soft cloth with water that feels comfortably warm to wrist; reapply as soon as it cools. Will require the full attention of parent for a full 10-minute period.

D. Give medication for 10 full days.

E. Tylenol or ibuprofen is of value only for the relief of discomfort or temperature control. Use only for these indications.

F. Node may not completely resolve for several weeks.

VIII. Follow-up

A. Telephone contact within 24 hours.

B. Return to office if no improvement within 48 hours.

C. Return immediately if node enlarges or if child seems toxic, dysphagic, or dyspneic.

IX. Complications

A. Suppuration of node.

B. Rarely, poststreptococcal acute glomerulonephritis or rheumatic fever.

X. Consultation/referral

A. Child under 2 years of age.

B. No improvement after 48 hours, or worsening of symptoms at any time.

C. Fluctuant node—may require incision and drainage.

D. Refer to dentist if dental abscess suspected.

E. Child is toxic, dehydrated, dysphagic, or dyspneic.

NOTES

CHILD ABUSE*

By definition child abuse is divided into four groups: physical abuse, emotional or physical neglect, emotional abuse, and sexual abuse.

Physical abuse may be present in a child with evidence of bodily bruises, lacerations, head trauma, human bites, burns, hematomas, fractures or dislocations, or bodily injury to the abdomen (evidenced by a ruptured liver or spleen or fractured ribs), all visible on physical exam.

Emotional and *physical neglect* are more difficult to identify, more subtle in their presentation, and more likely to have been going on for sometime. Such neglect implies the caretaker is unable to care for the child or protect the child from danger. Examples are the child who is emotionally distraught or the failure-to-thrive child, who is often suffering from an inadequate diet, shows signs of poor growth, is depressed and developmentally delayed, and who occasionally but not always is dirty and unkempt.

Emotional abuse is exemplified by the child who seems unable to relate to others and is apathetic, lacking any emotion because he is constantly berated, beaten, rejected, or ignored. Infants as well as older children can be emotionally abused.

Sexual abuse, the sexual exploitation of infants or children by an adult, may include exhibitionism, fondling or digital manipulation, masturbation, or vaginal or anal intercourse. The sexual abuser may be a stranger but more often is someone known to the family or even a member of the family. Father-daughter incest accounts for 75% of all cases of incest.

Child abuse is most often identified in the pediatric office; the nurse practitioner or pediatrician must be able to recognize the signs and symptoms of such abuse.

I. Physical abuse

A. Physical signs

1. Bruises. Explained or, often, unexplained welts or abrasions on the face, body, back, thighs. May also be several surface areas in different stages of healing, often recurring and suggesting the shape of the article used to inflict them (e.g., belt, whip).
2. Evidence of human bites.
3. Ocular insult.
4. Fractures or dislocations in various stages of healing.
5. Unexplained rupture of spleen, liver, or pancreas.
6. Neurological findings.
7. Signs of poisoning.
8. Unexplained burns. May appear on soles, palms, back, buttocks, or genitalia, often in pattern of cigarette, cigar, electric burner, or iron; rope burns around neck, body, or extremities.

B. Behavioral signs

1. Excessively aggressive or withdrawn.
2. Suspicious of adults.
3. Speaks in dull voice.

---

*This section was written by Rose Boynton.

4. Often feels he deserves the battering.
5. Lies very quietly during examination with vacant stare.
6. May not report injury inflicted by parent.
7. Seeks affection inappropriately.
8. Has poor self-esteem.

II. Physical neglect

A. Physical signs
   1. Failure to thrive (i.e., poor growth pattern, developmental delay, malnourishment).
   2. Inappropriate dress.
   3. Poor hygiene.
   4. Lack of supervision in dangerous activities, or abandonment.
   5. Absence of medical care; unattended physical problems.

B. Behavioral signs
   1. Excessive crying.
   2. In infants, ruminating behavior.
   3. Begging food.
   4. Poor school attendance, delinquency, falling asleep in school, stealing.
   5. Alcohol or drug abuse.
   6. States that "no one cares."

III. Emotional neglect

A. Physical signs
   1. Failure to thrive.
   2. Hyperactivity.
   3. Speech disorder.

B. Behavioral signs
   1. Developmental delays.
   2. Habitual sucking, rocking, ruminating, head banging, or destructive or antisocial behavior.
   3. Sleep disorders, repeated nightmares, constant waking to see whether parent is there.
   4. Phobias.
   5. Difficulty in learning, poor school performance.
   6. Inability to play for any length of time.
   7. Inappropriate adult behavior; not childlike.
   8. Wounding of self or attempted suicide.

IV. Sexual abuse

A. Physical signs
   1. Genital, urethral, vaginal, or anal bruising or bleeding.
   2. Swollen, red vulva or perineum.
   3. Positive cultures for sexually transmitted disease (e.g., gonococcus, venereal warts).
   4. Recurrent urinary tract infections.
   5. Recurrent streptococcus pharyngitis.

6. Recurrent abdominal pain.
7. Enuresis.
8. Encopresis.
9. Pregnancy.
10. Presence of foreign body in genital area.

B. Behavioral signs
1. Child knows and uses sexual terms.
2. Excessive sexual play.
3. Sleep disturbances (e.g., nightmares).
4. Appetite disturbances.
5. Avoidance behavior or excessive aggressive behavior.
6. Temper tantrums.
7. Poor school attendance, performance.
8. Excessive masturbation.
9. Running away.
10. Suicide attempts.

V. Role of medical provider

A. Identify and make diagnosis of child abuse.

B. Openly and candidly discuss abuse with parent.

C. Treat for medical injuries or neglect.

D. Report to Department of Welfare or Child Protection Unit, again notifying parent.
1. To protect child.
2. Initiate steps to ensure that the abuse will not recur.
3. Failure to report child abuse is a class A misdemeanor.

E. Request referral or consultation to medical or surgical staff, social worker, or other specialists as appropriate.

VI. Predisposing factors

Most abusive parents were themselves abused children and show little ability to cope with adult life. Many abusive caretakers are impulsive, immature persons who are unable to solve their own problems. They have trouble establishing meaningful relationships; they feel alone, stressed, and overwhelmed; and they are mistrustful of others and therefore unwilling to ask for help in caring for their children. Although they resent their own upbringing, they look for approval from other adults by repeating the abusive pattern.

Other factors that predispose a caretaker to perpetrate child abuse are mental illness, the inability to control temper, unrealistic expectations of a child at a specific age and, particularly, the inability to handle parental stress or stress caused by poverty, lack of a job, etc., and chronic illness of the child. The caretaker may not have bonded with the child at birth, and therefore feels insecure about his or her parenting abilities. Abuse may be seen in all social and economic backgrounds. In many cases, one parent is the active abuser while the other parent remains passive, thus allowing the behavior to continue.

VII. Management

A. A complete medical history must be outlined in the chart. Review the former medical record, especially outlining dates and occurrences of unexplained trauma, burns, or broken bones.

B. A thorough physical examination must be performed and appropriate laboratory work and x-ray studies requested.

C. Any positive physical findings should be photographed and a collaborating physician called in to verify the findings.

D. A social worker provides the necessary psychological workup, helping with the plan of care and contacting local agencies.

E. *Always* notify the parents and explain to them that you are reporting the diagnosis.

F. The severity of the child abuse determines the need for follow-up care. The primary concern in working with families involved in child abuse is protection of the child. The health care team determines the need for hospital care or the need to separate the child from the family.

G. After making the diagnosis and plan of care, report the findings to the appropriate agencies within 24–48 hours.

NOTES

COLIC

Characterized by periods of unexplained irritability and intense crying in healthy infants, apparently associated with abdominal pain.

I. Etiology

The cause is unknown but probably multifactorial. Precipitating factors include overfeeding, underfeeding, formula intolerance, failure to "burp," tension, or emotional problems in the family.

II. Incidence

Occurs during the first 1–2 weeks of life, most often in a first-born infant. Generally subsides by 3 months of age, but may continue for 5–6 months. Occurs with equal frequency in males and females in 10 to 20% of infants.

III. Subjective data

- **A.** Episodic, intense, persistent crying for periods up to 4–6 hours. Most often occurs in the late afternoon and evening.
- **B.** Legs drawn up to abdomen.
- **C.** Hands tightly clenched.
- **D.** Feet may be cold.
- **E.** Child passes flatus.
- **F.** Pertinent subjective data to obtain.
  1. Detailed dietary history—include amount and type of feeding.
  2. Detailed history of feeding techniques.
  3. If mother nursing, detailed history of her dietary intake.
  4. Detailed history of elimination pattern and any changes in elimination.
  5. Determine how long this has been going on.
  6. Determine duration and pattern of crying spells—how often do they occur? do they occur at a particular time of day?
  7. What have parents done to alleviate symptoms, and does anything seem to help?
  8. How are parents coping?
  9. What do parents think is wrong with the infant?
  10. Circumstances prevailing at time of conception.
  11. History of pregnancy, labor, and delivery.
  12. Family interaction: Is father supportive? is mother depressed? are parents having marital difficulties?
  13. In addition to being of diagnostic benefit, the history helps the parents unburden and feel supported.

IV. Objective data

- **A.** Temperature, weight, height, head circumference, chest circumference.
- **B.** Complete physical examination; include neurologic (may be marked response to Moro reflex). Abdomen may be distended and tense.
- **C.** Examine for testicular torsion; anal fissure; intestinal obstruction; incarcerated hernia; open safety pin; hair or thread wrapped around finger, penis, or toe.
- **D.** Observe

1. Maternal/child interaction.
2. Infant's reaction to stimuli (may be marked).
3. Infant's reaction to cuddling.

V. Assessment

A. Diagnosis is usually made by a history of repeated episodes, normal physical examination, and normal growth and development.

B. Differential diagnosis
   1. Anal fissure: bright blood in stool; fissure visualized in anus.
   2. Incarcerated hernia: sudden onset, swelling in groin, and ipsilateral scrotum.
   3. Testicular torsion: testis tense and tender; cord thickened and shortened.
   4. Poor feeding practices (over- or underfeeding): confirmed by history.
   5. Incorrect formula preparation: confirmed by history.
   6. Family tension: may be confirmed by interview.
   7. Poor coping ability: may be confirmed by interview.

VI. Plan

Management is varied and may not be successful but should include the following:

A. Immediate response to and understanding of parents' concern. Reassure parents that infant is not ill and that they are not responsible for the colic.

B. Formula
   1. Although there is no conclusive evidence that formula intolerance is a cause of colic, consider a formula change. (A slight difference in the fat source—polyunsaturated fats vs. saturated fats, or iron-fortified vs. plain—may help alleviate symptoms.)
   2. Soy formula may be given on trial basis if attacks are prolonged and there is a positive family history of allergies. May develop soy protein intolerance.
   3. Nutramigen: use if question of lactose and milk protein intolerance and infant does not improve with soy.
   4. Review amount and frequency of feedings and feeding techniques.

C. Breast-feeding
   1. Eliminate possible sources of distress from mother's diet—excess tea, coffee, cola, strong-flavored or highly spiced foods, chocolate, shellfish, excess milk.
   2. Review frequency of feedings and feeding techniques.
   3. Recommend supplementary feedings if weight gain is poor.

D. Abdominal warmth
   1. Place warm water bottle wrapped in a soft cloth on infant's abdomen.
   2. Put infant to sleep in prone position.

E. Rhythmic movement and singing. This helps eliminate tension in mother as well.
   1. Rocking chair.
   2. Carriage.

F. Feed 1–2 oz of warm water during attack.

G. Counsel parents regarding

1. Feelings of inadequacy and guilt.
2. Tension or stress in family or parent.
3. Feelings of inability to cope.
4. Changes in life-style with birth of infant.
5. Lack of rest and relaxation.

H. Environmental factors
1. Avoid overstimulation.
2. Prevent chilling.
3. Provide soft background noise (e.g., music).
4. Avoid sudden stimulation or startling of infant; approach infant slowly.

I. Pharmacologic management may be given a trial if other measures are not successful and mother is having a difficult time coping.
1. Mylicon drops: 0.3 ml four times a day.
2. Levsin drops at 4-hour intervals:

weight	dosage
2.3 kg (5 pounds)	3 drops
3.4 kg (7.5 pounds)	4 drops
5 kg (11 pounds)	5 drops
7 kg (15 pounds)	6 drops
10 kg (22 pounds)	8 drops

VII. Education

A. Explain the natural course of colic and that it generally subsides at 3 months of age; occasionally it lasts until 4 months, rarely until 5–6 months.

B. Explain that colic will not harm the baby physically or psychologically.

C. No specific treatment is guaranteed to produce an immediate "cure."

D. Feeding
1. Do not change formulas without consultation.
2. Do not discontinue breast-feeding; symptoms may become worse.
3. The addition of solid foods will not generally improve symptoms; it may exacerbate them.
4. Burp infant frequently during feeding.
5. Try to maintain a modified demand schedule for the benefit of both mother and infant. Stress consistency in routine and do not let infant sleep beyond usual feedings during the day.
6. Be very cautious about overfeeding. Attempts to comfort infant by too frequent feedings will cause overdistention of the bowel, resulting in more discomfort.
7. Nipple holes should allow a slow, steady stream.

E. Give medication only as directed. Call back immediately if vomiting occurs.

F. Mylicon drops relieve symptoms of excess gas in gastrointestinal tract by freeing it so that it can be eliminated more easily. Therefore, it may appear that the infant is "gassier."

G. Levsin is an antispasmodic that decreases abdominal discomfort. It may cause drowsiness.

H. Try a warm bath at the time baby is usually fussy rather than at "scheduled" bath time.

I. Encourage parents to go out on occasion. A reliable caretaker can cope with a crying baby for a few hours.

J. Encourage father to participate in care of infant and to relieve mother of some responsibilities.

K. The infant should not be left in his crib to "cry it out," he will become even more inconsolable.

L. Stress that it is not necessary to rush in and pick up the infant the moment he cries out, however. Give him an opportunity to go back to sleep. It may be helpful to soothe him by sitting by the crib and patting or rubbing his back. However, it will not spoil an infant to be given love and attention when he is distressed.

M. Reassure parents that a variety of emotions are within a normal range when they are unable to comfort an infant during repeated, prolonged crying episodes. Frustration, guilt, inadequacy, irritability, and even anger or hostility are emotions expressed by the most loving of parents.

VIII. Follow-up

A. Frequent follow-up is necessary to provide support and encouragement to the parents and to assess results. Formula changes, elimination diet in mother, and medication should be given an adequate trial and reassessed by telephone or return visit.

B. Daily telephone follow-up may be necessary for the first week if parents are tense and anxious; thereafter, weekly telephone follow-up is sufficient.

C. Return visit in 2 weeks; include detailed interval history, physical examination, assessment of growth and development.

D. If parents have adjusted well and infant is thriving, further return visits are at usual intervals. Weekly or biweekly telephone contact continues to be indicated.

IX. Complications

The most important complication is disruption of the mother/infant relationship.

X. Consultation/referral

A. Inadequate weight gain.

B. Maternal depression.

C. Abnormalities in physical examination.

D. Prolonged episodes; little response to treatment.

NOTES

NOTES

CONJUNCTIVITIS

Inflammation of the bulbar or palpebral conjunctiva or both.

I. Etiology

A. Viral. Predominantly adenoviruses.

B. Bacterial. *Staphylococcus aureus* is the most common bacterial cause. Other common pathogens are Koch-Weeks bacillus, *Streptococcus pneumoniae,* and *Hemophilus influenzae. Neisseria gonorrhoeae* and *Chlamydia trachomatis* are additional diagnostic considerations in the neonate.

C. Allergic. Allergens such as pollens, molds, animal dander, dust.

D. Chemicals and other irritants. Commonly seen after silver nitrate prophylaxis in newborns.

II. Incidence

Common in all age groups, but infants and young children are particularly susceptible. Bacterial conjunctivitis is highly contagious and therefore prone to epidemics.

III. Incubation period

A. Viral. 5–14 days.

B. Bacterial. 2–3 days.

IV. Subjective data

A. Photophobia.

B. Itching of eyes.

C. Burning of eyes.

D. Feeling of roughness under eyelids.

E. Discharge from eyes.

F. Eyelids stick together.

G. Eyelids swollen.

H. Pertinent subjective data to obtain

1. History of upper respiratory infection.
2. Any associated signs or symptoms, e.g., runny nose, sore throat, earache.
3. History of exposure to conjunctivitis.
4. Is conjunctivitis prevalent in the community?
5. History of swimming in a chlorinated pool or contaminated pond.
6. History of foreign body or trauma to the eye.
7. History of exposure to herpes simplex or concurrent cold sore.
8. History of exposure to volatile chemicals or other irritants.

I. No complaints of decreased vision.

V. Objective data

A. Viral conjunctivitis

1. Conjunctiva hyperemic.
2. Hypertrophy of lymphoid follicles in lower palpebral conjunctiva.
3. Tearing or mild mucopurulent discharge.
4. Pupils: normal and reactive to light.
5. Cornea: clear.

6. Vision: normal.
7. May have associated pharyngitis, preauricular adenopathy, and/or edema of lower eyelids.

B. Bacterial conjunctivitis
1. Conjunctiva mildly injected to markedly inflamed; discharge purulent or mucopurulent.
2. Pupils: normal and reactive to light.
3. Vision: normal.
4. Cornea: clear; check for ulcerations.
5. Eyelid margins: may be ulcerated.
6. Skin: occasionally impetigo is found on the face with a staphylococcal conjunctivitis.
7. Examine ears, nose, and throat for concomitant infection.

C. Allergic conjunctivitis
1. Conjunctiva edematous and moderately inflamed.
2. Watery or stringy mucoid discharge.
3. Vision: normal.
4. Associated symptoms of allergic rhinitis (see Allergic Rhinitis and Conjunctivitis).
5. Symptoms seem worse than inflammation would indicate.

D. Chemical conjunctivitis
1. Conjunctiva inflamed and edematous.
2. Tearing.
3. Diagnosis made by history of exposure.

E. Laboratory studies. Culture of conjunctival exudate should be done on all infants under 1 month of age.

VI. Assessment

A. Diagnosis is made by evaluation of subjective and objective data.
1. Viral conjunctivitis.
2. Bacterial conjunctivitis.
3. Allergic conjunctivitis.
4. Chemical conjunctivitis.

B. Differential diagnosis
1. Herpes simplex blepharitis: history of clinical findings of primary or secondary infection. Generally unilateral.
2. Herpetic keratitis: corneal inflammation and presence of dendritic figure on staining with fluorescein.
3. Trachoma (rare in the United States): upper eyelid and upper portion of globe more severely involved than lower; conjunctiva thickened, with papillary hypertrophy and formation of follicles.
4. Dacryostenosis: chronic tearing with or without discharge; generally unilateral; naris on affected side is dry.
5. Ophthalmia neonatorum: diagnosis established by culture of exudate.
6. Corneal abrasion/ulcer: severe pain and tearing, decreased vision, cornea may be hazy.

7. Iritis: moderate pain, no discharge, diminished vision, cornea may be cloudy, poor pupillary reaction.

VII. Plan

A. Viral conjunctivitis
   1. Usually associated with upper respiratory infection and self-limited.
   2. Medication of value only to prevent secondary infection.
      a. Sodium Sulamyd Ophthalmic Ointment or Solution 10%, 5 times daily.
      b. Cool compresses.

B. Bacterial conjunctivitis
   1. Sodium Sulamyd Ophthalmic Ointment or Solution 10%, 5 times daily.
      or
   2. Tobrex ophthalmic ointment or solution 2 to 4 times a day.
   3. Cool compresses.

C. Allergic conjunctivitis
   1. Treatment of underlying allergy and allergic rhinitis (see Allergic Rhinitis and Conjunctivitis).
   2. Cool compresses.
   3. Acular 0.5% (ketorolac tromethamine) ophthalmic solution:1 drop, 4 times a day.

D. Chemical conjunctivitis
   1. Immediately flush eye with copious amounts of tepid water, preferably normal saline.
   2. Consult with ophthalmologist for further treatment.

VIII. Education

A. Viral conjunctivitis lasts about 12–14 days. It is generally self-limited, but secondary bacterial infection may occur.

B. Bacterial conjunctivitis should respond to treatment within 2–3 days. Continue treatment for 1 week or for at least 3 days after symptoms have subsided; otherwise it may recur.

C. Cool, wet compresses: use cooled boiled water to moisten cotton ball; use a fresh cotton ball each time.

D. Wipe eyes gently from inner canthus to outer canthus to avoid spread to unaffected eye. Eyes should be cleaned before instillation of medication.

E. To instill ointment or drops, pull down inner canthus of lower eyelid toward center of eye; apply thin ribbon of ointment or drops to the "pocket." Do not allow applicator tip to touch eyelid or fingers.

F. Instillation of ointment will cause blurring of vision.

G. Continue medication for at least 2 full days after symptoms have disappeared.

H. Rubbing of eyes can cause spread to other eye.

I. Hygiene
   1. Keep child's facecloth and towels separate to avoid spread of infection.
   2. Use careful hand-washing technique to help prevent spread of infection.
   3. Keep child out of school until inflammation and discharge subside.

J. Acular helps stop the cycle of itching and rubbing that can create substantial irritation of the eyes.

IX. Follow-up

A. Call back if no improvement noted in 2–3 days.

B. Call back immediately if symptoms become worse or child complains of pain.

C. Call back if child initially responds to treatment but then seems worse; this may be an allergic reaction to the medication.

D. No routine follow-up is necessary if child responds well to medication. Resolution should be complete in 1 week for bacterial infections, 2 weeks for viral.

X. Complications

A. Blepharitis or corneal ulcers with bacterial conjunctivitis.

B. Secondary bacterial infection with viral conjunctivitis.

C. Sloughing of cornea or ulcer due to chemical irritation.

XI. Consultation/referral

A. Corneal ulcer.

B. Corneal inflammation.

C. Suspicion of herpes simplex.

D. No response to treatment within 3 days.

E. Complaints of pain, severe photophobia, or decreased vision.

F. Infants under 1 month of age.

G. Any irregularities of pupil size or reaction to light.

H. Chemical conjunctivitis.

NOTES

CONSTIPATION

A decrease in the frequency and bulk and/or liquid content of the stool. The term *constipation* refers to the character and consistency of the stool rather than to the frequency of bowel movements. Constipation is characterized by stools that are small, hard, and dry. Encopresis refers to the syndrome of fecal soiling or incontinence secondary to constipation or incomplete defecation.

I. Etiology

- **A.** Mechanical or anatomic (e.g., megacolon, anal stricture, obstruction).
- **B.** Psychological.
  - **1.** Disruption of child's routine.
  - **2.** Improper toilet training techniques, such as early, aggressive training.
  - **3.** Encopresis.
- **C.** Withholding. With a busy, active life-style, child ignores urge to defecate.
- **D.** Anal fissure.
- **E.** Dietary: too little fiber, too much milk.

II. Incidence

Frequently seen in childhood and adolescence, both as a chronic and as an occasional interruption of normal bowel patterns. It is often a familial complaint.

III. Subjective data

- **A.** Decrease in frequency of stools.
- **B.** Stools hard, dry, and small.
- **C.** Straining with bowel movement.
- **D.** Pain with stooling.
- **E.** Staining: intermittent or constant.
- **F.** Recurrent abdominal pain in approximately 60%.
- **F.** Pertinent subjective data to obtain
  - **1.** Usual pattern of elimination.
  - **2.** Description of stools.
  - **3.** Duration of constipation.
  - **4.** Frequency of episodes of constipation.
  - **5.** Detailed dietary history.
  - **6.** Use of laxatives.
  - **7.** Treatment tried and its effectiveness.
  - **8.** Psychosocial factors.
  - **9.** Availability of bathroom facilities and other factors, such as privacy.

IV. Objective data

- **A.** Abdominal examination.
  - **1.** Inspection for abdominal distention and bowel sounds.
  - **2.** Auscultation.
  - **3.** Percussion.
  - **4.** Palpation; stool palpable in colon.
- **B.** Anus: fissures.

C. Rectal examination.
   1. Hard stool in colon.
   2. Anal stricture.

V. Assessment

A. Diagnosis of constipation and its underlying cause is usually made by a detailed history.

B. Differential diagnosis
   1. Normal straining of infancy: stools are soft.
   2. Hirschsprung's: staining or soiling is rare; ampulla empty on rectal exam; history of constipation since birth.
   3. Encopresis: staining; feces in the rectal ampulla.

VI. Plan

A. If constipation is significant when the child presents, a pediatric Fleet enema may be indicated for immediate relief.

B. Retrain bowels.
   1. Encourage child to sit on toilet 20 minutes after meals.
   2. Explain gastrocolic reflex.

C. Stool softeners.
   1. Colace, 5 mg/kg/24 hours.
      or
   2. Maltsupex
      a. For child aged 1–12 months, 1/2 tsp bid—may increase to 1 tablespoon bid.
      b. For child aged 1–15 years, 1 tsp bid—may increase to 2 tablespoons bid.
      c. For child aged 5–15 years, 2 tsp bid—may increase to 2 tablespoons bid.
   3. Once stools are soft, daily dosage can be reduced.
   4. Continue use for 2–3 months until regular bowel habits are established.

D. Dietary changes: increase fiber, fluids, fruits, vegetables.

E. If child is toddler and not completely toilet trained, put him back in diapers and eliminate all pressure (e.g., from parents, grandparents, other caretakers).

F. Constipation with encopresis.
   1. Fleet enema.
   2. Mineral oil, 3 tsp tid or qid. Give until stools are loose to the point of incontinence, then decrease dosage gradually until child has 2–3 loose stools daily.
   3. "Toilet" at regular intervals.
   4. Colace, 5–10 mg/kg/24 hours, as maintenance once regular bowel habits have been established.
   5. Increase dosage of water-soluble vitamins (vitamin B complex and vitamin C) while on mineral oil.
   6. High roughage diet: bran, cereals, vegetables, fruits.
   7. Do not put pressure on child; treatment must be approached in a calm, relaxed manner.

G. Anal fissure.
   1. Stool softeners as above.

2. Sitz baths.

VII. Education

A. Avoid laxatives and enemas.

B. Every person's bowel habits are unique to him; a daily bowel movement may not be the norm for everyone.

C. Dietary changes.

1. Increase water intake.
2. Increase high-residue foods (green vegetables and fruits).
3. Include bran and whole-grain products in diet.
4. Reduce intake of cheese and milk, which may be constipating.

D. Gastrocolic reflex is a mass movement of colon contents occurring about 20 minutes after a meal.

E. With a busy life-style, the child may not take time to go to the bathroom.

F. A bathroom may not be available for the child when he needs it.

G. Make bathroom time relaxed and unhurried.

H. Keep special books—such as normally forbidden comic books—for relaxation in the bathroom.

I. If child is a small preschooler, toilet may be too big; instead, use a small, portable "john."

J. Stool softeners are not laxatives and are not habit forming. They prevent excessive drying of stool and are not effective if child is withholding.

K. Mineral oil may be put in juice or cola.

L. If away from home, child may not use bathroom facilities because of unfamiliarity with them or their lack of cleanliness or privacy.

M. Review toilet training techniques (see p. 165).

1. When to start: child indicates readiness.
2. How to proceed.

N. Explain physiology of constipation to parent:

1. Because of discomfort from either a hard stool or an anal fissure, child withholds stool.
2. Stool collects in the rectum and, over time, rectum dilates and propulsive peristaltic action decreases.
3. As volume of rectum increases, sensation decreases.
4. Constipation becomes self-perpetuating and often more severe with time.
5. In encopresis, because of the enlarged rectal vault, the external anal sphincter relaxes, allowing loose or mushy stool to leak out around firm stool in rectum. Child has no sense of need to defecate and little or no control over leakage.

O. Water-soluble vitamins are B vitamins (thiamine, riboflavin, nicotinic acid, pyridoxine) and vitamin C.

P. Because excesses of water-soluble vitamins are excreted in the urine, the danger of toxicity is low.

VIII. Follow-up

A. Telephone call in 1 week to report; repeat telephone contact at intervals indicated by scope of problem.

B. If child old enough, have him make phone calls himself.

C. With chronic constipation or encopresis, recheck every month until rectal vault has returned to normal size.

D. Treatment for constipation or constipation with encopresis may take from as little as 6 months to as long as 2–3 years.

IX. Complications

A. Encopresis.

B. Anal fissure.

C. Impaction.

X. Consultation/referral

Constipation with encopresis: refer for psychological evaluation if child has poor response to treatment or exhibits emotional problems in other areas.

NOTES

DIAPER RASH—PRIMARY IRRITANT

Erythema, scaling, and/or ulceration of skin in the diaper area.

I. Etiology

A. The result of prolonged contact of urine and feces with the skin leading to maceration and chemical irritation (from urea and intestinal enzymes).

B. Consider neglect; carelessness; sensitivity from contact reactions to plastic, rubber, disposable diapers, and laundry products.

II. Subjective data

A. Reddened diaper area.

B. Sores in diaper area.

C. Baby itchy, uncomfortable; cries when voiding.

D. Baby irritable.

E. History of use of inappropriate laundry products, change in diapers (disposable), change in family situation, strong odor of ammonia.

F. Detailed history of treatment used.

III. Objective data

A. One or a combination of the following will be present in the diaper area:
   1. Erythema.
   2. Papules.
   3. Vesicles.
   4. Oozing.
   5. Ulcerations.
   6. Burned or scalded appearance.

B. Check urethral meatus in circumcised male; ulceration is frequently present.

C. Inspect entire child.
   1. Intertriginous areas may be irritated if general hygiene is poor.
   2. Legs and heels may be affected from contact with wet diapers.
   3. Eczema or other skin disease may be present.

IV. Assessment: Differential diagnosis

A. Candidiasis: beefy red, shiny; sharply demarcated borders with satellite lesions.

B. Atopic dermatitis: by detailed history and involvement of other areas (e.g., chest, face, neck, extremities).

C. Allergic contact dermatitis (sensitivity to disposable diapers, laundry products): by detailed history.

D. Psoriasis: scaling papules and plaques with inflammation. Often a positive family history.

V. Plan

A. Mild—erythema only. Apply one of the following at each diaper change:
   1. Caldesene medicated powder.
   2. Dyprotex medicated diaper rash pads.
   3. Desitin cream.

B. Erythema, papules.
   1. Hydrocortisone cream, 1%—3 times a day.

C. Intense erythema, vesicles, ulcerations.
  1. Neosporin Cream tid.
  2. Burow's solution—apply compresses for 20 minutes tid.

D. Ulceration of meatus.
  1. Neosporin Cream tid.
     or
  2. Garamycin Cream 3 times a day.

Note: Do not give refills for hydrocortisone cream. Corticosteroids should not be used indiscriminately.

VI. Education

A. Primary concern is prevention.

B. Frequent diaper changes.
  1. Wash diaper area at each change.
  2. Do not use packaged wipes.

C. Apply petroleum jelly to penis of circumcised male at each diaper change.

D. Omit diapers as often as possible.

E. Use plastic pants for social occasions only.

F. Do not use cornstarch; it can be metabolized by microorganisms.

G. Use Caldesene medicated powder on a routine basis.

H. Diaper laundry.
  1. Diaper service is generally acceptable.
  2. Home laundering.
     a. Use mild soap (e.g., Ivory Snow).
     b. Do not use bleach, fabric softeners in wash, or softener sheets in dryer.
     c. Put through rinse cycle twice.
     d. Use vinegar—1 oz/gal of water—in final rinse.

I. Disposable diapers.
  1. Switch to another brand if sensitivity is suspected.
  2. Fold plastic away from body.
  3. Tear small holes in plastic to decrease humidity in diaper area.

J. Diet.
  1. Increase fluids.
  2. Include cranberry juice if child is 12 months of age or older—changes pH of urine, making it less irritating.
  3. Exclude all other juices.
  4. Do not add any new foods.

K. Watch for sensitivity to Neosporin cream—erythema, edema, scaling, itching.

L. Wet dressings cool and dry skin.

M. Use soft, clean cloth for compresses. Moisten and reapply every 10 minutes.

VII. Follow-up

A. Call if no improvement in 2 days or immediately if rash is worse.

B. If ulceration of meatus, check for full stream when voiding.

C. Call if any question of sensitivity to Neosporin.

VIII. Complications

Secondary bacterial infection.

IX. Consultation/referral

Failure to respond to treatment after 10 days.

NOTES

DIARRHEA—ACUTE

An increase in the frequency and fluid content of stools. Usually self-limited in older children and adolescents, but potentially-life threatening in infants.

I. Etiology

A. Causes
   1. Diet.
   2. Inflammation or irritation of the gastrointestinal mucosa.
   3. Gastrointestinal infection—viral, bacterial, parasitic.
   4. Antibiotic associated.
   5. Psychogenic disorders.
   6. Nongastrointestinal disease ("parenteral" diarrhea).
   7. Mechanical or anatomic conditions.

B. Pathophysiologic reactions
   1. Disturbance of normal cell transport across the intestinal mucosa, as in sugar malabsorption.
   2. Increase in intestinal motility due to an excess of prostaglandins and serotonin.
   3. Decrease in intestinal motility causing an increase in bacterial colonization.
   4. Decrease in surface area available.
   5. Nonabsorbable molecules in the intestine.
   6. Excessive secretion of water and electrolytes because of increased intestinal permeability.

II. Incidence

A common symptom throughout childhood. Diet is the most common cause of acute diarrhea in early infancy. In older infants and children, infections of both the gastrointestinal tract and other systems are the most common causes.

III. Subjective data

A. Temperature may be elevated.

B. Lethargy.

C. Anorexia.

D. Increase—sudden or gradual—in the number of stools.

E. Decrease in the consistency of stools.

F. Increase in the fluid content of stools (watery stools).

G. Crampy abdominal pain.

H. Pertinent subjective data to obtain
   1. Usual pattern of elimination—description of stools.
   2. Last accurate weight.
   3. Type of onset (e.g., rapid, with explosive, watery stools).
   4. Duration of diarrhea.
   5. Frequency of stools.
   6. Description of stools—bloody, purulent, foul smelling, mucoid.
   7. Associated vomiting.

8. Localized abdominal pain.
9. Antibiotic therapy—concurrent or recent course.
10. Epidemiologic data: exposure to others with GI infection—e.g., home, daycare, school.
11. Detailed dietary history to determine overfeeding, malnutrition, or foods that may cause diarrhea.
12. Infant on formula: ascertain type of formula.
13. Breast-fed infant: check mother's diet and medication intake.
14. Introduction of new foods in diet.
15. Previous history of allergic response to foods.
16. Family history of atopy.
17. Ingestion of suspected contaminated foods.
18. History of travel.
19. Use of laxatives.
20. What treatments have been tried and how effective they have been.
21. Psychosocial factors creating stress in the child's environment.
22. Urinary output: assess for symptoms of urinary tract infection; change in output.

IV. Objective data

A. Weight.

B. Assess state of hydration (see Appendix D, Clinical Signs of Dehydration).

C. Temperature: elevation may be due to infection or related to the degree of dehydration.

D. Abdominal examination.

1. Inspection: abdominal distention.
2. Auscultation: hyperactive bowel sounds.
3. Percussion: increased tympany.
4. Palpation: may be slight, generalized tenderness; no local or rebound tenderness, masses, or organomegaly.

E. Ears, nose, throat, chest, glands: examine for signs of associated infection.

F. Skin: examine for rash.

V. Assessment

Diagnosis of acute diarrhea in children and infants generally can be made with a careful history. It is usually a diagnosis of exclusion. A stool culture or test for ova and parasites is not indicated unless the history or clinical picture is indicative of a more complex problem. A hemocult stool test can be readily done and should be negative for red blood cells.

A. Infectious diarrhea. Diagnosis made by history of exposure and positive stool culture.

1. Nonbacterial. Abrupt onset; vomiting is common; fever is rarely present; there is often an associated upper respiratory infection. Stools are loose with an unpleasant odor.
2. Salmonella. Onset 6–72 hours after ingestion of contaminated foods such as milk, eggs, or poultry or from contact with infected animals. Severe abdominal cramps and loose, slimy, sometimes bloody, green stools with a characteristic odor of rotten eggs are the diagnostic clinical features.

3. Shigella. Abrupt onset of fever, abdominal pain, and vomiting. Watery, yellow-green, relatively odorless stools, which may contain blood, occur shortly after onset. Transmitted by ingestion of infected foods or person-to-person contact.
4. *Escherichia coli.* Gradual onset of slimy, green, "pea soup" stools with a foul odor. Fever and vomiting are not predominant symptoms. Major cause of traveler's diarrhea, or "Montezuma's revenge."
5. Giardiasis. Commonly waterborne, seen endemically and epidemically in daycare centers and communities with inadequate water treatment facilities. Symptoms include anorexia, nausea, abdominal distention, and crampy abdominal pain. Stools are pale, greasy, bulky, and malodorous. Onset may be sudden or gradual. Cysts may not always be found in a stool specimen.

B. Parenteral diarrhea. Concurrent infection of another system (respiratory tract, urinary tract).

C. Diarrhea due to food or drug sensitivities. Indicated by history.

D. Starvation diarrhea. Frequent scanty, green-brown stools; history of decreased food intake for 3–4 days.

VI. Plan

Primary treatment of diarrhea is aimed at resting the intestine and keeping the child well hydrated.

A. Nursing infants
1. Continue nursing.
2. Offer 1–2 oz of water between feedings.
3. Do not give any foods or juices.
4. With concurrent vomiting, give 5 ml of water or oral rehydration solution every 5 minutes.

B. Bottle-fed infants 3–18 months of age.
1. First 24 hours.
   a. Discontinue formula or milk.
   b. Oral rehydration solution (Pedialyte, Ricelyte, or Lytren): give 1–2 oz/lb of body weight divided into frequent feedings of 3–4 oz each.
   c. With concurrent vomiting, give 5 ml of water or oral rehydration solution every 5 minutes.
2. Second day.
   a. Isomil or ProSobee: use half strength; give amount of infant's usual feeding. If infant refuses Isomil or ProSobee, try half-strength formula or milk.
   b. Consult with office if diarrhea has not improved.
3. Third day.
   a. Full-strength Isomil or ProSobee or full-strength formula.
   b. Diet: slowly introduce usual diet beginning with bland solids:
      (1) Rice cereal.
      (2) Banana.
      (3) Jell-O.
      (4) Soup.
   c. If diarrhea recurs, resume half-strength formula and proceed again through dietary plan as listed above.

C. Children
   1. First 24 hours.
      a. Give clear liquids only: water, oral rehydration solution, weak tea, Jell-O water, Gatorade, popsicles.
      b. Give 1–2 oz every hour.
   2. Second day.
      a. If diarrhea has improved, add bland solids:
         (1) Rice cereal.
         (2) Banana or banana flakes, applesauce.
         (3) Jell-O.
         (4) Saltines.
         (5) Toast and jelly.
      b. If diarrhea has not improved, consult with office. A stool culture may be indicated.
   3. Third day.
      a. With improvement of diarrhea, gradually add more bland solids.
      b. Avoid milk, fried foods, vegetables, fruits, and meat.

D. Salmonella:
   1. Antimicrobial treatment of mild illness does not shorten clinical course.
   2. Consult and treat systemically if disease appears to be progressing systemically in infants, or if child is immunocompromised.

E. Shigella:
   1. Trimethoprim-sulfamethoxazole: 8 mg/kg trimethoprim and 40 mg/kg sulfamethoxazole per day in 2 divided doses.
   2. Bacteriologic cure will be achieved in 80% of children after 48 hours.

F. *E. Coli:*
   1. Trimethoprim-sulfamethoxazole: 8 mg/kg trimethoprim & 40 mg/kg sulfamethoxazole per day in 2 divided doses.

G. Giardiasis:
   1. Flagyl:
      a. Children—15–20 mg/kg/day in 3 divided doses.
      b. Adolescents and adults: 250 mg tid.

   or

   2. Atabrine:
      a. Children—6 mg/kg/day in 3 divided doses.
      b. Adolescents and adults—100 mg tid.

VII. Education

A. Discontinue milk, juices, and foods.

B. Do not use boiled skim milk (hypernatremia may result from high solute load).

C. Too frequent feedings may exacerbate diarrhea by stimulating the gastrocolic reflex.

D. Use petroleum jelly or Desitin on perianal area to prevent excoriation.

E. Use careful hand-washing technique to help prevent spread of infectious diarrhea. Keep child home from school to prevent spread.

F. Do not continue clear liquids any longer than 24 hours.

G. Childhood diarrhea can be treated effectively by resting the gastrointestinal tract and then slowly resuming a normal diet, but the plan has to be followed carefully.

H. Call back immediately if child is not taking liquids, is vomiting, or has any signs of dehydration (see Appendix D, Clinical Signs of Dehydration).

I. Sweetened juices and soda can increase the severity of diarrhea (hyperosmotic fluids draw more fluid into intestinal lumen).

J. Incubation period for viral diarrhea is 1 to 3 days (mean 2 days).

K. Duration of diarrhea is generally 3 to 7 days.

L. Transmission is via fecal-oral route.

VIII. Follow-up

A. Telephone follow-up in 8–12 hours if child is not dehydrated and retains liquids. Have caretaker call back sooner if child refuses liquids or is vomiting.

B. Continue to maintain daily telephone contact until diarrhea has subsided, giving mother dietary instructions at each stage.

C. With infants, check weight daily. Continue follow-up until preillness weight is reestablished.

IX. Complications

With simple diarrhea, dehydration is the major complication.

X. Consultation/referral

A. Any child with signs of dehydration.

B. Bloody diarrhea.

C. Diarrhea in a child who is taking antibiotics (e.g., ampicillin, erythromycin) or iron.

D. Infant under 3 months of age.

E. Diarrhea persisting over 3–4 days.

NOTES

DYSMENORRHEA-PRIMARY

Painful menstruation without demonstrable pelvic disease. Occurs 1–3 years after menarche when ovulation is established.

I. Etiology

Recent data demonstrate that prostaglandins which are released during the breakdown of the endometrium are higher in dysmenorrheic females. The prostaglandins act as pain mediators and stimulate uterine contractility. Dysmenorrhea is not usually associated with the onset of menses although some adolescents experience discomfort with the first cycles (generally an ovulatory).

II. Incidence

An estimated 75% of all adolescent girls complain of one or more symptoms of dysmenorrhea. It is the most common gynecologic complaint in this age group and the leading cause of short-term school absenteeism in females.

III. Subjective data

A. Onset of one or more of the following symptoms during or prior to menstruation. Pain usually starts within 1–4 hours of onset of menses but can occur 1–2 days prior to menses. Symptoms persist for 24–48 hours following beginning of menstrual flow, less frequently for 2–4 days.
   1. Premenstrual tension, including irritability or emotional lability, headache.
   2. Abdominal cramps.
   3. Nausea, vomiting, anorexia.
   4. Constipation, diarrhea.
   5. Weight gain.
   6. Fluid retention, bloating (3–5 lbs in the 4–7 days prior to onset of menses).
   7. Syncope.
   8. Vaginal discomfort.
   9. Suprapubic pain radiating to back and thighs.

B. Pertinent subjective data to obtain
   1. Detailed menstrual history:
      a. Age at menarche?
      b. Are menses regular?
      c. Heavy flow?
      d. Duration of menses?
      e. When did cramping start in relation to menarche?
   2. Where is the pain? What is it like?
   3. When does pain or cramping occur?
   4. How long does pain last?
   5. Are there any premenstrual symptoms (e.g., bloating, irritability)?
   6. Does she have mittelschmerz?
   7. Is this what she expected to happen with menses? Did mother or sisters have dysmenorrhea?
   8. Does she miss school because of dysmenorrhea? If so, how often and how many days? Does she miss other activities (e.g., parties, sports events)?

9. What treatment has been used? How effective has it been?
10. What is adolescent's understanding of the menstrual cycle?
11. What is her relationship with her mother like?
12. Is she sexually active? Some adolescents will use a complaint of dysmenorrhea as an entry to the health care system when they either want, or want to discuss, birth control.

Note: A detailed menstrual history should be obtained from every adolescent female presenting for routine health care. Discussion should include questions about discomfort relating to menses.

IV. Objective data

A. Weight, height, blood pressure.

B. Mild cramps on first day: complete physical examination, including inspection of external genitalia for hymenal abnormalities, is appropriate for 13- to 16-year-old age group who are not sexually active.

C. Moderate to severe cramps: complete physical examination, including pelvic exam; if unable to complete pelvic exam, rectoabdominal exam should be done to rule out pelvic pathology. Include careful palpation of uterosacral ligaments for tenderness or nodules (suggestive of endometriosis).

D. Include pelvic exam, pap smear, and cultures for adolescents who are sexually active.

E. Pelvic ultrasound to rule out uterine or vaginal anomalies. (Will not detect endometriosis.)

V. Assessment

A. Diagnosis of primary dysmenorrhea can be made by history typical for primary dysmenorrhea and negative findings on physical examination.

B. Differential diagnosis. Secondary dysmenorrhea: atypical history and positive findings on physical examination. Adnexal tenderness and masses or nodules of uterosacral ligaments.

VI. Plan

The goals of treatment are to allay anxiety and provide symptomatic relief of pain.

A. Reassurance

1. Simple explanation of the menstrual process and anatomy.
2. The pain is not "in her head" as may have been suggested.
3. Pain can be managed; she does not have to anticipate pain every month.

B. Pharmacologic management. Begin with the simplest treatment and progress to stronger medications as needed. Use one of the following:

1. Aspirin: 300–600 mg every 4 hours as needed.
2. Anaprox: 550 mg stat, followed by 275 mg every 6 hours or 550 mg bid. Maximum dose: 1,375 mg/24 hours.
3. Orudis: 25–50 mg every 6 to 8 hours. May increase dosage to 75 mg every 6 to 8 hours. Maximum dose: 300 mg/24 hours.
4. Motrin: 400 mg every 6 to 8 hours. Increase to 600 mg or 800 mg every 6 to 8 hours, if necessary. Maximum dose: 3200 mg/24 hours.
5. Ponstel: 500 mg initially, then 250 mg every 6 hours as needed for pain; do not exceed 1 week of therapy.

Note: For severe dysmenorrhea associated with vomiting, one of the above medications may be started 1–2 days prior to menses if not sexually active.

6. Birth control pills

a. Pelvic examination and Pap smear prior to starting treatment.
b. Indicated for severe dysmenorrhea associated with vomiting and with unsatisfactory response to analgesics and antiprostaglandins.
c. Tri Norinyl #28 or Ortho-Novum 7:7:7 #28: use for 3 months, discontinue for 3–6 months, and resume for another 3 months. Patient will usually continue to have relief for 1–2 months between use of birth control pills because of anovulation. If cramps recur, try antiprostaglandin before starting birth control pills again.
d. Use of birth control pills helps distinguish organic pathology. If cramps become worse while patient is on birth control pills, refer for laparoscopy to rule out endometriosis.

7. Compazine: 5 mg every 4 hours at onset of menses to control vomiting.

C. Local measures. Heating pad on abdomen.

VII. Education

A. Dysmenorrhea is not abnormal. It does not mean that there is any physical abnormality or disease present, nor is it a psychosomatic illness.
B. Dysmenorrhea is an indication that ovulation is occurring. Stress the positive future aspects of motherhood.
C. Dysmenorrhea may be more severe during times of stress.
D. If fluid retention or bloating is a problem, decrease salt intake for 10 days before menses.
E. Continue with regular routine as much as possible. Some discomfort may persist once on medication, but if pain is under control, do not forego activities.
F. Increased exercise (e.g., jogging, bicycling, ice skating) on a regular basis has been of value in decreasing menstrual pain. Competitive athletes have fewer ovulatory cycles and therefore less dysmenorrhea.
G. Showers, baths, and shampoos during menses will not increase discomfort or cause cramps.
H. Medication
1. Aspirin taken with a cup of coffee or tea may be quite effective. The caffeine potentiates the effects of aspirin.
2. Take antiprostaglandins with food to minimize gastrointestinal side effects.
3. Continue antiprostaglandins for 2–3 days only.
4. Do not use medication longer than necessary.
5. After 1–2 years on a birth control pill regimen of 3 months on and 3 months off, cramps often improve spontaneously.
6. When on the birth control pill, flow will be lighter.
7. Give mother and child complete information on birth control pill, and have them read booklet that comes with prescription packet.
8. Stress importance of calling the office immediately if there are any questions regarding side effects.
9. Take all medication as directed. Do not take more than prescribed.

VIII. Follow-up

A. Have patient call after next menstrual period to report effectiveness of treatment.

B. Return visit in 3–4 months to evaluate effectiveness of medication and to maintain encouragement and support.

C. Follow-up visit every 3 months while on birth control pills with a complete physical, including pelvic examination, every 6 months.

IX. Complications

A. Vomiting causing inability to retain medication.

B. Psychological stress.

X. Consultation/referral

A. Questionable or abnormal findings on physical examination or history.

B. Severe dysmenorrhea prior to institution of pharmacologic therapy.

C. No response to prescribed treatment.

D. Inability to retain medication because of vomiting.

NOTES

ENURESIS

The involuntary passage of urine, usually occurring at night (nocturnal enuresis) in a child over 5 years of age. It is subdivided into two classifications—primary and secondary. Primary enuresis is that occurring in a child who has never been dry at night for a period of greater than a week. Secondary enuresis is that occurring in a child who has been dry at night for a prolonged period and subsequently loses bladder control. Diurnal enuresis is enuresis occurring during the day.

I. Etiology

A. Primary nocturnal enuresis
   1. Immature development of bladder with resultant small capacity.
   2. Immature arousal mechanism for non-REM sleep.
   3. Psychological problems, such as regression after the birth of a sibling.
   4. Neurologic causes: myelomeningocele, mental retardation.
   5. Urologic lesions or anomalies.
   6. Diabetes mellitus or diabetes insipidus.

B. Secondary nocturnal enuresis
   1. Psychological problems.
   2. Developmental delays.
   3. Urinary tract infection (UTI).
   4. Diabetes mellitus.
   5. Diabetes insipidus.

II. Incidence

A. Approximately:
   1. 10–15% of 6-year-olds.
   2. 5% of 10-year-olds.
   3. 3% of 12 year-olds.
   4. 1% of 15-year-olds.

B. Enuresis is more common in boys than in girls.

C. There is a familial tendency toward enuresis. It is more prevalent in large families and in lower socioeconomic groups.

III. Subjective data

A. Primary. Bed-wetting one or more times a night at least once a week without having achieved bladder control at night.

B. Secondary. Bed-wetting one or more times a night at least once a week after having achieved bladder control at night.

Note: As part of the history obtained at the well child visit, every child should be asked if he has any urinary symptoms and if he ever wets his pants or the bed.

C. Pertinent subjective data to obtain
   1. Has child ever been dry? If so, when did onset of wetting occur.
   2. How frequently does child wet the bed?
   3. When does wetting occur—late evening, early am?

4. What do parents do about bed-wetting? How do they feel about it? Do they see it as a problem?
5. Is there a history of bed-wetting in the family—siblings or parents?
6. How does the child feel about wetting the bed?
7. Is there a family history of diabetes mellitus?
8. Has child awakened up with sore muscles or bitten tongue suggesting nocturnal seizures?
9. Does child have a full stream when voiding?
10. What is the daytime voiding pattern: frequency, volume of urination, dribbling, diurnal enuresis? (Frequent, small-volume voidings, dribbling, and diurnal enuresis suggest primary enuresis.)
11. Has the child complained of frequency, urgency, pain, or burning on urination?
12. Has the child been dry when sleeping away from home?
13. Determine whether there are any psychosocial problems (indicative of secondary enuresis):
    a. New baby in the family.
    b. Death of a family member.
    c. Illness or hospitalization of the child or a family member.
    d. Divorce or separation of parents.
    e. School problems.
    f. Loss of a pet.
14. Obtain accurate history of hours of sleep and child's bedtime routine. Does he have regular sleep habits and sufficient sleep? Does he have a large amount of fluid at bedtime? Does he void before going to bed?

IV. Objective data

A. Physical examination is generally within normal limits. Significant neurologic deficits would present with history or findings in addition to nocturnal enuresis and would probably already have been identified.

1. Complete physical and neurologic examination.
    a. Check for constant dribbling.
    b. Check genitalia for external anomalies.
    c. Check rectal sphincter tone.
    d. Check skin for cafe au lait spots.
    e. Check spine for bony defects, masses, hairy tufts.
    f. Check abdomen for masses or enlarged kidneys.
    g. Check gait.
2. Measure height, weight, blood pressure to rule out chronic occult urinary tract disease.

B. Laboratory tests. Urinalysis and culture of clean-voided specimen.

V. Assessment: Differential diagnosis

A. UTI: positive urine culture.

B. Diabetes mellitus: urine positive for glycosuria and acetonuria.

C. Diabetes insipidus: specific gravity under 1.006.

D. Glomerulonephritis, pyelonephritis, cystitis, urethritis.

1. Urine positive for proteinuria.
2. Microscopic examination positive for erythrocytes and leukocytes.

VI. Plan

A. Before any treatment for enuresis is attempted, the child must want to be dry and the parents must be willing to participate in the treatment.

B. A voiding volume of under 200–300 ml will not be sufficient for child to remain dry at night.

C. Management should not be attempted until psychosocial issues and pressures within the family have been ruled out or issues have been resolved.

D. Do not attempt management when any stress is anticipated, such as a family move or birth of a sibling.

E. Primary enuresis. The following are three commonly used, acceptable methods of management:

1. Bladder-stretching exercises
   a. Have mother measure volume of urine several times.
   b. Once daily, have child hold urine as long as he can after the desire to void is felt.
   c. Encourage increased fluid intake, particularly during the time child is holding urine.
   d. Measure voiding volume after child has achieved his maximum ability to control his desire to urinate.
   e. Once child has increased his bladder capacity, have him practice starting and stopping urine stream.
2. Pharmacologic therapy.
   a. Imipramine (Tofranil): the drug most frequently used. It has an atropine-like effect on the bladder, increasing the capacity by increasing sphincter tone and decreasing the tone of the muscle that causes bladder contraction. Imipramine is an antidepressant and may interfere with natural sleep pattern and depth. Do not use in children under 6 years of age.
      (1) Initially 15–25 mg hs, increased to a maximum dosage of 50 mg in children under 12 years of age and 75 mg in children over 12 years of age.
      (2) Continue treatment for 6–8 weeks, and taper dosage over 4–6 weeks to avoid relapse.
      (3) If child wets during the early night hours, give 25 mg of imipramine at 4:00 P.M., and repeat dose at bedtime.
   a. DDAVP: an antidiuretic hormone that decreases urine production. It is used intranasally in children age 6 and older.
      (1) Initially 20 mcg intranasally at at bedtime. Administer one spray per nostril.
      (2) Subsequent dosage: May be adjusted up to 40 mcg if child does not respond.
      (3) Use lowest dose possible. May be adjusted down to 10 mcg.
3. Behavioral treatment
   a. Pad and bell technique:
      (1) Studies report an initial success rate of 75%. The alarm system is a pad of two conductive layers with an insulating cloth in between.

The child sleeps on the pad. When he wets and soaks through the insulating cloth, an electrical circuit is completed, causing the bell to ring.

(2) When the bell rings, awakening the child, he should go to the bathroom to finish voiding.

(3) Child or parent then changes the bed and resets the alarm.

(4) Treatment with this method may take from 5–12 weeks.

(5) If there is no improvement after 10 weeks, stop treatment. Another trial may be undertaken in 3 months.

(6) There is a relapse rate of 20–40% with this method. If relapse occurs after cessation of treatment, retreatment with the pad and bell is successful in most instances.

c. Sleep Dry Alarm or Wet Stop.

(1) Moisture sensor is attached by Velcro patch sewn on underpants. Alarm unit attaches to pajama top with Velcro.

(2) At onset of voiding, alarm goes off to awaken child.

(3) Sleep Dry Alarm program includes instructions and motivational materials (charts, stars).

F. Secondary enuresis. Therapy must be specific to the etiology.

1. Psychosocial problems or stressful situations

a. Counseling.

(1) Explanation of enuresis to parents and child.

(2) Discontinuance of pressure and punishment.

(3) Development of a plan with child and parents that will work for them.

(4) Contact school principal or nurse regarding school problems.

b. Imipramine: see E.2 above for dosage.

2. Developmental lag

a. Behavioral conditioning.

b. Gold star chart.

3. UTI. See Urinary Tract Infection.

4. Diabetes mellitus. Refer to physician.

5. Diabetes insipidus. Refer to physician.

VII. Education

A. Do not attempt management unless child is willing and is over 8 years of age.

B. Primary enuresis is a self-limited problem.

C. Avoid punishment, embarrassment, or shaming the child.

D. Do not be too aggressive in approach.

E. Avoid causing anxiety in other family members or child.

F. Involve child in treatment plan.

G. Bladder stretching.

1. When increasing fluid intake, child may have more frequent enuresis and may have daytime accidents.

2. It may take several months for child to achieve a voiding volume of 240–300 ml.

3. Generally, when voiding volume of 300 ml is achieved, child will be able to sleep through the night without voiding. Some children, however, need a greater volume before becoming dry at night.

H. Do not diaper child.

I. If child is willing, restrict fluids after dinner.

J. Have child void before going to bed.

K. If child has no difficulty going back to sleep, it is sometimes helpful for parents to get child up to void before they go to bed.

L. Make a chart or calendar on which to record bladder capacity and wet and dry nights. Encourage child to keep the chart. Use gold stars for dry nights.

M. Imipramine

1. Most common side effects seen in enuretic children on imipramine are irritability, sleep disorders, fatigue, gastrointestinal disturbances, and nervousness. Other reported reactions include constipation, convulsions, anxiety, emotional instability, syncope, and collapse.

2. Keep imipramine out of reach of small children.

N. DDAVP

1. An antidiuretic hormone.

2. Decreases urine production.

3. Nasal spray bottle accurately delivers 50 doses of 10 mcg each. Discard remaining medication after 50 doses.

O. Pad and bell technique

1. Do not use alarm system that has an electric shock; use only the type that has a bell.

2. Check batteries on apparatus frequently; electrolysis of urine may result from weak batteries, producing topical burns and preventing alarm bell from ringing.

P. Wet Stop and Sleep Dry have moisture sensors in underpants which, when activated by even a few drops of urine, trigger alarms. Child is awakened before bed is wet and voiding is completed. Also, the alarms are located near the child's head so that he responds to it more readily.

1. Wet Stop Alarm. Available from Palco Labs, 1595 Soquel Drive, Santa Cruz, CA 95065.

2. Sleep Dry Alarm. Follow instructions with program. Available through Star-Child/Labs, P.O. Box 404, Aptos, CA 95001-0404.

Q. Alarms have the highest cure rate—about 70%.

VIII. Follow-up

A. Primary enuresis

1. Telephone contact in 2 weeks. Have child call back to report his progress.

2. Return visit in 1 month. Have child bring in chart.

3. Continue follow-up at 2- to 4-week intervals for encouragement.

4. Follow-up may alternate between telephone calls and office visits.

B. Secondary enuresis

1. Counseling contract should be individualized. Initially, follow-up should be at least every 10–14 days. Encourage child to call and report successes.

2. Return visits at least monthly while on imipramine.

3. With behavioral conditioning and gold star chart, follow recommendations in A above.
4. UTI: see Urinary Tract Infection.

IX. Complications

A management plan that is too vigorous or stressful may result in psychological problems or increase stress for the family.

X. Consultation/referral

A. Diurnal enuresis, dribbling.
B. Identification of significant psychological problems, child abuse.
C. UTI.
D. Genitourinary abnormality.
E. Failure to improve with adequate trial of bladder retention or behavioral conditioning.

NOTES

ENVIRONMENTAL CONTROL FOR THE ATOPIC CHILD

With mild or questionable atopy, aggressive environmental control may be disruptive to the family and home environment. The health care professional should select portions of environmental control applicable to the individual child. In many children, environmental control results in significant improvement. When discussing environmental control, it is important to keep in mind that the removal of a family pet can cause an emotional upheaval for both the child and his family.

I. Indications for environmental control

A. Positive skin tests for environmental allergens.

B. Pollen sensitivity.

C. Clinical history of significant symptoms of allergy, including food sensitivity.

II. Commonly encountered allergens in the home

A. Animals—cat, dog, guinea pig, hamster, gerbil.

B. Plants, flowers.

C. Jute, horse hair—carpet padding.

D. Kapok—pillows, upholstery, stuffed animals.

E. Feathers, down—pillows, upholstery.

F. Wool—blankets, clothing.

G. House dust; in addition to containing the allergen, dust contains bacteria, mites, kapok, dander, horse hair.

H. Cosmetics—talcum powder, perfumes.

I. Molds—found in bathroom, shower stall, tile grout, basement, garage, attic, books, wallpaper, foam rubber pillows.

J. Smoke—cigarettes, wood stoves.

III. General measures for the home

A. Damp dust daily.

B. Use vacuum cleaner with an effective filtration system. Do not vacuum when child is in room.

C. Steam cleaning of carpeting should be done routinely. Dust mites have sticky feet and vacuuming does not remove them from carpeting.

D. Use air conditioner rather than fan. Air conditioning allows house to be closed to decrease exposure to outdoor allergens. It also lowers humidity.

E. Hot air ducts and returns should be covered with filters or cheesecloth. Vacuum ducts weekly.

F. Replace air conditioner and furnace filters regularly.

G. Shades and cotton curtains are preferable to venetian blinds and draperies.

H. Avoid wool rugs and blankets.

I. Paint walls or use washable wallpaper.

J. Kitchen, bathroom, and laundry should be adequately ventilated. Clean tile, grout, under sink, and behind toilet frequently.

K. Keep windows closed during pollen season.

L. Keep humidity below 50%. Dust mites thrive at 50% or above.

M. Use hot water laundering to kill mites. They cannot be washed away.

N. Pet.

1. The recommendation to remove a family pet may be very difficult to implement, but it is a sound prophylactic measure even in the absence of a positive skin test because sensitivity frequently develops in an atopic child.
2. If giving up the family pet is a problem, try to keep animal outside as much as possible and restricted to one area in the house.
3. If pet dies, advise parents not to replace it. (Snakes are acceptable for an atopic child.)

O. Do not give child chores such as dusting or mowing the lawn.

P. Plants may harbor mold. They should be removed.

Q. Discourage smoking and use of a woodstove or fireplace.

R. Keep child out of attic and cellar.

S. Air purifiers or filters need to be considered only if symptoms remain severe when all other environmental control measures are taken. Dust and dust mites settle quickly so even high efficiency particulate air filters are not effective for them. They are effective only for air borne particulate material.

T. Cleaning products:

1. Chlorine bleach—for bathrooms, cellars, other damp areas.
2. Ammonia—for general cleaning.
3. Club soda—spot remover.
4. Vinegar—removes mold.
5. Baking soda—for carpets and refrigerator.

IV. Environmental control for child's room

A. Remove everything from room and closet except large pieces of furniture. Rugs should be removed also.

B. Vacuum mattress and box spring, and cover with plastic. Zipper of plastic case can be covered with adhesive tape.

C. Wash walls, woodwork, ceiling, floor, and windows.

D. Paint walls or cover with washable wallpaper. Do not use wall hangings; paint murals on walls instead.

E. Install washable, synthetic window shades.

F. Dust and wax furniture; damp dust drawers.

G. Seal off forced hot air ducts and returns. Use an electric heater if necessary.

H. Carefully screen all items returned to room.

I. Use Dacron pillows.

J. Use cotton or Dacron blankets, bedspreads, sheets, and curtains. Do not use mattress pads or quilts.

K. Use wood or plastic chairs and tables. Avoid stuffed or wicker furniture.

L. Do not use venetian blinds or louvered doors.

M. Lamps should have plastic shades.

N. Return clothes to closet and drawers. Do not store woolens, flannels, or unnecessary items of clothing.

O. Books, stuffed animals, sports equipment, old shoes, and "collections" are dust and mold collectors and should not be in the room the child sleeps in.

P. To maintain dust-free room:

1. Keep door closed to minimize dust entering room.

2. Daily.
   a. Damp dust.
   b. Damp mop.
3. Weekly.
   a. Clean room thoroughly.
   b. Vacuum mattress and box spring.
   c. Wash all bedding and curtains.

V. School

A. Child should not sit near blackboard or handle erasers.
B. Caged pets such as hamsters or gerbils should not be in school room.
C. Concrete slab floors covered with carpeting may harbor molds.
D. Molds may grow on plants or dried arrangements.
E. Outdoor gym class may be a problem during pollen season.

NOTES

ERYTHEMA INFECTIOSUM (FIFTH DISEASE)

A mild viral illness that is characterized by a three-stage exanthem. The first is a slapped-cheek appearance, the second a maculopapular rash on the trunk and extremities which becomes a reticular, lacey rash and in the third stage has periodic evanescence and recrudescence. The disease is of importance primarily because maternal infection during pregnancy can cause spontaneous abortions, stillbirths, and asymptomatic intrauterine infection. This risk, however, is presumed to be only 1–2% of those infected.

I. Etiology

Human parvovirus B19. It is referred to as "fifth disease" because it was the fifth childhood exanthem described, the others being measles, rubella, scarlet fever, and roseola.

II. Incidence

Community outbreaks are common, most frequently in late winter and in spring. The highest incidence is seen in school-aged children between 5 and 15 years of age. Over 60% of adults are immune because of prior disease

III. Incubation period

4–14 days.

IV. Communicability

Transmitted by droplet infection. Most infectious prior to onset of rash. Secondary spread occurs in about 50% of close contacts.

V. Subjective data

A. History of mild systemic symptoms of a nonspecific viral illness which is often identified only in retrospect.
   1. Fever—low grade.
   2. Headache.
   3. Chills.
   4. Malaise.
   5. Myalgia.
   6. Pharyngitis.
   7. Conjunctivitis.

B. Symptoms last for 2 to 3 days and are followed by an asymptomatic period of 4 to 7 days.

C. Rash—predominant presenting complaint seen 17 to 18 days after exposure. This is the third stage of the disease.

VI. Objective data

Objective findings vary according to phase of illness.

A. Prodromal phase. Duration 1 to 4 days.
   1. Mildly erythematous pharynx and/or conjunctiva.

B. Second stage. Duration 4 to 7 days.
   2. Asymptomatic.

C. Third stage. Exanthem appears in three stages.
   1. First stage.
      a. Typical "slapped-cheek" appearance which appears 4 to 7 days after resolution of systemic symptoms. Fiery red rash on cheeks with circumoral pallor.

2. Second stage.
   a. Appears 1 to 4 days after onset of facial rash.
   b. Erythematous maculopapular discrete rash on trunk and extremities.
   c. Fades as central clearing occurs leaving a lacy, reticulated rash.
3. Third stage.
   a. 1- to 3-week duration.
   b. Lacy, reticulated rash characterized by periodic evanescence and recrudescence.
   c. Fluctuations in intensity are associated with environmental changes such as elevated temperatures and sun exposure.

VII. Assessment

A. Diagnosis is generally easily made by the appearance of the characteristic exanthem.

B. Differential diagnosis. Atypical cases may be confused with other viral exanthems such as measles, rubella, and enteroviruses or with drug reactions or other allergic responses.

VIII. Plan

A. There is no specific treatment.

B. Acetaminophen or ibuprofen for associated myalgias.

IX. Education

A. Most contagious prior to onset of rash, therefore isolation is not necessary once rash appears.

B. Avoid contact with pregnant women until the rash begins to fade.

C. Erythema infectiosum contracted during pregnancy can result in spontaneous abortion, stillbirth, and asymptomatic intrauterine infection.

D. Fetal abnormalities have not been associated with B19 viral infections during pregnancy.

E. Blood tests to determine diagnosis are generally used only for pregnant women and people who have blood disorders or who are immunocompromised

F. About 50–60% of adults have serologic evidence of past infection.

G. Avoid contact with people with hemolytic anemias.

H. In school related outbreaks, a 25% attack rate is the norm.

I. Exacerbation of rash can be precipitated by exposure to heat or sun.

J. Rash may recur for weeks to months.

X. Complications

Generally none.

XI. Follow-up

None required.

XII. Referral

Children with hypoplastic anemias.

NOTES

EXTERNAL OTITIS

An inflammation of the external auditory canal, commonly known as "swimmer's ear," that is characterized by inflammation, pruritus, and pain.

I. Etiology

A. Bacterial: Pseudomonas, Streptococcus, Pneumococcus.

B. Fungal: Candida, Aspergillus.

C. Maceration, trauma, or excessive dryness of the lining of the ear canal causes it to be susceptible to superimposed infection.

D. Excess cerumen.

E. Secondary to tympanic membrane perforation with purulent drainage.

II. Incidence

It is most often seen in the summer, particularly in areas where swimming in fresh water is popular. It is seen year-round, but most often in adolescents who shampoo daily and where year-round swimming pools are available. It is not unusual to find external otitis in an infant who has a bottle in bed because of milk dribbling into the ear canal, keeping it moist and providing a medium for bacterial growth.

III. Subjective data

A. Pain in the ear.

B. Pain on movement of earlobe or when ear is touched.

C. Pain when chewing.

D. Sensation of itching or moisture in ear canal.

E. Discharge from ear.

F. Pertinent subjective data to obtain

1. Has child put anything in his ears?
2. History of use of cotton swabs to clean ear canals.
3. History of swimming, particularly in fresh water.
4. History of frequent showers and/or shampoos.
5. History of use of hairsprays.
6. History of otitis media with perforation.
7. History of use of earplugs.
8. Previous history of otitis externa.

IV. Objective data

A. Pain on movement of pinna or application of pressure on tragus.

B. Exquisite tenderness of canal on insertion of speculum.

C. Canal.

1. Edematous.
2. Erythematous.
3. Exudative; exudate may have foul odor.

D. Tympanic membrane.

1. May not be clearly visualized because of edema and exudate in canal.
2. May be inflamed with a widespread external otitis.
3. May be perforated if otitis externa is secondary to otitis media.

E. Pinna: may be inflamed and edematous.

F. Adenopathy: preauricular, postauricular, cervical.

V. Assessment

A. Diagnosis is confirmed by the characteristic inflammation and edema of the ear canal.

B. Differential diagnosis

1. Otitis media with secondary otitis externa: history of acute otitis media with perforation.
2. Foreign body: by history and visualization of foreign body.
3. Abscess in ear canal: mass visualized in canal.

VI. Plan

A. External otitis involving only the ear canal.

1. Coly-Mycin S Otic: 4 drops in affected ear tid or qid for 10 days.
   or
2. Cortisporin Otic: 4 drops in affected ear tid or qid for 10 days.
3. Aspirin, acetaminophen, or codeine for pain.

B. Do not order generic eardrops. They have been associated with increased complaints of pain on instillation, resulting in decreased compliance.

C. External otitis with fever, tympanic membrane involvement, cellulitis of pinna, or tender postauricular adenopathy should be treated with systemic antibiotics as well.

1. Ear drops as in A above. Order suspension if tympanic membrane is perforated or not visualized.
2. Augmentin: 40 mg/kg/day in 3 divided doses for 10 days.
   or if penicillin allergic:
3. Ceclor: 40 mg/kg/day in 3 divided doses.
4. Aspirin, acetominophen, or codeine for pain (see Drug Index).

D. Recurrent external otitis.

1. Follow initial treatment plan above. After final recheck, use one of the following for prophylaxis during the swimming season:
   a. Otic Domeboro Solution: 5 drops in each ear after swimming.
      or
   b. V-Sol Otic Solution: 5 drops in each ear after swimming.
2. In external otitis, the pH of the canal changes from acid to alkaline, creating a favorable environment for bacterial and mycotic overgrowth. Domeboro and V-Sol are antibacterial and antifungal with an acid pH and are effective in preventing recurrences.

VII. Education

A. Explain etiology to child and parent.

B. Medication.

1. Acute pain should subside within 24–48 hours of treatment.
2. Call office if no apparent response to medication.
3. Ear drops contain an antibiotic as well as cortisone to decrease inflammation.
4. Side effects of ear drops may be a local stinging or burning sensation or a rash where drops have come in contact with the skin.
5. For instillation of drops, child should lie on his side with the affected ear up. Pull tip of auricle up and back, and then instill drops without allowing

dropper to touch ear. Child should remain in this position for at least 5 minutes.

6. With more extensive involvement and treatment with systemic antibiotics, medication should be taken for 10 full days even if child seems better.

C. Ear canal must be kept dry.

1. No swimming.
2. No shampoos (without protection).
3. No showers.
4. Do not use cotton in ears; it will retain moisture.
5. Do not use earplugs.
6. Lamb's wool is water repellent and can be used to occlude canal for shampoos.
7. Silly Putty may be used after the acute phase to keep canal dry while bathing or shampooing; it forms a malleable external plug.
8. Do not use cotton swabs.

D. Recurrences are not uncommon, especially in adolescents who swim, shower, or shampoo daily. Many of them also use cotton swabs to dry and clean their ears. Suggest instillation of 2–3 drops of alcohol to dry ears after showering or swimming.

VIII. Follow-up

A. Recheck in 48–72 hours if there is marked cellulitis and tympanic membrane is not visualized.

B. Recheck immediately if suspected sensitivity to ear drops or child complains of increase in pain.

C. Recheck in 10 days. If not completely resolved, continue medication and precautions. Recheck again in 10 days.

IX. Complications

A. Local reaction to ear drops (cutaneous reaction to neomycin).

B. Recurrent external otitis.

X. Consultation/referral

A. Symptoms worse after 24 hours of treatment.

B. No response to treatment in 48–72 hours.

C. External otitis not markedly improved at 10-day recheck—will require culture and sensitivity.

D. Foreign body in ear canal not readily removed.

NOTES

NOTES

FEVER CONTROL

A common presenting symptom in pediatrics and a cardinal sign of illness. Most fevers in children are seen in conjunction with an acute infectious process. Fever control is secondary to identification and treatment of its underlying cause.

There is controversy over whether all fevers should be actively treated. Fever is actually a protective measure and in itself not harmful. Some experts contend that hyperpyrexia may be helpful in halting replication of a virus and some studies have demonstrated that fever of a moderate degree can enhance immunologic response. High body temperatures, however, can diminish or reverse this effect and a rapid increase in body temperature has been implicated as a triggering mechanism in febrile convulsions. Also, a child is generally more comfortable when his fever is reduced. For these last three reasons, fevers of over 102°F rectally should probably be treated once the etiology is established.

Elevation of temperature does not correlate with the severity of its cause (e.g., a neonate with sepsis may be hypothermic).

I. Subjective data

- **A.** History of exposure.
- **B.** Diseases prevalent in the community.
- **C.** Fever pattern.
  - **1.** Continuous.
  - **2.** Remittent.
  - **3.** Intermittent.
  - **4.** Recurrent.
- **D.** How high has the temperature been?
- **E.** Duration of fever.
- **F.** Determine accuracy of parent's method of assessing temperature.
- **G.** Does child seem sick?
- **H.** Is there any change in level of sensorium?
- **I.** Are there other associated symptoms?
  - **1.** Respiratory.
  - **2.** Gastrointestinal.
  - **3.** Genitourinary.
  - **4.** Musculoskeletal.
  - **5.** Central nervous system.
- **J.** History of drug ingestion.
- **K.** History of decreased liquid intake.
- **L.** Determine what treatment has been used and its effectiveness.

II. Objective data

- **A.** Complete physical examination to determine infectious etiology, include weight.
- **B.** Activity level.
- **C.** Level of sensorium.

D. Assess state of hydration (see Appendix D, Clinical Signs of Dehydration).

E. Toxicity.

F. Laboratory tests as indicated by history and physical findings.

1. Urinalysis and culture.
2. Throat culture.
3. CBC.
4. Blood culture.
5. CSF examination.
6. Stool culture.

III. Plan

A. Assess parent's ability to take and interpret temperature correctly.

B. Oral temperature for most children 5 years of age and older.

1. Place thermometer under tongue and leave it there for 4 minutes with lips closed.
2. If child has had anything to eat or drink or has been chewing gum, wait for 10 minutes before taking his temperature.

C. Rectal temperature. Lubricate rectal thermometer with K-Y jelly or petroleum jelly, and gently insert 2.5 cm into rectum. Leave in place for 3–4 minutes.

D. Axillary temperature. Place thermometer high in axilla and hold arm close to body; remove shirt so that skin surfaces are touching. Leave in place for 4–5 minutes.

E. Normal temperature values

Oral	98.6°F ± 0.4–0.5°F
Rectal	99.4°F ± 0.4–0.5°F
Axillary	97.6°F ± 0.4–0.5°F

Fever peaks at about 6 P.M. and is at its lowest point at about 4 A.M.

F. With temperature elevation, for each degree of fever

1. Pulse increases 10 beats/minute. The increase may be higher in bacterial infections. Increased intracranial pressure, meningitis, and salmonellosis are associated with a decreased pulse rate.
2. Respirations increase 2 cycles/minute. Increased intracranial pressure, pulmonary disease, and acid-base disturbance produce greater elevations.

G. Hydration

1. Encourage liquids to prevent dehydration; clear liquids are easiest to retain.
2. Give small amounts frequently.
3. Try tea, cola, ginger ale, Popsicles, ice chips, Jell-O, ices, half- or full-strength juices.

H. Sponging or bathing

1. Every 2 hours if necessary for 30 minutes maximum.
2. Use tepid water—water that feels comfortable to the parent's wrist. Do not use alcohol or ice water. Chilling effect can cause shivering, which can increase body temperature. Rubbing with alcohol can cause toxicity through inhalation of fumes.
3. Rub skin briskly with a washcloth or towel to dry. Brisk rubbing increases skin capillary circulation and heat loss.

4. Cold sponging is generally recommended only for heat illness (hyperthermia).

I. Clothing
   1. Clothe lightly to enhance heat loss through skin by radiation.
   2. Avoid overdressing or covering with blankets, which will decrease radiation and cause further elevation of temperature.

J. Activity. Encourage rest; activity can increase body temperature.

K. Antipyretics for rectal temperatures over 102°F.
   1. Use with caution.
   2. Can mask fever.
   3. Will not cure disease.
   4. Do not use if child is dehydrated.
   5. Acetaminophen:
      a. 15 mg/kg every four hours.
      b. Do not exceed 60 mg/kg/day. Give adequate dose for weight.
      c. Acetaminophen half-life is significantly prolonged in infants and newborns. Use at a reduced dosage and with caution.
   6. PediaProfen or Children's Advil Susp. (100 mg/5ml).
      a. 5 mg/kg every 6 to 8 hours for fevers 102.5°F or less.
      b. 10 mg/kg every 6 to 8 hours for fevers over 102.5°F.
      c. Maximum daily dose: 40 mg/kg.
      d. Do not use for infants under 6 months.

IV. Follow-up

A. Dependent on degree of fever and etiology. With no established diagnosis, telephone contact should be maintained every 12–24 hours. Even if child does not seem sick, parents may be anxious without definite diagnosis.

B. Child should be reevaluated if fever continues beyond 24 hours, if signs of toxicity occur, or if any signs or symptoms of infection occur.

V. Consultation/referral

A. Fever persisting over 5 days (fever of undetermined origin).

B. Acute high fever or prolonged high- or low-grade fever.

C. Infant under 6 months of age.

D. Child with a stiff neck, petechiae, swollen or inflamed joints, or dehydration.

E. Tachypnea out of proportion to temperature elevation.

F. Fever associated with seizure.

NOTES

NOTES

FROSTBITE

Cellular injury due to cold characterized by pallor and numbness of the affected area.

I. Etiology

A. Exposure to cold temperatures, usually for a prolonged period of time.

B. The severity of frostbite is influenced by the following:

1. Duration of exposure.
2. Intensity of cold exposure determined by both temperature and windchill factor.
3. Rate and method of rewarming.

II. Incidence

A. Seen in winter months, especially in young children who do not have proper supervision while playing in the snow, in skiers, and in winter sports enthusiasts (e.g., mountain climbers, winter campers).

B. The parts most subject to cold trauma are the hands, feet, and face—particularly the cheeks, nose, and ears.

III. Subjective data

A. Often asymptomatic.

B. Numbness.

C. Prickling sensation.

D. Pruritus.

E. Stiffness.

F. Skin white and cold.

G. Complaints of pain in mild or moderate frostbite.

H. Pertinent subjective data to obtain to aid in assessing degree of frostbite:

1. Previous history of frostbite in same area.
2. Duration of exposure.
3. Cold intensity—temperature and wind velocity.
4. If treated, how was rewarming accomplished?

IV. Objective data

Degree of frostbite cannot be accurately assessed prior to thawing.

A. Mild

1. Skin pale and cold.
2. Edema.
3. Area feels frozen on the surface, but gentle pressure reveals soft tissue underneath.

B. Moderate to severe

1. Skin pale and cold.
2. Edema.
3. Area feels solidly frozen on deep palpation.
4. Blister and bulla formation 24–48 hours after thawing.
5. Necrosis of subcutaneous tissues 24–48 hours later.

V. Assessment

A. Diagnosis of frostbite is made by history of exposure and appearance of white, cold skin in affected area.

1. Mild. Erythema and edema of part after thawing; sometimes becomes purple. No significant tissue damage.
2. Moderate to severe. After thawing, area becomes hyperemic, then blue, purple, or black and edematous. Blister and bulla formation occurs in 24–48 hours. With severe frostbite, lack of formation of blebs is indicative of inadequate circulation and necrosis of underlying tissue.

B. Investigate possible parental neglect in young children with moderate to severe frostbite.

VI. Plan

A. Do not attempt rewarming if there is danger of refreezing.

B. Check body temperature to rule out hypothermia.

C. Loosen all constricting garments.

D. Remove all wet clothing in contact with skin.

E. Do *not* rub or massage affected area.

F. Rewarming. Warm gradually. Rapid rewarming increases cell metabolism and without adequate blood supply (due to vasoconstriction), can damage cells.

1. Immerse part in whirlpool or agitated water at 100–105°F; monitor water temperature with a thermometer.
2. For face or ears, use warm, moist soaks, changing frequently to maintain temperature at 100–105°F; monitor water temperature.
3. Continue rewarming for about 20 minutes (until area is unfrozen).
4. Use analgesics as necessary: aspirin, acetaminophen, or codeine. Rewarming is a painful process.
5. Elevate affected part.

G. General measures

1. Provide dry clothing.
2. Adjust environmental temperature.
3. Encourage warm liquids.

H. Assess degree of involvement

1. Mild or first-degree of small area: may be followed at home with a careful follow-up plan.
2. Mild with extensive involvement or moderate to severe: consult with physician for treatment and admission to hospital.

I. Sterile, loose dressing to necrotic areas.

VII. Education

A. Never rewarm with dry heat (e.g., oven or fireplace).

B. Do not rub frostbitten area; it will cause further tissue damage.

C. Protect area from trauma—use padding when indicated.

D. Avoid smoking, which causes peripheral vasoconstriction, decreasing blood flow to skin.

E. Keep part elevated.

F. Watch carefully for blistering or tissue damage.

G. Do not puncture blisters.

H. Do not expose part to extremes in temperature.

I. Paresthesia of injured area is common. Expect some burning, prickling, or tingling sensations.

J. Expect future hypersensitivity to cold and increased susceptibility to repeated frostbite of injured area.

K. Use face mask, earmuffs, mittens, or heavy boots as applicable for protection.

L. Prevention

1. Avoid alcohol and cigarettes during cold exposure.
    a. Nicotine causes vasoconstriction, inhibiting flow of blood to periphery.
    b. Alcohol causes peripheral vasodilation, which increases rate of heat loss from the skin.
2. If suspicious of potential frostbite, warm by natural body heat (e.g., place hands in groin or axilla). Do not use snow, ice, or dry heat.
3. If frostbite has occurred, do not thaw until possibility of refreezing is eliminated.
4. Wear several layers of loose, warm clothing. This protects better than one heavy, well-fitting garment.
5. Do not scrub face, shave, or use after-shave lotion prior to anticipated exposure.
6. Mittens generally offer more protection than gloves.
7. Wet skin increases the cooling and freezing rate. Wet clothing causes conductive heat loss from the part covered.
8. Use "buddy" system when out in severe cold; check each other's noses, faces, and ears for evidence of frostbite.
9. If exposure planned, take extra socks and mittens.

VIII. Follow-up

A. Recheck by phone in 24 hours.

B. Return to office if any blisters appear.

C. Return to office if any signs of infection.

IX. Complications

A. Necrosis of affected area with subsequent infection.

B. Area has increased susceptibility to frostbite.

X. Consultation/referral

A. Moderate to severe degrees of frostbite—appearance of blisters or bulla.

B. Any question of parental neglect.

NOTES

NOTES

HAND-FOOT-AND-MOUTH DISEASE

A contagious viral disease characterized by fever and vesicular lesions of the mouth, palms of the hands, and soles of the feet.

I. Etiology

Coxsackie virus A, an enterovirus.

II. Incidence

A highly infectious disease generally occurring among children in epidemic form; seen mainly in summer. Enteroviral infections with other manifestations may be prevalent in the community concurrently (herpangina, gastroenteritis).

III. Incubation period

3–6 days.

IV. Communicability

Highly communicable. Spread by fecal-oral route and possibly by respiratory route. The virus can maintain activity for days at room temperature.

IV. Subjective data

A. Abrupt onset of fever—around 101°F.

B. Sore throat; dysphagia.

C. Anorexia.

D. Occasionally headache and abdominal pain.

E. A rash on the palms of the hands and the soles of the feet may or may not be noted.

F. Convulsions may occur with onset of fever.

V. Objective data

A. Elevated temperature.

B. Hyperemia of anterior tonsillar pillars.

C. Vesicles on an erythematous base on anterior tonsillar pillars; also, on soft palate, tonsils, and uvula. Vesicles rapidly ulcerate, leaving shallow ulcers.

D. Maculopapular rash and vesicles on palms of hands and soles of feet, as well as interdigital surfaces.

VI. Assessment

A. Diagnosis. Classic case easily diagnosed by clinical picture.

B. Differential diagnosis

1. Herpangina: clinical picture similar, but no lesions on hands and feet.
2. Gingivostomatitis (herpes simplex); gingival and buccal mucosa involved; no lesions on hands and feet.

VII. Plan

A. Treatment is symptomatic.

B. Warm saline mouth rinses.

C. Acetaminophen or PediaProfen for elevated temperature and discomfort (see Drug Index for dosage and administration).

D. Tepid baths for elevated temperature.

E. Force fluids.

1. Cold, bland liquids.
2. Try Popsicles, Jell-O, sherbet.

VIII. Education

A. Call back if child will not take fluids or is vomiting.
B. Fever will last 1–4 days.
C. Do not overdress; keep child cool.
D. Be alert for dehydration (see Appendix D, Clinical Signs of Dehydration).
E. Transmitted by direct contact with nose and throat secretions, stools, and blood of infected child.
F. Keep child isolated until temperature is normal for 24 hours.
G. Highly contagious, at least during acute phase.
H. There is no prophylaxis.
I. Carbonated drinks, citrus juices, hot, spicy foods, and the like should be avoided, since they may increase discomfort.
J. Do not be concerned about dietary intake during acute stage, but do force fluids.
K. Prognosis is excellent—disease is self-limited.
L. Immunity to infecting strain is generally conferred after one attack.
M. Lesions may persist for a week or more.

IX. Follow-up

A. Maintain daily telephone contact if temperature is markedly elevated.
B. Generally no follow-up visit is necessary.

X. Consultation/referral

A. Signs of dehydration.
B. Hand-foot-and-mouth disease in an infant.
C. Prolonged course—no improvement within 5–6 days.
D. Febrile convulsions.

NOTES

HERPANGINA

A communicable viral disease characterized by the abrupt onset of fever and vesicular eruptions of the anterior tonsillar pillars.

I. Etiology

Coxsackie virus A, an enterovirus.

II. Incidence

A highly infectious disease generally occurring among infants and children in epidemic form; seen mainly in summer. Other types of Coxsackie viruses may be present in the community at the same time.

III. Incubation period

3–5 days.

IV. Subjective data

A. Abrupt onset of fever up to 105°F (40.5°C).

B. Dysphagia occurring within 24–36 hours.

C. Sore throat after temperature elevation.

D. Anorexia.

E. Occasionally, headache and abdominal pain.

F. Convulsions may occur with abrupt onset of fever.

V. Objective data

A. Elevated temperature.

B. Hyperemia of anterior tonsillar pillars.

C. Vesicles on an erythematous base on anterior tonsillar pillars; also, but less frequently, on soft palate, tonsils, and uvula.

D. Vesicles ulcerate rapidly, leaving shallow ulcers.

E. There is no involvement of gingival or buccal mucosa.

VI. Assessment

A. Diagnosis. Classic case easily diagnosed by the clinical picture.

B. Differential diagnosis

1. Hand-foot-and-mouth disease: clinical picture similar, but small, grayish papulovesicular lesions on palms of hands and soles of feet.
2. Acute gingivostomatitis (herpes simplex): gingival and buccal mucosa involved.

VII. Plan

A. Treatment is symptomatic.

B. Warm saline mouth rinses.

C. Acetaminophen or PediaProfen for elevated temperature and discomfort.

D. Chloraseptic gargle for children over 6 years of age only; may be used every 2 hours.

E. Tepid baths for elevated temperature.

F. Force fluids—cold, bland liquids; also try Popsicles, Jell-O, sherbet. Avoid carbonated beverages or acidic juices.

G. Soft, bland diet—try yogurt, puddings.

VIII. Education

A. Call back if child will not take fluids or is vomiting.
B. Fever will last 1–4 days.
C. Tepid water for baths; air dry or rub briskly with towel.
D. Do not overdress; keep child cool.
E. Be alert for dehydration (see Appendix D, Clinical Signs of Dehydration).
F. Transmitted by direct contact with nose and throat secretions, stools, and blood of infected child.
G. Keep child isolated until temperature is normal for 24 hours.
H. Highly contagious, at least during acute phase.
I. There is no prophylaxis.
J. Carbonated drinks, citrus juices, hot, spicy foods, and the like should be avoided, since they may increase discomfort.
K. Do not be concerned about dietary intake during acute stage, but do force fluids.
L. Prognosis is excellent—herpangina is self-limited.
M. Immunity to infecting strain is generally conferred after one attack.

IX. Follow-up

A. Maintain daily telephone contact during acute phase.
B. Generally no follow-up visit is necessary.

X. Complications

A. Febrile convulsions.
B. Dehydration.

XI. Consultation/referral

A. Signs of dehydration.
B. Prolonged course—child not improved in 5 days.
C. Febrile convulsions.

NOTES

HERPES SIMPLEX TYPE 1

A recurrent viral infection characterized by multiple small, grouped vesicles on an erythematous base on the skin or mucous membranes.

I. **Etiology**

Herpes simplex virus type 1 (HSV-1) in its recurrent form. The primary herpes simplex infection is often seen in children as acute herpetic gingivostomatitis (see Herpetic Gingivostomatitis). The virus remains latent in the sensory ganglia and can be activated by a number of triggering factors or excitants throughout life. Emotional stress, exposure to sun, drugs, menses, trauma, febrile illness, and systemic infections have been identified as factors responsible for activating the virus.

HSV-1 also causes 5 to 15 percent of initial episodes of genital herpes.

II. **Incidence**

Seen in all age groups; affects approximately 7% of the population. Incidence of herpes simplex lesions is related to susceptibility and exposure to triggering factors.

III. **Incubation period**

2–12 days.

IV. **Communicability**

At least as long as lesion is present.

V. **Subjective data**

A. Burning or tingling sensation several hours prior to appearance of lesion.
B. "Cold sore" on lip and/or sore anywhere on body.
C. Generally no systemic symptoms unless fever or infection is the triggering factor.
D. Frequently a past history of herpetic gingivostomatitis.
E. Frequently a history of a similar lesion following exposure to same triggering factor.
F. Pertinent subjective data to obtain. Any symptoms of ocular involvement, such as photophobia, pain (herpetic keratitis), or inflammation of the eyelid (herpes simplex blepharitis).

VI. **Objective data**

A. Lesion progresses through the following stages; may be seen at any stage.
   1. Collection of small transparent vesicles on an erythematous base.
   2. Vesicles become cloudy and purulent.
   3. Vesicles dry and become crusted; may crack and bleed. Base is edematous and erythematous.
B. Lesion generally found at the mucocutaneous junction of the lips or nose but may be found anywhere on the body; consistently at the same site with recurrent infections.
D. Herpetic whitlow (infection of the finger) may be found on finger or thumb of child—particularly one who sucks a finger or thumb.
C. Regional, tender lymphadenopathy often present.
D. Inspect entire body.

VII. **Assessment**

A. Diagnosis usually made by characteristic appearance of lesion (grouped vesicles) and history of similar lesion or herpetic gingivostomatitis.

B. Differential diagnosis. Impetigo: lesions often similar; presence of yellow or honey-colored crust on lesion is indicative of bacterial superinfection.

VIII. Plan

One of the following may be tried. There is no documentation that these treatments are of value in decreasing healing time, but they may give symptomatic relief.

A. Idoxuridine ointment (Herplex): apply to lesion hourly for 1 day, then qid until lesion is healed.

B. Blistex or petroleum jelly: apply to lesion as often as desired to soothe and protect from cracking.

C. Bacitracin or Neosporin ointment: apply to lesion 4 times a day for prevention or treatment of bacterial superinfection.

D. Zovirax ointment is not generally indicated for the treatment of simple, uncomplicated HSV infection in non-immunocompromised host. It may help select out resistant strains. It can, however be prescribed for particularly large or unsightly lesions or to speed the healing process in certain circumstances—i.e., for a bride, for a health care worker, or other such cases.

IX. Education

A. Latent virus in sensory ganglia can be activated by stress, sun exposure, drugs, menses, trauma, fever, or infection.

B. Incubation period is 2–12 days.

C. Recurrences are common and are usually at the same site.

1. Recurrent lesions are less painful than the original herpetic gingivostomatitis.
2. Recurrent lesions are preceded by a burning or tingling sensation, which may last for several hours.

D. Lesions may be spread by autoinoculation. In a young child concurrent lesions may be found on fingers or thumb (particularly if child is a finger or thumb sucker). Lesions may also be spread to labia via autoinoculation.

E. Lesion does not leave a scar but may cause temporary depigmentation.

F. Lesion is self-limited, lasting 8–14 days.

G. Transmitted through direct contact with saliva.

H. Communicable at least as long as lesion is present.

I. Do not allow child near newborns, children with eczema or burns, or persons on immunosuppressive therapy.

J. Prevention. There is no cure for recurrent herpes simplex, but many methods have been attempted to prevent or abort lesions. The most effective method is to avoid known triggering factors if possible.

1. For lesions activated by sun exposure, liberal use of sun-screening agents (e.g., Sundown) has been effective for some persons.
2. Application of ice to lesion may be of benefit in aborting the lesion if used as soon as tingling or burning sensation is felt.
3. Fluorinated corticosteroid creams used at the onset of tingling have been felt to be useful in diminishing the severity of the lesion by decreasing the inflammatory response. Such creams are contraindicated for use on the face, since they may cause telangiectasia.
4. Zovirax ointment is not indicated for the prevention of recurrent HSV.

X. Complications

A. Secondary bacterial infection.

B. Eczema herpeticum in a child with atopic dermatitis: characterized by irritability, high temperature (104°F), and generalized lesions (crops of vesicles at site of eczematous skin lesions).

C. Erythema multiforme may occur in 3 to 4 days after a recurrence.

XI. Consultation/referral

A. Neonates or infants.

B. Suspicion of herpetic keratitis or herpes simplex blepharitis (photophobia, pain).

C. Children with atopic dermatitis.

D. Newborns or children with atopic dermatitis, with burns, or those who are immunocompromised exposed to herpes simplex.

NOTES

HERPES SIMPLEX TYPE 2

One of the most common sexually transmitted diseases, characterized by painful vesicular lesions of the genitals. An acute infection or reactivation of latent herpes.

I. Etiology

Herpesvirus hominus type 2; occasionally type 1, especially in primary infections. Seventy-five percent of type 1 (HSV-1) infections involve the face and skin above the waist. Approximately 75% of type 2 (HSV-2) infections involve the genitalia and skin below the waist. Either can, however, be found at either site.

HSV-2 persists in a latent form following infection. Reactivation occurs in about 80% of cases with variable frequency. Recurrence rate generally decreases after the first year.

II. Incidence

Primarily seen in persons beyond the age of puberty. It is one of the most common sexually transmitted diseases.

III. Incubation

A. Three to 12 days following exposure. Maximum may be as long as several weeks; minimum is 32 hours.

B. Recurrent herpes: 24 hours following precipitating cause.

IV. Communicability

A. Primary infection: 15–42 days.

B. Recurrent infection: 6 days.

C. Virus is present in the lesions during the prodromal period; highly contagious during prodromal.

V. Subjective data

A. Primary infection

1. Tenderness of genital area prior to appearance of lesions.
2. Lesions on vulva or penis.
3. Severe pain in genital area.
4. Swollen glands.
5. Fever may be present with associated symptoms of headache, malaise, and myalgia.
6. Discharge from lesions of vulva or penis.
7. Inability to void, or burning and stinging on urination.
8. May have lesions or "sores" at other sites.

B. Recurrent infection

1. Burning or tingling sensation of several hours duration prior to appearance of lesions.
2. Lesions are less painful than in primary infection; may be pruritic.
3. Urethral or vaginal discharge.
4. Lesions are fewer in number than in primary infection and are generally external.

VI. Objective data

A. Primary herpes

1. Edema, erythema, and exquisite tenderness of vulva or penis. Uncircumcised males may present with more severe involvement.
2. Multiple discrete or grouped vesicular lesions with subsequent erosion in 1 to 3 days producing gray-white ulcerations.
3. Lesions are found on the labia, vagina, and/or cervix in females and external genitalia in males.
4. Lesions may occur at other sites from autoinoculation—on buttocks, thighs, fingers, pharynx, conjunctiva.
5. Discharge from vagina or penis.
6. Tender inguinal adenopathy.
7. Bladder may be distended.

B. Recurrent herpes

1. Discrete or clustered vesicles on an erythematous base; lesions are generally external.
2. Mucoid discharge if cervical, vaginal, or urethral involvement.
3. Inguinal adenopathy not a significant finding.

VII. Assessment

A. Diagnosis is generally made from the history and typical appearance of the lesions. There may be a history of exposure. If diagnosis is in doubt, a culture of the vesicle fluid may be done.

B. Differential diagnosis

1. Traumatic lesions.
2. Scabies.
3. Chancroid.

VIII. Plan

There is no prophylaxis or cure for herpes simplex type 2; treatment is aimed at pain control.

A. Topical: 5% acyclovir ointment (Zovirax) 6 times a day for 1 week. Begin therapy within 6 days of onset.

B. Sitz baths.

C. Dry heat (hair dryer).

D. With urinary retention, advise females they may void with less pain while in the tub. (Catheterization may be necessary.)

E. Topical anesthetics

1. Benzocaine aerosol: use as needed.
   or
2. Lidocaine jelly 2% qid.

F. Betadine 1% 3–4 times a day; apply with cotton balls.

G. Zovirax capsules: for severe primary herpes or to shorten duration of recurrent episodes.

1. Primary herpes: 1 capsule 5 times a day every 4 hours for 10 days.
2. Recurrent herpes: 1 capsule 5 times a day every 4 hours for 5 days. Initiate therapy at first sign of recurrence.
3. Chronic suppressive therapy for recurrent herpes: 400 mg (two 200 mg capsules) 2 times a day for up to 12 months.

H. Treatment should include evaluation for other sexually transmitted diseases.

IX. Education

A. Avoid indiscriminate sexual practices.

B. Avoid sexual contact with person with active lesions. Genital ulcers are of particular concern because they provide a portal of entry for the HIV virus.

C. Virus is shed during prodrome and can also be shed when entirely asymptomatic.

D. There is no prevention (other than safe sex) or cure for herpes simplex type 2.

E. Zovirax ointment will help decrease healing time and in some cases, decrease the duration of viral shedding and duration of pain. It will not prevent transmission of the virus to other persons or prevent recurrences.

F. Zovirax orally shortens the viral shedding time. In some patients it may decrease the duration of pain and new lesion formation. With frequent recurrences (6 or more episodes a year), administration of Zovirax may prevent or reduce severity and/or frequency of recurrences.

G. Although benzocaine aerosol may be used frequently for comfort, caution patient that it may be a skin sensitizer.

H. Stress hygiene, particularly careful hand-washing to avoid spread of virus.

I. Use finger cot or rubber glove to apply ointment to avoid autoinoculation of other areas or transmission to other people.

J. Primary attack lasts 2–6 weeks.

K. HSV-2 persists in a latent form following infection. Reactivation occurs in about 80% of cases with variable frequency.

L. Recurrent attack lasts a few hours to 10 days.

M. Recurrent attacks are less frequent as patient becomes older.

N. Advise patient that recurrent episodes are heralded by burning or tingling sensation prior to eruption of lesions. Virus can be transmitted during this time; avoid intercourse.

O. If herpes simplex type 1 caused initial attack, recurrences are unlikely to occur in genital area.

P. Pap smear should be done yearly because of increased incidence of dysplasia and carcinoma of cervix.

X. Complications

A. Secondary infection.

B. Urinary retention.

XI. Follow-up

A. Call stat if unable to void.

B. Return if question of secondary infection.

C. Annual Pap smears.

XII. Referral

A. Pregnant woman.

B. Patient with urinary retention.

NOTES

HERPES ZOSTER

An acute viral infection affecting the dorsal root ganglion cells. It is self-limited and localized and is characterized by a vesicular eruption and neurologic pain.

I. Etiology

Varicella zoster virus. After an attack of chickenpox, the virus remains latent in the dorsal root ganglia. Varicella is the manifestation of the VZV in a nonimmune host and herpes zoster is the recrudescence of the latent virus in a partially immune host.

II. Incidence

Relatively rare under 10 years of age, but can occur at any age. There is an increased incidence in patients with malignancies or on immunosuppressive therapy.

III. Incubation period

2–3 weeks.

IV. Subjective data

- **A.** Usual history of varicella.
- **B.** History of itching, tenderness, or pain in area about 3–5 days prior to rash. Prodromal pain can be quite severe and can mimic cardiac or pleural disease, acute abdomen or vertebral disease.
- **C.** Rash.
  1. Erythematous maculopapular rash that progresses to vesicles within 24 hours.
  2. Generally on trunk, face, or back.

V. Objective data

- **A.** Rash: small, grouped vesicles on an erythematous base.
- **B.** Distribution.
  1. Appears first at a point near the central nervous system along a dermatome or two adjacent dermatomes.
  2. Ends at midline of body.
  3. Generally on trunk (over 50%), trigeminal (10–20%), lumbosacral and cervical (10 to 20%).
  4. Generally unilateral.
  5. A few vesicles may be outside the dermatome.
- **C.** Successive crops of lesions may appear.
- **D.** Pain with rash is less frequent in children than in adults.
- **E.** Occasionally a generalized rash will occur.
- **F.** Regional lymphadenopathy.

VI. Assessment

- **A.** Diagnosis is made by the distribution and characteristic appearance of the rash as well as by the associated pain. It may be confirmed by cytologic smear of vesicle.
- **B.** Differential diagnosis
  1. Coxsackie viruses: distribution of rash differs; lesions do not crust.

2. Multiple insect bites: generally do not follow path of dermatome or have the characteristic appearance (small group of vesicles).

VII. Plan

A. Treatment is symptomatic.

B. Calamine lotion.

C. Cool compresses with Burow's solution 1:20.

D. Acetaminophen for pain (children do not always have sensory changes, so analgesics may not be indicated).

E. Infected lesions: Neosporin or bacitracin ointment 3 times a day.

F. Zovirax capsules: 800 mg 5 times daily for 7 days.

VIII. Education

A. Successive lesions appear for up to one week.

B. Eruption usually clears in 14–21 days; if vesicles appear over a period of 1 week, clearing may take up to 5 weeks.

C. Lesions become pustular and dry and crust over.

D. Transmitted by both direct and indirect contact. Approximately 15% of susceptible (nonimmune) persons will contract varicella.

E. Avoid exposure of children with malignancies or persons on immunosuppressive therapy.

F. Postherpetic neuralgia may persist once lesions have healed.

G. There is no prevention for herpes zoster.

H. Compresses: use cool soft cloths 4 times a day.

I. Zovirax reduces viral shedding time and the duration of new lesion formation. It also shortens the times to complete lesion scabbing, healing, and the cessation of pain.

IX. Follow-up

A. Generally not indicated for typical case.

B. Return immediately if there are any symptoms of ocular involvement.

C. Recheck in 5 days if there is secondary bacterial infection.

X. Complications

A. Secondary bacterial infection.

B. Rarely, ocular complications.

XI. Consultation/referral

A. Patients with lesions on the tip of the nose, since there is a possibility of keratoconjunctivitis.

B. Patients with hemorrhagic or bullous lesions.

C. Patients with disseminated herpes zoster.

D. Patients on immunosuppressive therapy.

NOTES

HERPETIC GINGIVOSTOMATITIS

An acute primary herpes simplex infection characterized by painful vesicular lesions and ulcers of the oral mucosa.

I. **Etiology**
Herpes simplex virus (type 1) in its primary form.

II. **Incidence**
Gingivostomatitis is the most frequent manifestation of the primary form of herpes simplex. It is the most common cause of stomatitis in children under 5 years of age.

III. **Incubation period**
2 to 12 days with a mean of 6–7 days.

IV. **Communicability**
Highly infectious throughout course of illness which takes 4 to 5 days to evolve and at least an additional 7 days for resolution. It is transmitted by saliva and by contact with infected skin or mucous membranes.

V. **Subjective data**

A. History of exposure to a child or adult with cold sores or stomatitis.

B. Fever: 104–105°F.

C. Irritability.

D. Malaise.

E. Sore throat and mouth.

F. Gums red and swollen.

G. Painful sores in the mouth.

H. Drooling.

I. Foul odor to breath.

J. Not eating; taking liquids poorly.

VI. **Objective data**

A. Fever.

B. Vesicular lesions:

1. On or around lips, along gingiva, on anterior tongue, and on hard palate. May be seen over entire buccal mucosa.
2. Appear on chin and face.
3. Vesicles rupture leaving a grayish ulceration on an erythematous base.

C. Gingival edema, erythema, and bleeding.

D. Enlarged tender cervical and submandibular glands.

E. Increased salivation.

F. Foul odor to breath.

G. Occasional vesicular lesion on a sucked thumb or finger.

H. Rarely may occur as a generalized vesicular eruption.

I. May also rarely have herpetic vulvovaginitis from handling genital area with contaminated hands.

VII. **Assessment**

A. Diagnosis is usually made by clinical findings.

B. Differential diagnosis

1. Herpangina: no lesions on buccal mucosa, posterior pharyngeal lesions only.
2. Hand-foot-and-mouth disease: oral lesions not on buccal and gingival mucosa; rash present on hands and feet.
3. Varicella: if the rare type of gingivostomatitis with generalized vesicular reaction.

VIII. Plan

A. Acetaminophen or PediaProfen for fever or pain (see Drug Index for dosage and administration).

B. One of the following for discomfort:

1. Gly-Oxide Liquid to clean lesions 4 times a day (after meals and at bedtime).
2. Viscous Xylocaine: 1 tbsp (15 ml or 300 mg) swished around mouth every 4 hours.
3. Chloraseptic Mouthwash (for children over 6 years of age) every 2 hours as needed.

C. Force fluids—cold, bland liquids.

D. Tepid baths every 2 hours as needed.

IX. Education

A. Alert parent to signs of dehydration—decreased urine output, elevated temperature, decreased tears, dry mucous membranes, increased thirst, lethargy (see Appendix D, Clinical Signs of Dehydration).

B. Give cold liquids or semisolids.

1. Try Popsicles, sherbet, ice cream, Jell-O.
2. Maintain hydration with frequent sips.
3. Use straw to minimize contact with lips and gums.

C. Do not give carbonated beverages or citrus juices.

D. Do not be concerned about solid food during acute phase.

E. Do not allow child to swallow Chloraseptic Mouthwash or Viscous Xylocaine.

F. Gly-Oxide: place 10 drops on tongue and swish around mouth; do not swallow or rinse.

G. Tepid water for baths; air dry or rub briskly to increase skin capillary circulation and heat loss.

H. Dress child lightly.

I. Duration of illness: 1–3 weeks.

1. Duration of acute phase: 4–9 days.
2. Ulcers heal spontaneously in 7–14 days.

J. Following primary infection, the herpes simplex virus remains latent in sensory neural ganglia innervating sites originally involved. Therefore recurrences occur in identical regions but are less severe than primary infections.

K. Recurrent infection appears as a cold sore or fever blister occurring on the mucocutaneous junction.

L. In adolescents, exudative pharyngitis with typical herpetic lesions on the tonsils may be caused by the HSV-2 virus due to oral/genital sex.

Note: Highly communicable throughout course of illness. Do not expose to newborns, children with eczema, children on immunosuppressive therapy, or children with burns.

X. Follow-up

A. Recheck in 2 days by telephone.

B. Call immediately if liquid intake decreases or signs of dehydration or secondary bacterial infection appear.

C. Call immediately if complaints of eye problems.

XI. Complications

A. Dehydration.

B. Keratitis.

C. Conjunctivitis.

XII. Consultation/referral

A. Newborns and infants.

B. Dehydration in child of any age.

C. Generalized skin eruption.

D. Signs or symptoms of ocular involvement—photophobia, pain, inflammation, or ulceration of cornea.

NOTES

HORDEOLUM

A hordeolum, or "sty," is a localized infection of a sebaceous gland of the eyelash follicle.

I. Etiology

Causative organism is usually *Staphylococcus aureus.*

II. Incidence

Occurs frequently in children.

III. Subjective data

A. Localized swelling, tenderness, and inflammation of margin of eyelid.
B. May complain of a bump or pimple on eyelid.
C. Generally unilateral.
D. Visual acuity is not affected.

IV. Objective data

A. Localized erythema, edema, and pain near the lid edge.
B. Abscess may point at lid margin.
C. May have purulent drainage along lid margin.

V. Assessment

A. Diagnosis is made by clinical picture of erythema, pain, and swelling.
B. Differential diagnosis
   1. Chalazion: a chronic granulomatous infection of the meibomian gland that is relatively painless.
   2. Conjunctivitis: conjunctival erythema; mucopurulent discharge; foreign body sensation. No localized swelling.
   3. Blepharitis: chronic scaling and discharge with matting of the eyelashes; not localized.

VI. Plan

A. Hot, moist compresses for 15–20 minutes every 2–3 hours.
B. 10% Sodium Sulamyd Ophthalmic Ointment (sodium sulfacetamide) 4–5 times daily during acute stage.
C. Assess visual acuity. Child may rub eyes repeatedly with a refraction error.

VII. Education

A. For moist compresses, use a soft cloth and water as warm as child can tolerate.
B. Medication
   1. To instill ophthalmic ointment, gently pull down lower lid and apply a thin ribbon of ointment.
   2. Side effects to ointment are rare, but call back immediately if child complains of burning or stinging.
   3. Vision may be blurred temporarily following administration of ointment.
C. Use thorough hand-washing technique after soaks and instillation of medication to prevent spread.
D. Keep fingers away from eyes.
E. Never squeeze a sty.

F. Inflammation generally subsides after 5–6 days.

G. Continue treatment for several days following resolution of lesions.

VIII. Follow-up

A. Return immediately if symptoms get worse.

B. Return in 48 hours if no response to treatment.

C. Return if lesion becomes larger and points.

D. Return in 6 days if lesion is not resolved.

E. Return for evaluation if problem is recurrent.

IX. Complications

A. Conjunctivitis.

B. Cellulitis.

X. Consultation/referral

A. If lesion is well localized to assess need for incision and drainage.

B. No response to treatment after 48 hours.

C. Lesion not resolved after 6 days.

D. Recurrent sties: may indicate immunologic deficit or systemic disease (e.g., diabetes).

E. Cellulitis: may require systemic antibiotics.

NOTES

IMPETIGO

Purulent infection of the skin characterized by honey-colored, crusted lesions or bullae surrounded by narrow margin of erythema.

I. Etiology

Most common causative organism is *Staphylococcus aureus.* Earlier research suggested that most crusted impetigo was streptococcal in origin. It now appears that most crusted as well as bullous impetigo is caused by *Staphylococcus aureus.*

Streptococcal impetigo is always crusted. Bullous impetigo is virtually never strep. Secondary impetigo (superimposed on a preexisting condition such as atopic dermatitis) is nearly always staphylococcal.

II. Incidence

Primary bacterial skin infection in children seen in all age groups. Predisposing factors include poor hygiene and antecedent lesions such as chickenpox, scabies, insect bites, or trauma.

III. Incubation period

1–3 days.

IV. Communicability

Under 48 hours once therapy is initiated; weeks to months if untreated.

V. Subjective data

A. Sores
   1. Mainly on the head (particularly around the nares and mouth) and extremities. May occur anywhere on body.
   2. Begin as macules, which develop into vesicles and then become pustular.

B. Pruritus, which may spread the infection.

C. Often a history of minor trauma (e.g., insect bites, scratches, scabies, or herpes simplex) providing entry to the organism.

D. History of exposure to impetigo.

VI. Objective data

A. Nonbullous
   1. Lesion appears as clear vesicle on an erythematous base and rapidly becomes pustular. Pustule ruptures, enlarges, and spreads. The characteristic honey-colored adherent crust is formed. Satellite lesions are common.
   2. Inspect entire body—lesions may be multiple.
   3. Check for regional adenopathy.

B. Bullous
   1. Lesions are rapidly formed—fragile bullae filled with clear fluid, which progresses to cloudy fluid prior to rupture. These bullae heal centrally, leaving a crusted arcuate or annular formation. Recently ruptured bullae have an erythematous, shiny base. Older lesions are dry and not erythematous.
   2. Inspect entire body.
   3. Check for regional adenopathy.

VII. Assessment

A. Diagnosis
   1. Usually made by clinical picture of oozing vesicles and honey-colored adherent crusts.

2. Routine culturing of lesions not indicated but recommended if lesions are extensive or severe.

B. Differential diagnosis (all of the following may become secondarily impetiginized).

1. Herpes simplex.
2. Contact dermatitis.
3. Eczema.
4. Seborrhea.
5. Fungal infection.

VIII. Plan

A. Local treatment may be adequate when only one or two lesions are present.

1. Remove crusts by gentle washing with warm water and an antiseptic soap or cleaner such as Betadine.
2. Apply topical antibiotic ointment.
    a. Neosporin ointment for crusted lesions. Apply 4–5 times a day.
    b. Bactroban ointment (prescription required) for bullous lesions. Apply 3 times a day.
3. Follow up with a telephone check in 24 hours. If other lesions have appeared or clearing has not begun, institute systemic treatment.
4. Systemic treatment is used for multiple lesions, widely separated lesions (e.g., one on the face and one on the buttocks), or lesions that are not showing rapid response to local therapy. Administer one of the following:
    a. Dicloxacillin 25 mg/kg/day in 4 divided doses.
    or
    b. Erythromycin, 30–50 mg/kg/day in 4 divided doses.

IX. Education

A. Continue medication for 10 full days; do not stop because lesions have cleared.

B. Spread occurs cutaneously as well as systemically.

C. Bullous impetigo is more likely to spread.

D. Incubation period is 1–3 days.

E. Not communicable after 48 hours on antibiotic therapy.

F. Use separate towel, washcloth, etc., to prevent spread.

G. Wash linen and clothing in hot water.

H. Keep fingernails short to minimize spread caused by scratching.

I. Check contacts and other family members.

J. Child should not return to school until lesions are clear or he has been on antibiotics for 48 hours.

K. Transmitted by direct and sometimes indirect contact.

X. Follow-up

A. Call office if no improvement is noted within 24 hours after treatment has been started.

B. Call immediately if dark-colored urine, decreased urinary output, or edema is noted.

C. Return in 3 days if not markedly improved.

XI. Complications

Acute glomerulonephritis, the most important complication, occurs with nephritogenic strains of streptococci. There is no conclusive evidence that early, vigorous treatment will prevent glomerulonephritis.

XII. Consultation/referral

A. Signs or symptoms of acute glomerulonephritis.

B. No response to treatment after 4–5 days.

C. Bullous impetigo in newborn or infant.

NOTES

INFECTIOUS MONONUCLEOSIS

An acute, self-limited viral infection characterized by fever, malaise, sore throat, generalized lymphadenopathy, splenomegaly, and increased numbers of atypical lymphocytes and monocytes in the peripheral blood.

I. Etiology

Epstein-Barr virus, a herpesvirus. Infectious mono is an initial or primary EBV infections. EBV produces other clinical disorders as well.

II. Incubation period

2–7 weeks.

III. Communicability

Low to moderate contagion. Transmitted by close contact, especially by oropharyngeal secretions. Because it is spread by the oral-pharyngeal route, kissing may well be the chief mode of spread in adolescents and young adults. Viral shedding via saliva occurs in 90% of patients in the first week of illness and continues for many months.

The period of communicability is not known because 10–20% of healthy, seropositive individuals, shed virus intermittently.

IV. Incidence

Can occur at any age but is most commonly diagnosed in adolescents and young adults (15–22 years of age). Incidence in males and females is equal but peak incidence in females is 16 years and in males 18 years.

V. Immunity

One attack is felt to confer immunity although following the initial EBV infection, the virus regularly produces infection of the B lymphocytes for life.

VI. Subjective data

- **A.** Malaise.
- **B.** Fever—gradual onset.
- **C.** Headache.
- **D.** Sore throat.
- **E.** Swollen glands.
- **F.** Abdominal pain.
- **G.** Anorexia, nausea, vomiting.
- **H.** Excessive fatigue.
- **I.** Jaundice (rare).

VII. Objective data

- **A.** Early in disease (first few days):
  1. Tonsils enlarged and erythematous; small areas of patchy gray exudate.
  2. Pharynx inflamed.
  3. Petechiae at junction of hard and soft palate. Seen at the middle to end of first week of illness.
  4. Bilateral posterior cervical adenopathy—nontender.
  5. Fever: 101–103°F
  6. Periorbital edema.
- **B.** After 3–5 days of presenting complaints, the following may be found in addition to the above:

1. Tonsillar exudate becomes more extensive with large patches.
2. Pharyngeal edema.
3. Tender anterior and posterior cervical adenopathy.
4. Axillary and inguinal adenopathy.
5. Erythematous maculopapular rash.
6. Jaundice.
7. Splenomegaly in approximately 75% of patients.
8. Hepatomegaly in approximately 50% of patients.

C. Laboratory tests
1. WBCs generally 10,000–20,000/mm^3.
2. Lymphocytes over 50%, with numerous atypical lymphocytes and monocytes.
3. Monospot test: positive after 7–10 days of illness.
4. Heterophil antibody test: titer of 1:112 significant, 1:160 diagnostic (may be negative for first 7–10 days of illness and in young children).
5. Throat culture to rule out streptococcal pharyngitis, a bacterial infection frequently associated with infectious mononucleosis.

VIII. Assessment

A. Diagnosis is made by the history, clinical findings, and positive laboratory results.

B. Differential diagnosis
1. Streptococcal pharyngitis: positive throat culture.
2. Blood dyscrasias, especially leukemia: pancytopenia and blast cells present.
3. Measles: preceded by a 3–4 day prodrome of cough, coryza, and conjunctivitis; pathognomonic Koplik's spots are present; negative immunization history.
4. Viral exanthems: clinical course differs; extensive lymphadenopathy very rare.
5. Viral hepatitis: clinical picture similar, but fewer atypical lymphocytes and lacks positive heterophil; liver function tests are abnormal.

IX. Plan

A. Symptomatic.
1. Rest according to degree of illness, until afebrile.
2. Liquids.
3. Acetaminophen or ibuprofen for elevated temperature or discomfort.
4. Warm saline gargles.
5. No contact sports.

B. Treat concurrent streptococcal pharyngitis with penicillin or erythromycin (see protocol, p. 356). Do not use ampicillin. It causes an allergic-type rash in approximately 80% of patients treated.

C. Corticosteroids do not generally affect the course of the disease. However, they are indicated if upper respiratory obstruction by enlarged, infected tonsils is impending.

Note: Acyclovir has not been proven to modify the clinical course of uncomplicated infectious mono although it has good in vitro activity against EBV.

X. Education

A. Infection is self-limited.

B. Treatment is symptomatic.

C. Isolation is unnecessary.

D. Throat may be very sore.

E. Gargle: 1 tsp of salt in a glass of warm water, as often as necessary.

F. Encourage fluids.

  1. Avoid orange juice or carbonated beverages if sore throat is a problem.
  2. Use cool, bland liquids.

G. Rest.

  1. Encourage bed rest when febrile.
  2. Encourage frequent rest periods.

H. Patient may feel an overwhelming fatigue, which may persist for as long as 6 weeks.

I. Strenuous activity and contact sports should be avoided while splenomegaly persists.

J. Avoid alcoholic beverages because of the possibility of liver involvement.

K. Encourage a well-balanced diet as soon as anorexia subsides.

L. Acute phase lasts 1–2 weeks; fatigue generally resolves in 2–4 weeks.

M. Complete recovery may take 3–6 weeks.

N. Call office if rash or jaundice appears.

O. Patient should not donate blood.

XI. Follow-up

A. Diagnosis may not be confirmed on the first visit, even with a high index of suspicion; therefore, patient may need to be seen in 24–48 hours for confirmation of the diagnosis or reevaluation.

B. Monospot or heterophil antibody test becomes positive 1 week after onset of illness.

C. Recheck weekly until patient is completely recovered and splenomegaly no longer persists.

D. More frequent telephone contacts may be necessary during acute phase, particularly if throat is so sore that drinking is a problem.

XII. Complications

A. Splenic rupture.

B. Neurologic

  1. Guillain-Barré syndrome.
  2. Aseptic meningitis.

XIII. Consultation/referral

A. Marked toxicity, splenomegaly, or respiratory compromise (may require prednisone).

B. Markedly enlarged tonsils and difficulty swallowing (may require prednisone).

C. Jaundice.

NOTES

INTERTRIGO

An inflammatory dermatosis occurring where two moist skin surfaces are in opposition.

I. Etiology

A. Skin rubbing on skin in the presence of heat and moisture leads to maceration and inflammation.

B. *Candida albicans* can be causative agent or may be secondarily involved.

II. Incidence

Seen most often in summer, but can be present at any time of year in obese children and overdressed infants.

III. Subjective data

A. Complaints of red rash in body folds—mild to severe.

B. Complaints of soreness and/or itching.

C. There may be no presenting complaint; nurse practitioner may find on routine physical examination.

IV. Objective data

Inspect entire body; areas most often involved in infants and children are neck creases, axillae, umbilicus, inguinal area, and crease of buttocks.

A. Mild. Mild erythema.

B. Moderate

1. Oozing.
2. Moderate erythema.

C. Severe

1. Oozing and crusting.
2. May be purulent.
3. Intense erythema.

V. Assessment: differential diagnosis

A. Eczema: by detailed history and appearance of rash.

B. Candidiasis: by detailed history and typical appearance of moist, red, sharply demarcated borders with satellite lesions.

C. Bacterial: culture pustules, if present.

VI. Plan

A. Wash area with mild soap and water 3–4 times a day; gently pat dry.

B. Mild to moderate

1. Caldesene Medicated Powder: apply liberally; gently brush away excess.
   or
2. Calamine lotion (soothing and drying).

C. Moderate to severe

1. Domeboro solution compresses to exudative areas 3–4 times a day for 2–3 days.
2. 1% Hydrocortisone cream 3 times a day.

D. Candidiasis

1. Nystatin cream 3 times a day.
   or

2. If areas are very moist, nystatin powder 3 times a day.
3. Domeboro solution compresses 3–4 times a day for 2–3 days.

VII. Education

A. Dry carefully after bathing.
B. With a drooling baby, keep neck dry; avoid plastic bibs.
C. Clothing
  1. Use loose cotton clothing.
  2. Avoid wool, nylon, synthetics.
  3. Do not overdress, but do use cotton undershirt to help keep body folds separated.
D. Do not let plastic on disposable diapers come in contact with skin.
E. Try to keep environment cool and dry. Use dehumidifier, fan, air conditioner.
F. Laundry.
  1. Use mild soap (e.g., Ivory Snow).
  2. Do not use bleach or fabric softeners.
G. Powder
  1. Use powder with caution to avoid inhalation by infant or child. Do not shake on from can; shake into hand and apply.
  2. Do not let powder accumulate in creases.
  3. Do not use cornstarch; it may be metabolized by microorganisms.
H. Medication
  1. Avoid prolonged use of corticosteroid creams.
  2. Apply hydrocortisone cream sparingly.
  3. Dissolve 1 packet of Domeboro powder in 1 pt of warm water; keep in covered container.
  4. Use soft cloth for compresses.
I. Dietary counsel if obesity is a problem.

VIII. Follow-up

A. Telephone follow-up in 5–7 days.
B. Return in 1 week if no improvement is noted. May require a fluorinated corticosteroid cream (e.g., Kenalog) if severely inflamed.

IX. Consultation/referral

A. No response to treatment after 2 weeks.
B. Recurrent or persistent intertrigo for evaluation of diabetes.

NOTES

IRON DEFICIENCY ANEMIA

A hypochromic, microcytic anemia that is characterized by a lowered hemoglobin content of red blood cells and decreased numbers of red blood cells. It is the most common hematologic disease of infancy and childhood.

I. Etiology

Insufficient available iron for hemoglobin synthesis because of

A. Inadequate iron stores at birth due to prematurity, maternal or fetal bleeding, or maternal iron deficiency.

B. Insufficient dietary iron to meet requirements of expanding blood volume during periods of rapid growth.

C. Iron loss.

1. Occult gastrointestinal blood loss (e.g., in cow's milk intolerance).
2. Hemorrhage.

II. Incidence

A. Rarely seen in the full-term infant under 6 months of age, since the iron stores available at birth are adequate to meet the infant's needs for the first 3–6 months.

B. Iron deficiency anemia is the leading cause of anemia between 6 months and 2 years. It is common also during the adolescent years because of rapid growth and often inadequate dietary iron.

III. Subjective data

A. Mild

1. Pale appearance.
2. Diminished energy level.
3. May be asymptomatic and discovered in routine screening.

B. Moderate to severe

1. Pallor.
2. Listlessness, fatigue, irritability.
3. Anorexia.
4. Weight gain usually satisfactory in early deficiency—"milk baby"; poor growth rate in chronic, untreated cases.
5. Delayed development.
6. Slow growth of nails.
7. Pica (especially of ice).
8. Increased incidence of infections.

C. Pertinent subjective data to obtain

1. History of prematurity.
2. Detailed dietary history may reveal the following:
   a. Excessive milk intake—greater than 1 qt/day.
   b. Lack of iron-fortified formula or iron supplement in first year of life.
   c. Diet low in solid foods with high iron content.
   d. Poor appetite; "picky" eater.
   e. Increased intake of "junk" foods.

3. History of iron deficiency anemia or other types of anemia in siblings or parents.
4. History of blood loss.
5. History of chronic infection (e.g., diarrhea).

IV. Objective data

A. Mild
   1. Palpebral conjunctiva may be pale.
   2. Physical findings normal.

B. Moderate to severe
   1. Pallor.
   2. Listlessness.
   3. Splenomegaly in 10–15% of children.
   4. May be obese or underweight.
   3. In marked iron deficiency anemia:
      a. Poor muscle tone.
      b. Heart murmur.
      c. Spoon-shaped nails.

C. Laboratory tests
   1. Order the following:
      a. CBC with red cell indices.
      b. Reticulocyte count.
      c. Blood smear.
      d. Lead level.
   2. Findings in iron deficiency anemia (see Appendix E for normal red blood cell values):
      a. Hematocrit below normal value for age.
      b. Low hemoglobin: less than one-third the hematocrit.
      c. Low serum iron: below 30 μg/100 ml (normal 90–150 μg/100 ml).
      d. Elevated total iron binding capacity: 350–500 μ/100 ml (normal 250–350 μg/100 ml).
      e. Red cells on smear are microcytic and hypochromic.
      f. Reticulocyte count is low, normal, or slightly elevated.
      g. Decreased mean corpuscular hemoglobin: 12–25 μg.
      h. Decreased mean corpuscular volume: 50–80 μ^3.
      i. Low mean corpuscular hemoglobin concentration: 25–30%.

V. Assessment

A. Diagnosis is made by blood values consistent with findings identified as diagnostic for iron deficiency anemia and by the response to therapeutic doses of iron.

B. Differential diagnosis
   1. Thalassemia trait: normal or increased serum iron; no response to iron therapy.
   2. Lead poisoning: elevated lead level and FEP.
   3. Chronic infection: evidence of infection on history or physical examination.

VI. Plan

A. Establish etiology—deficient diet, blood loss, intestinal malabsorption.

B. The aim of therapy is to achieve normal hemoglobin values and to replenish iron stores in the marrow.

C. Pharmacologic therapy

1. Elemental iron in doses of 4–6 mg/kg/day.

 a. Ferrous sulfate is the most effective and least expensive oral therapy (see Drug Index for dosage and administration).

 (1) Fer-in-Sol, 75 mg (15 mg elemental iron)/0.6 ml dropper.

 or

 (2) Feosol Elixir (44 mg elemental iron/5 ml).

 b. Continue treatment for at least 3 months after normal hemoglobin level is reached to replenish body stores.

2. Vitamin C: 35 mg/day for infants; 40 mg/day for children. Supplement if child is not on multivitamins and if dietary history is deficient in vitamin C (no citrus fruits, potatoes, or vegetables such as cabbage, cauliflower, broccoli, spinach, tomatoes).

D. Dietary recommendations

1. Iron-fortified formula (supplemented with 12 mg/L) for infants.

2. Foods high in iron:

 a. Best sources: liver, dried pinto and kidney beans; Cream of Wheat; dry baby cereal.

 b. Good sources: beef, veal; dried prunes, apricots, raisins; spinach and other leafy, dark green vegetables; egg yolks; nuts; fortified cereals.

3. If milk intake is excessive, decrease to 24 oz a day.

VII. Education

A. Give iron in 3 divided doses between meals.

B. Absorption of iron is decreased if given with meals or with milk.

C. Iron may be given with juice.

D. Iron can stain teeth; give through a straw if possible. Follow medication with water, rinsing mouth, and/or toothbrushing.

E. Iron may cause gastrointestinal upset—cramps, nausea, diarrhea, or constipation. It is best to give on an empty stomach, but if it is causing distress, consider giving with meals.

F. Stools may be black or green.

G. Keep iron out of reach of children. It is highly toxic in large doses.

H. Strive for a diet high in vitamin C to ensure optimal absorption of iron from foods.

I. Iron intake is a function of caloric intake. There are approximately 6 mg of iron per 1,000 calories.

J. Avoid whole cow's milk in infants under one year. Blood loss induced by protein in cow's milk is not related to lactose intolerance or milk allergy.

K. Iron losses increase in rapid pubertal growth and with heavy menses.

L. Athletes are particularly vulnerable. Twenty percent of runners have positive tests for fecal blood. Also, excess perspiration produces increase loss of iron in perspiration.

M. Iron therapy generally produces rapid recovery.

N. Continue iron therapy for 3 months after hemoglobin and hematocrit return to normal to replace marrow iron stores. A medication reminder chart may be helpful.

VIII. Follow-up

A. Marked or symptomatic anemia (hemoglobin 2 gm or more below lower limits of normal):

1. Repeat reticulocyte count and hemoglobin in 1–2 weeks. (Reticulocyte count should rise in 3–5 days and reaches a peak 7–10 days after therapy is initiated. Hemoglobin begins to increase during the first 7–10 days of therapy.)

2. Repeat hemoglobin and hematocrit after 1 month.

   a. If normal, continue treatment for 3 months, and recheck at completion of therapy.

   b. If below normal, continue treatment (stress dosage and compliance), and recheck in 1 month. Consult with physician if below normal at this time. If normal, continue treatment for 3 months, and recheck at completion of therapy.

B. Mild anemia (hemoglobin 1–2 gm below lower limits of normal): repeat reticulocyte count and hemoglobin in 1 month.

1. If normal, continue treatment for 3 months, and recheck at completion of therapy.

2. If below normal, continue treatment (stress dosage and compliance), and recheck in 1 month. Consult with physician if below normal at this time. If normal, continue treatment for 3 months, and recheck at completion of therapy.

IX. Complications

A. Progressive anemia.

B. Intercurrent infection.

X. Consultation/referral

A. Marked, symptomatic anemia.

B. Infants under 6 months of age.

C. Noncompliance with oral pharmacologic therapy.

D. Normal hemoglobin levels not achieved after 2 months of therapy.

NOTES

NOTES

LYME DISEASE

A tick-borne illness associated with widespread immune-complex disease. It has three stages, each with multiple clinical features, not all of which are apparent in each patient. It can affect the dermatologic, cardiac, neurologic, and musculoskeletal systems. The hallmark of the disease is erythema chronicum migrans, an annular expanding skin lesion.

This protocol deals primarily with the identification and treatment of stage 1 since recognition of the clinical picture and treatment at stage 1 prevents the subsequent manifestations of stages 2 and 3.

I. Etiology

A spirochete, *Borrelia burgdorferi,* which is transmitted by *Ixodes dammini,* a tiny deer tick. The cycle of transmission depends on the interaction of immature deer ticks and the white-footed mouse—their primary hosts.

II. Incidence

Primarily occurs in northeast, midwest, and western United States. Onset of illness is generally between May and November with most cases seen in June and July. All ages and both sexes are affected.

It is endemic in areas where the adult female deer tick can feed on deer, virtually the sole blood source for the adult tick. The larval ticks subsequently feed on infected mice. After feeding for a 2 day period which is when infection by *Borrelia* is suspected to occur, they lie dormant over winter. They molt to the nymph stage in the spring. This is the stage when the ticks tend to bite humans.

The risk of developing Lyme disease after a tick bite in an endemic area is low—approximately 5%.

III. Incubation period

3–32 days.

IV. Subjective data

- **A.** First stage—7–10 days after inoculation.
  - **1.** Rash:
    - **a.** Round, red rash that enlarges.
    - **b.** Clear in center.
    - **c.** May have one or several lesions.
    - **d.** Nonpruritic, nonpainful.
  - **2.** Associated symptoms:
    - **a.** Chills, fever.
    - **b.** Headache, backache.
    - **c.** Malaise.
    - **d.** Fatigue, often severe and incapacitating.
    - **e.** Conjunctivitis.
- **B.** Second stage—2 weeks to months after bite.
  - **1.** Heart palpitations, chest pain.
  - **2.** Dizziness.
  - **3.** Shortness of breath, dyspnea.
  - **4.** Generalized swollen glands.

5. Neurological complications—meningitis, cranial neuritis, peripheral neuropathy, encephalitis.

C. Third stage—weeks to years after onset if untreated. (Generally 2–6 months after vector bite.)
   1. Joint pains—particularly knees.
   2. Less commonly—memory loss, mood swings, inability to concentrate.

V. Objective data

A. Characteristic rash: erythema chronicum migrans (ECM)
   1. Seen at site of tick bite 3–30 days after inoculation.
   2. Occurs most commonly on thighs, groin, and axilla.
   3. Occurs in 80–90% of cases.
   4. An annular, expanding lesion of at least 6 cm to as many as 60 cm.
   5. As lesion expands, it looks like a red ring and and generally has central clearing.
   6. Center may be intensely erythematous and indurated in early lesions.

B. Secondary and migratory annular lesions.
   1. Smaller.
   2. Centers are not indurated.
   3. May occur anywhere on body but generally spare palms, soles, and mucous membranes.

C. Regional lymphadenopathy.

D. Neck pain and stiffness.

E. Hepatosplenomegaly.

F. Malar flush.

G. Urticaria.

H. Except for ECM, physical exam of limited value.

VI. Assessment

A. Diagnosis
   1. Clinical diagnosis is most readily made by evaluation of ECM—the hallmark of Lyme disease—by history of associated flu-like symptoms, by epidemiologic data, and by serologic testing.
   2. Lyme titer: Not accurate until 3 weeks after exposure. Indirect fluorescent antibody (IFA) and an ELISA test are available but tests are not standardized. ELISA has slightly greater specificity and sensitivity. Both false positives and false negatives occur. Diagnostic help is most needed during stage 2 or 3 when patient has attained a peak antibody rise. Since antibodies remain elevated for years, missing the diagnostic rise in stage 1 can be problematic in making an association between positive titer and symptoms in stages 2 and 3.

VII. Plan

A. Prophylactic antimicrobial therapy is not routinely indicated after a tick bite in endemic areas. In most cases, experts advise judiciously waiting for symptoms of Lyme disease or the appearance of erythema migrans unless patient is immunocompromised.

B. Antimicrobial treatment at stage 1 shortens stage 1 and aborts stages 2 and 3. Regardless of treatment, signs and symptoms disappear in 3 to 4 weeks. However, dermatologic manifestations often recur.

C. Children through age 9:
  1. Phenoxymethyl penicillin (Pen V) 250 mg every six hours for 21–30 days. (50 mg/kg/day in divided doses)
     or
  2. Amoxicillin 250 mg every eight hours for 21 to 30 days. (25–50 mg/kg/day in divided doses, maximum 1–2 gm/day) or, if penicillin allergic
  3. Erythromycin 250 mg every six hours for 21 to 30 days. (30 mg/kg/day in divided doses)

D. Ages 9 and up:
  1. Tetracycline (preferred therapy) 250 mg PO every 6 hours for 21–30 days.
     or
  2. Doxycycline 100 mg PO every twelve hours for 21–30 days.
     or
  3. Amoxicillin 500 mg PO every eight hours for 21–30 days.

E. Stages 2 and 3 should be treated with antibiotics as indicated above. Persistent arthritis, carditis, meningitis, or encephalitis require IV or IM antibiotics and hospitalization.

VIII. Education

A. Prompt removal of ticks is the best method of prevention. A minimum of 24 hours of attachment and feeding is necessary for transmission to occur.

B. Examine children's bodies after playing outside, hiking, etc.

C. Shower or bathe after expected exposure.

D. Scalp, axillae, and groin are often preferred sites for tick attachment.

E. Avoid tick infested areas.

F. Areas of risk must be suitable for both mice and ticks to live in—generally wooded areas and overhanging brush although they have been found in grass.

G. Dress for protection
  1. Light-colored clothing so that ticks can be easily spotted.
  2. Long sleeved shirts.
  3. Tuck cuffs of pants into socks or boots.
  4. Check clothes for ticks.

H. Wash and dry clothing in high temperatures.

I. Use tick repellant containing DEET or Permethrin.

J. Use DEET sparingly in young children as seizures have been reported coincident with its use.

K. Identify tick
  1. *Ixodes dammini*—pinhead sized.
  2. Oval body with no apparent segmentation and no antennae.
  3. Body covered with leathery, granulated cuticle.
  4. Hard ticks have a scutum, or hard shield, on their backs.
  5. Stages:
     a. Larvae—less than 2–3 mm long with 6 legs.
     b. Nymphs—4–8 mm long with 8 legs (stage at which they generally infect humans.
  6. Unfed ticks are flat; ticks that have recently fed are engorged.

L. Tick removal
  1. Do not handle tick with bare hands—infectious agents may enter through breaks in the skin.
  2. Use blunt tweezers.
  3. Grasp tick close to skin and pull with steady, even pressure.
  4. Do not squeeze, crush, or puncture tick. (Body fluids may contain infected particles.)
  5. Disinfect bite site.
  6. Flush tick down toilet or submerse in alcohol.

M. Rash
  1. ECM and secondary lesions generally disappear within days once treatment is started.
  2. If untreated, lesion may persist for months and recur for up to one year after onset.

IX. Follow-up

A. Recheck in 24–48 hours by telephone.
B. Call immediately if symptoms exacerbate.
C. Recheck Lyme titer if nonresponsive to medication.
D. Convalescent titers may be done to monitor progress of disease.

X. Complications

A. Cardiac complications: Seen 4–83 days (median 21 days after onset of ECM in approximately 8% of untreated cases.
B. Lyme arthritis:
C. Neurologic: Bell's Palsy, Guillain-Barré, polyradiculitis.

XI. Consultation/Referral

A. Stages 2 and 3.

NOTES

MARGINAL BLEPHARITIS

Chronic inflammation of the eyelid margins with accumulation of yellowish scales. Often associated with seborrheic dermatitis.

I. **Etiology**
Seborrhea (see Seborrhea of the Scalp). May be associated with *Staphylococcus aureus.*

II. **Incidence**
Seen in all age groups but most often seen in infancy and adolescence. Often occurs in conjunction with seborrhea of the scalp.

III. **Subjective data**

A. Scaling and inflammation of the eyelid margins.

B. Crusting, itching, or burning may be present.

C. May be asymptomatic, identified on routine physical examination.

IV. **Objective data**

A. Yellowish, oily scales on eyelashes.

B. Lashes often matted.

C. Eyelashes may not grow.

D. Inflammation, scaling, and exudate on eyelid margins.

E. Mild conjunctivitis may be present.

F. Ulcerations of lid margins if severe.

G. Check entire body for presence of seborrhea elsewhere, particularly on the scalp and eyebrows.

V. **Assessment**
Diagnosis easily made by typical appearance.

VI. **Plan**

A. Warm, moist compresses 4 times a day to remove crusts and scales.

B. Sodium Sulamyd ointment hs; use 4 times a day if inflammation is present.
or

C. Ilotycin ophthalmic ointment at bedtime; use 4 times a day if inflammation is present.

D. Treat concurrent seborrhea of the scalp according to protocol.

VII. **Education**

A. Use warm, moist compresses for 10 minutes.

B. Use soft facecloth for compresses.

C. Pull down lower eyelid, and apply a thin ribbon of ointment along inner margin of lower lid.

D. Continue treatment for 1 week after symptoms have cleared.

E. Use of ointment may cause temporary blurring of vision.

F. Sodium Sulamyd may cause stinging or burning if child is sensitive to it.

G. Problem is chronic.

H. Treatment will control the condition but generally will not effect a complete cure.

I. Once cleared, teach parent or child to be alert for symptoms of recurrence so treatment can be instituted early. Warm compresses should be used immediately if symptoms recur.

J. Does not affect visual acuity.

VIII. Follow-up

A. Return in 3–4 days if no improvement is noted or symptoms seem worse.

B. Call back immediately if any reaction to medication occurs.

IX. Consultation/referral

A. No response to treatment after 1 week.

B. Refer to ophthalmologist for monitoring of intraocular tension with intermittent or chronic use of steroid therapy.

NOTES

METATARSUS ADDUCTUS

A positional deformity characterized by a concavity of the medial border of the foot.

I. **Etiology**
Caused by uterine position.

II. **Incidence**
Frequently seen in the newborn; most commonly as a flexible deformity.

III. **Subjective data**

A. Generally detected on physical examination of the neonate.

B. If missed in the newborn, subjective findings would include a complaint by the parents of toes turning in. Often, a concurrent complaint of bowlegs.

IV. **Objective data**

A. Forefoot adducted on the hind foot with the heel in a normal position.

B. Lateral border of the foot angulated at the base of the fifth metatarsal—a convex lateral border.

C. Flexible deformity: foot assumes a normal position when lateral border of the foot is scratched.

D. Rigid deformity: deformity cannot be corrected past the midline.

E. Carefully check hips and legs for other postural deformities (e.g., tibial torsion).

V. **Assessment: Differential diagnosis**
Talipes equinovarus: this includes plantar flexion of the foot at the ankle joint, inversion deformity of the heel, and forefoot adduction.

VI. **Plan**

A. Rigid deformity. Refer to orthopedist for probable serial casting.

B. Flexible deformity

1. Exercising by parent—6 times a day: place thumb along lateral border of foot; with other hand on distal medial border, apply pressure to straighten lateral border, and hold in position for a slow count of 10.
2. Use equinovarus prewalkers or reverse-last shoes if deformity persists despite exercise or if parent does not do exercising routinely. Order for involved foot only, and leave on 24 hours a day initially. Gradually decrease time as deformity improves.
3. Straight-last shoes: persistence of deformity on weight bearing is an indication for straight-last shoes once child is walking.
4. Spontaneous correction occurs in 85% of infants without treatment.

VII. **Education**

A. Explain that problem is caused by intrauterine position.

B. Explain that it is correctable but that treatment plan must be followed.

C. Demonstrate exercise, and have parent return demonstration.

D. Equinovarus prewalkers or reverse-last shoes:

1. Leave on for prescribed length of time.
2. Remove for bath.
3. Remove several times a day to check foot for pressure and to exercise.

4. Buy pajamas slightly large so that shoe will fit underneath.
5. Use white cotton sock under shoe. Buy correct size so there will be no wrinkles under shoe.
6. Shoe must be firmly laced and securely strapped if it is to be effective.

E. Nurse practitioner should recognize that a busy mother may feel pressured by the additional time it takes to do exercising and provide support and encouragement.

VIII. Follow-up

A. First recheck should be at office visit at 2–3 weeks of age. If easily corrected, continue exercises until next visit. If no improvement is noted, stress exercising.

B. Second recheck should be at 6–7 weeks of age. If no improvement is noted at this time, reverse-last shoes should be used.

C. Routine follow-up should be included at each well child visit. Check carefully for persistence of deformity, both at rest and on weight bearing. Reverse-last shoe may be used for several months. If there is marked improvement after 1 month of use, shoe may be left off for longer periods of time.

IX. Consultation/referral

A. Refer to orthopedist if rigid deformity—one that cannot correct past the midline.

B. Refer to orthopedist at 4 to 6 months of age if no improvement of flexible deformity with conscientious exercising by parent.

NOTES

MILIARIA RUBRA (HEAT RASH)

"Heat rash," or "prickly heat," characterized by an erythematous papular rash, distributed in areas where sweat glands are concentrated.

I. Etiology

Heat and high humidity from external environment cause sweating that leads to swelling and plugging of the sweat gland orifice. The duct becomes distended and breaks, leaking sweat into the skin, thereby causing the irritation.

II. Incidence

Infants and children are most prone. Seen most often in the summer months and in obese and overdressed infants.

III. Subjective data

A. Pruritus.
B. Fine, red, raised rash.
C. Pustules may be present in neck and axillae.
D. History of overdressing.
E. History of predisposing environmental factors (e.g., hot spell in summer or house kept too warm).

IV. Objective data

A. Rash is erythematous and vesiculopapular. Lesions are pinhead size and may coalesce on an erythematous patch or remain isolated.
B. Distribution: found in areas of sweat gland concentration and areas of friction (e.g., neck, axillae, face, shoulders, chest, antecubital and popliteal fossae).
C. Check entire body; intertrigo may be present as well.

V. Assessment

A. Diagnosis made by appearance and history (hot, humid environment).
B. Differential diagnosis
   1. Contact dermatitis: distribution different according to contact; edematous; erythematous; vesicular; history of contact.
   2. Viral exanthems: accurate history would reveal elevated temperature and other prodromal signs or symptoms.
   3. Candidiasis: shiny, intensely inflamed, sharply defined border with satellite lesions.

VI. Plan

A. Treatment is symptomatic.
   1. Keep environment cool and dry; use air conditioner, fan, and/or dehumidifier if possible.
   2. Tepid to cool baths tid; may use baking soda in bath.
   3. Caldesene powder: apply frequently.
   4. Clothing.
      a. Light, absorbent cotton clothing.
      b. Do not overdress baby.
      c. Use a cotton shirt to keep body folds separated.
      d. Omit plastic pants, disposable diapers, and plastic bibs.
   5. Use cotton mattress pad over plastic covered mattress.

B. Severely inflamed miliaria. 1% Hydrocortisone cream 3 times a day (do not order refills).

VII. Education

A. Powder.

1. Do not allow child or baby to play with powder.
2. Use powder with caution near face to avoid inhalation.
3. Shake into hand to apply. Do not shake from can directly onto infant or child.
4. Do not let powder accumulate in creases.
5. Do not use cornstarch; it encourages bacterial and fungal overgrowth.

B. Use hydrocortisone cream sparingly.

C. Use mild or hypoallergenic soap (Neutrogena or Lowila).

D. Laundry: avoid harsh detergents, bleach, and fabric softeners.

E. Keep baby's fingernails short.

F. If rash is on the back of the neck, advise mother not to wear irritating fabrics (wool, nylon, synthetics) when feeding baby.

G. Do not put baby to sleep in the sun.

VIII. Follow-up

A. Telephone follow-up in 4–6 days.

B. If no improvement is noted by parents, try calamine lotion 4 times a day for soothing and drying effect.

C. Return for reevaluation if above treatment measures are unsuccessful.

IX. Consultation/referral

No improvement with treatment or exacerbation of rash.

NOTES

MOLLUSCUM CONTAGIOSUM

A benign viral disease of the skin with no systemic manifestations. It is characterized by waxy, umbilicated papules.

I. Etiology

Poxvirus.

II. Incubation period.

Generally between 2 and 7 weeks but may be as long as 6 months.

III. Communicability

The period of communicability is unknown and infectivity is low although occasional outbreaks have occurred. It is contracted by direct contact, fomites, and autoinoculation. Humans are the only known source of the virus.

IV. Subjective data

- **A.** Complaints of "warts" or bumps.
- **B.** May be 1 or 2 to hundreds of lesions.
- **C.** Occasional complaints of infected lesions.
- **D.** Often asymptomatic and found on physical exam.

V. Objective data

- **A.** Papules—1–5 mm in diameter.
  - **1.** Pearly white or skin colored.
  - **2.** Waxy.
  - **3.** Umbilicated.
  - **4.** Isolated or in clusters.
- **B.** Distribution
  - **1.** Face.
  - **2.** Trunk.
  - **3.** Lower abdomen.
  - **4.** Pubis, penis.
  - **5.** Thighs.
  - **6.** Mucosa.
- **C.** No associated systemic manifestations.

VI. Assessment

Diagnosis is usually made by the characteristic appearance of the lesions. Diagnosis can be confirmed by scraping lesions and viewing molluscum bodies under magnification. Warts are the most common differential diagnosis.

VII. Plan

- **A.** Curettage: remove each lesion with a sharp curet.
- **B.** Trichloracetic acid 30%: apply to base of each lesion avoiding surrounding skin.
- **C.** Occlusal-HP:
  - **1.** Apply to lesion.
  - **2.** Cover with tape.
  - **3.** Remove tape after 12 hours.
- **D.** Retin-A gel 0.01%: apply to lesions once daily.

E. Infected lesions:
   1. Hot soaks 5–6 times a day for 10 minutes.
   2. Neosporin ointment.

F. Genital lesions: rule out sexual abuse.

VIII. Education

A. Lesions are generally self-limited and may last for 6 to 9 months but can last for years.

B. Treatment prevents spread by autoinoculation.

C. Restrict direct body contact with infected child to prevent spread.

D. Can be spread by contact with contaminated surfaces.

E. Children with atopic dermatitis are prone to development of widespread lesions.

F. Although many lesions can be and are picked off by children, they may become secondarily infected.

IX. Follow-up

A. Recheck in office in one week.

B. Call if inflammatory reaction to local medication.

X. Complications

A. Secondary infection.

B. Reaction to local treatment.

XI. Consultation/referral

A. Question of sexual abuse.

B. Multiple, widespread lesions nonresponsive to treatment.

NOTES

MYCOPLASMAL PNEUMONIA

An acute infection of the lungs characterized by cough and fever. Symptoms are generally milder than those of bacterial pneumonia. Mycoplasmal pneumonia is the so-called walking pneumonia.

I. **Etiology**
Mycoplasma pneumoniae, the smallest known pathogen that can live outside of cells.

II. **Incidence**
The most common cause of pneumonia in school-age children and adolescents, occurring in about 5 per 1,000 school-aged children annually. It is the most common cause of nonbacterial pneumonias in all age groups. Peak incidence is in the fall and early winter but it does occur sporadically year round.

III. **Incubation period**
14–21 days.

IV. **Subjective data**
- **A.** Insidious onset.
- **B.** Headache.
- **C.** Chills.
- **D.** Low-grade temperature.
- **E.** Malaise.
- **F.** Cough—initially nonproductive, dry, hacking.
- **G.** Sore throat.
- **H.** Occasionally, ear pain.
- **I.** Anorexia.
- **J.** History of exposure to mycoplasmal pneumonia or other respiratory illnesses (pharyngitis, cough, earache).

V. **Objective data**
- **A.** Fever variable, generally low grade.
- **B.** Lethargy.
- **C.** Child does not appear particularly ill.
- **D.** Chest findings are variable.
  1. Decreased percussion note (rare).
  2. Decreased tactile and vocal fremitus (rare).
  3. Diminished breath sounds.
  4. Few scattered rales to severe bilateral involvement.
  5. Expiratory wheezing may be heard.
  6. Lower lobes are involved more frequently than are upper lobes.
- **E.** X-ray findings are variable but are more extensive than would be expected from clinical signs.
  1. Increase in bronchovascular markings.
  2. Unilateral peribronchial infiltrate or lobar consolidation although multilobe involvement does occur.
- **F.** Laboratory test.
  1. Cold agglutinins are helpful in diagnosis but are nonspecific.

a. Cold agglutinins are seen in influenza, Infectious mono, and other nonbacterial infections.

b. Cold agglutinin titer develops in about 50% of children with mycoplasmal pneumonia.

c. Titer rises 8–10 days after onset and peaks in 12–25 days.

d. Titer of 1:256 is suggestive of mycoplasma.

2. Culture and serologic testing takes too long to be useful in determining treatment.

VI. Assessment

A. Diagnosis of mycoplasma pneumonia is based on typical features:

1. Patient age.
2. Patient nontoxic.
3. History of slowly evolving symptoms.
4. Fine rales heard on auscultation.
5. Low-grade fever.

B. Differential diagnosis. Mycoplasmal pneumonia cannot be distinguished from other atypical pneumonias by clinical signs. (See also Differential Diagnosis of Viral Croup, Bronchiolitis, Pneumonia, and Bronchitis.)

VII. Plan

A. Antibiotics. Since *M. pneumoniae* is the predominant cause of antibiotic-responsive pneumonia in the school-aged child, therapy should be instituted if the diagnosis is suspected.

1. Erythromycin, 40–50 mg/kg/day in 4 divided doses.
   or
2. Tetracycline (in children over 12 years of age), 250 mg 4 qid.

B. Acetaminophen for temperature over 101°F; use sparingly, since temperature in part indicates response to pharmacologic therapy.

C. Rest.

D. Increased fluids.

E. Cool mist vaporizer.

F. Cough suppressant as indicated—Benylin Cough Syrup.

VIII. Education

A. Give antibiotic for 10 full days.

B. Antibiotics shorten the course of the illness but generally do not produce a dramatic response as in bacterial pneumonias.

C. Do not give antihistamines.

D. Encourage fluids to help keep secretions from thickening.

E. Transmitted directly by oral and nasal secretions and indirectly by contaminated articles.

F. Use careful hand-washing technique.

G. An attack probably confers immunity for a year or longer; no permanent immunity is conferred.

H. If child has trouble coughing up secretions, place him prone with head lower than feet, and percuss chest with cupped hands.

I. Call immediately if child has difficulty breathing or if he becomes restless or anxious; these symptoms are indicative of anoxia.

J. Duration of illness is about 2 weeks. A night cough persists longer.

IX. Follow-up

A. Call back daily until improvement is noted.

B. Recheck if no improvement in 48 hours.

C. Recheck in 10 days.

D. Call if any question of sensitivity to medication.

X. Complications

Rare.

XI. Consultation/referral

A. Infants.

B. Toxic child.

C. Respiratory distress or cyanosis.

D. No clinical improvement after 48 hours of therapy.

NOTES

OTITIS MEDIA—ACUTE

An acute infection in the middle ear characterized by middle ear effusion leading to partial or complete obstruction of the eustachian tube. It is associated with acute signs of illness.

I. Etiology

Major causative organisms are *Streptococcus pneumoniae* (approximately 31%), *Hemophilus influenzae* (22%), and *Moraxella catarrhalis* (7%). A small percentage of cases are due to beta-hemolytic streptococci.

II. Incidence

Otitis media is the second most common organic disease seen in pediatric practice. (Upper respiratory tract infection is the most common.) The incidence corresponds to the incidence of acute upper respiratory infection.

The peak prevalence of otitis media is in the 6 to 36 month age group. There is an increased incidence in children with cleft palate and with Down's syndrome. Approximately 93% of all children have at least one episode by age 7.

The diagnosis, treatment and follow-up of otitis media comprise up to 33% of pediatric office visits. The incidence declines at about 6 years of age.

III. Subjective data

- **A.** Rhinorrhea.
- **B.** Malaise.
- **C.** Irritability.
- **D.** Restlessness.
- **E.** Pulling or rubbing ear.
- **F.** Pain in ear.
- **G.** Purulent discharge from ear.
- **H.** Temperature may be elevated to 101–102°F.
- **I.** Diarrhea or vomiting.
- **J.** Pertinent subjective data to obtain
  1. History of upper respiratory infection.
  2. Previous history of ear infections.
  3. Family history of allergies.
  4. Does hearing seem normal?
  5. Does the child take a bottle to bed, or is he fed supine with a propped bottle or flat on mother's lap?

IV. Objective data

- **A.** Fever.
- **B.** Rhinorrhea.
- **C.** Tympanic membrane—characteristics in otitis media:
  1. Discharge suggests perforation of eardrum.
  2. Contour: fullness, bulging, or loss of concavity, which results in diminished or absent landmarks.
  3. Color.
     - **a.** Intense erythema.
     - **b.** Abnormal whiteness can result from scarring or the presence of pus in the middle ear.

4. Luster: generally dull with loss of light reflex, but dullness in itself is not indicative of otitis media.
5. Bulla may be seen on eardrum.
6. Perforation or scarring may be present.
7. Mobility decreased or absent.

D. Include evaluation for the following:
1. Mastoid tenderness.
2. Adenopathy.
3. Pharyngitis.
4. Lower respiratory tract involvement.

V. Assessment

A. Diagnosis is confirmed by the characteristic findings of the tympanic membrane (TM).

B. Differential diagnosis
1. Hyperemia of the TM from crying or high temperature: TM is bright, landmarks are evident, and mobility is normal.
2. Eustachian tube obstruction: causes transient pain, but TM is normal.
3. Serous otitis: TM is not inflamed and will not move inward with positive pressure, although it may move outward on negative pressure. Air bubbles may be visualized behind TM.
4. External otitis: diffuse inflammation of the ear canal with or without exudate; pain on movement of pinna. TM may be inflamed with widespread involvement.

VI. Plan

A. Antimicrobials
1. Amoxicillin, 20–40 mg/kg/day in 3 divided doses every 8 hours for 10 days.

   or if allergic to amoxicillin:
2. Trimethoprim (TMP)-Sulfamethoxazole (SMX)—(Bactrim or Septra)—8 mg TMP and 40 mg SMX/kg/day given in divided doses every 12 hours for 10 days.

   or
3. Erythromycin, 40 mg/kg/day given in 4 divided doses every 6 hours, plus sulfisoxazole, 100–150 mg/kg/day given in 4 divided doses for 10 days

   or for resistant organisms or patients who are allergic to the first line drugs:
4. Augmentin, 40 mg/kg/day in three divided doses every 8 hours for 10 days (dosage based on amoxicillin component).

   or
5. Cefaclor, 40 mg/kg/day given in 3 divided doses every 8 hours.

Note: In an acute episode of otitis media, amoxicillin is the drug of choice for initial therapy. However, a significant number (approximately 17%) of *H. influenzae* and *Moraxella catarrhalis* are ampicillin resistant (usually beta-lactamase-producing organisms). The rationale for the subsequent antimicrobial therapy, if otitis media does not respond to amoxicillin, is that these antimicrobials are beta-lactamase inhibitors. Because they are generally more expensive and have more side effects than amoxicillin, these antimicrobials are not generally used as a first line of defense. Cefaclor is best reserved for children with amoxicillin and sulfa allergies. It is very effective but is also more expensive and has more potential for significant hypersensitivity reactions.

B. Antihistamines and decongestants.

1. These drugs have been widely used to attempt to open the eustachian tube, but the efficacy of their use has not been proved. Therefore, it is advisable not to order them routinely but to order them only for symptomatic relief.
2. Use an antihistamine/decongestant such as Actifed or Dimetapp for children with known allergic rhinitis.
3. Use a decongestant such as Sudafed (see Drug Index) for children with acute nasal congestion.

C. Acetaminophen for elevated temperature and/or pain (see Drug Index).

D. Auralgan Otic Solution 4 times a day for relief of pain and reduction of inflammation if TM is not perforated.

E. Record review with each incidence of otitis. Question parent about interval visits to emergency room or other health care provider. Follow-up plan may need to include prophylaxis.

VII. Education

A. Encourage fluids. Baby may not suck because of pain. Offer small amounts frequently by teaspoon or shot glass.

B. Medication.

1. Give medication for 10 full days.
2. If child cannot retain medication, call back immediately.
3. Side effects of antimicrobials are diarrhea, rash, and fever.
4. Side effects of antihistamine and decongestant preparations are lethargy and hyperactivity.
5. If using Auralgan: fill canal with medication; do not touch ear with dropper; use cotton pledget in meatus after instilling. Use only for pain; discontinue use once pain has subsided, do not use if eardrum is ruptured, and do not use for future ear infections until ear has been evaluated.

C. Improvement should be noted within 24 hours of treatment.

D. Child may return to school once temperature has been normal for 24 hours.

E. There is no evidence that otitis media is transmitted person-to-person. It is, rather, the viral infections predisposing a child to otitis that are transmitted person to person.

F. Child may have temporary difficulty hearing. Notify school if applicable.

G. Complete resolution of middle ear effusion may require 8–12 weeks.

H. Explain disease process to parent. Reassure that earache did not occur because child went out without a hat on or because the ears got wet during shampoo.

I. Explain postural factors implicated in otitis media. Discontinue bottle in bed or horizontal feedings.

J. Stress importance of follow-up. Recognize that treatment of an episode of otitis media can be very expensive, and if there are recurrences or two children in the same family have otitis media, parents may be concerned about the cost and may not return unless they understand why it is necessary.

K. Explain that there will be an increased incidence of otitis with new exposures when child enters day care or kindergarten.

L. Concurrent viral infections significantly interfere with the resolution of otitis media.

VIII. Follow-up

A. Call back if child vomits medication or if side effects to medication occur.

B. Return if child is not improved in 24 hours or if there is persistent fever, pain, or discharge.

C. Return visit in 10 days for recheck. Include otoscopic examination, pneumatic otoscopy, and audiogram, as well as tympanometry or acoustic otoscopy if available.

D. If symptoms have not improved within 48 hours or otitis is not resolved in 10 days, retreat for resistant organisms. Include subsequent follow-up in another 10 days in plan.

E. General guidelines for chemoprophylaxis:

1. Three episodes in six months or 4 in one year.
2. Chemoprophylaxis should be continued during period of peak incidence of viral respiratory infections.
3. Recheck every 2 to 4 weeks (according to office protocol) if child on chemoprophylaxis.
4. Chemoprophylaxis:

a. Sulfisoxazole, 50 mg/kg/day in 2 divided doses.
or
b. Amoxicillin 20 mg/kg/day in a single daily dose.

IX. Complications

A. Recurrent otitis media.

B. Perforation of tympanic membrane.

C. Mastoiditis.

D. Meningitis.

E. Reaction to medication.

X. Consultation/referral

A. Infants under 3 months of age.

B. No improvement within 24 hours.

C. Failure of tympanic membrane to regain normal appearance after 20 days of treatment.

D. Cases of frequent recurrences (e.g., three in one season) should be referred for chemoprophylaxis. Give one-half therapeutic dose of amoxicillin, sulfisoxazole, or trimethoprim sulfamethoxazole to suppress colonization.

E. Persistent diminished hearing.

F. Myringotomy with tube insertion must be considered in a child with:

1. Persistent middle ear effusion between recurrent episodes of acute otitis media.
2. Consistent hearing loss of >15dB for longer than 3 months.
3. An effusion present for greater than 3 months.

NOTES

PEDICULOSIS CAPITIS, CORPORIS, AND PUBIS

Pediculosis capitis: human lice that live in the hair. Pediculosis corporis: human lice that live on the body and in seams of clothing. Pediculosis pubis: human lice that live in pubic hair and may also infest the eyebrows, eyelashes, beard, moustache, and hair of the trunk.

I. Etiology

A. Capitis: *Pediculus humanus capitis* (head louse).

B. Corporis: *Pediculus humanus corporis* (body louse).

C. Pubis: *Phthirus pubis* (pubic, or "crab," louse).

D. These lice, which are in the order Anoplura, are ectoparasites. They are sucking lice and are completely dependent on their host's blood for nourishment. They are transmitted by close personal contact as well as by clothing and bedding. Since they are obligate parasites, they cannot survive away from their hosts for more than 10 days. However, most pubic or head lice that are on fomites are dead or dying, so the danger of spread from toilet seats, for example, is minimal.

II. Incidence

Occurs without regard to socioeconomic status, age, or sex. However, infestation is seen most frequently in areas of overcrowding where sanitation facilities and hygiene are poor. In general, lice are more common among children than adults and females than males. Pubic lice are commonly found on adolescents who are engaged in multiple sexual relationships. Head lice are common among elementary school children. Blacks are rarely infested.

III. Incubation period for ova

Variable depending on temperature, but averages 8 or 9 days. Ova may lie dormant for up to 35 days. Ova develop to adulthood in 10 to 15 days and generally live for 30 days. Newly hatched nymphs must feed within 24 hours to survive.

IV. Subjective data

A. Pediculosis capitis

1. Pruritus of scalp.
2. "Bugs" in head.
3. "Dandruff" that sticks to hair.
4. History of exposure.

B. Pediculosis corporis

1. Pruritus of body.
2. Multiple bite and scratch marks, particularly on upper back, around the waist, and on upper arms.
3. History of exposure.

C. Pediculosis pubis

1. Pruritus of pubic area; most intense at night.
2. Multiple bite and scratch marks in pubic area.
3. "Bugs" in pubic hair, in eyebrows, and/or in axillae.

V. Objective data

A. Pediculosis capitis

1. Lice on scalp; most commonly found behind the ears and the back of the head.

2. Ova visualized as whitish ellipsoids on hair shafts; these are firmly attached and difficult to remove. These are the usual signs of infestation.
3. Bites on scalp.
4. Scratch marks on scalp; these may be secondarily infected.
5. Occipital and cervical adenopathy.

B. Pediculosis corporis
1. Body lice are rarely found.
2. Lice in seams of clothing.
3. Bite marks where lice have fed, generally on upper back, waist, and axillae.
4. Excoriations from scratching.
5. Secondary infections in areas of excoriations.
6. Regional adenopathy.
7. Occasionally, nits on body hair.

C. Pediculosis pubis
1. Lice attached to pubic hair.
2. Lice may also be found in eyebrows and axillae.
3. Ova visualized as whitish ellipsoids firmly attached to hair shaft.
4. Bite marks on abdomen, lower thighs, and genital area. (Bluish-grey, faint purpuric-like lesions.)
5. Excoriations from scratching.
6. Secondary infections in areas of excoriation.
7. Inguinal adenopathy.
8. Rule out sexual abuse if found in child.

VI. Assessment

Diagnosis is made by the characteristic signs and symptoms and by history of exposure; with head and pubic lice diagnosis is generally made by observation alone.

VII. Plan

A. Follow selected treatment plan. Do not overtreat. Chemical irritation from medication or hypersensitivity to the bite of the louse may result in persistent itching and may be misinterpreted as treatment failure. Order only enough medication for the treatment schedule.

B. For all infestations, all family members and other close contacts should be examined and treated if any evidence of lice or nits is found. All sexual contacts should be treated simultaneously.

C. Pediculosis capitis
1. Nix Creme Rinse (permethrin 1%).
   a. Shampoo and rinse hair; towel dry.
   b. Apply Nix Creme Rinse, thoroughly saturate hair and scalp.
   c. Allow Nix to remain on hair for 10 minutes, then rinse.
   d. Nits may be combed out for cosmetic reasons (Nix is ovicidal).
   e. Advantages
      (1) Ovicidal.
      (2) Active for 14 days following treatment.
      (3) Action of rinse is not affected by shampooing.

(4) 99.2% effective.
(5) Minimal systemic absorption.
(6) No potential for sensitization.

or

2. Kwell shampoo (gamma-benzene hexachloride). Do not prescribe for pregnant women or children under 2 years of age.
   a. Thoroughly wet hair and scalp with Kwell Shampoo.
   b. Add small amount of water and work in shampoo until good lather forms.
   c. Continue shampooing for 4 minutes.
   d. Rinse thoroughly.
   e. Towel dry.
   f. Fine-comb nits from hair after treatment.
   g. Repeat application in 7 days (Kwell is not ovicidal).

D. Pediculosis corporis
1. Since body lice are rarely found on the body except when they are feeding, clothing and bedding are the main foci of treatment.
2. Kwell cream or lotion (gamma-benzene hexachloride).
   a. Bathe or shower thoroughly.
   b. Apply cream or lotion to affected hairy areas and surrounding skin and to suspect areas.
   c. Leave medication on for minimum of 12 hours and maximum of 24 hours.
   d. Shower or bathe thoroughly with soap and warm water.
   e. Bed linen and clothing must be changed and laundered or dry cleaned.
   f. Application may be repeated in 4 days if necessary.

   or

3. RID.
   a. Bathe or shower thoroughly.
   b. Apply RID to all infested areas and suspect areas until wet; do not apply to eyelashes or eyebrows.
   c. Allow to remain on for 10 minutes.
   d. Bathe or shower thoroughly with soap and warm water.
   e. Bed linen and clothing must be changed and laundered or dry cleaned.
   f. If necessary, treatment may be repeated once only in 24 hours.
4. Clothing. (See Education.)

E. Pediculosis pubis
1. Kwell lotion (gamma-benzene hexachloride).
   a. Shower and towel dry.
   b. Apply sufficient quantity to thinly cover skin and hair of pubic area and, if involved, the thighs, trunk, and axillae.
   c. Rub into skin.
   d. Leave lotion on for minimum of 12 hours and maximum of 24 hours.

   - **e.** Shower thoroughly.
   - **f.** Repeat treatment in 7 days.

   or

2. Kwell shampoo.
   - **a.** Apply sufficient shampoo to thoroughly wet hair and skin of affected and adjacent hairy areas.
   - **b.** Add small amount of water, working shampoo into hair and skin until lather forms.
   - **c.** Continue shampooing for 4 minutes.
   - **d.** Rinse thoroughly.
   - **e.** Towel dry.
   - **f.** Repeat application after 7 days if living lice were found on exam.

F. Oral antihistamine; rarely indicated if treatment has been effective.

1. Tacaryl.

   or

2. Benadryl.

G. Infected lesions. Follow protocol for Impetigo (see p. 294).

VIII. Education

A. Infestation with lice can be a traumatic emotional experience for both the child and his family. Education and support are important in helping them cope with the problem.

B. Lice are highly contagious and can affect all social classes.

C. Most head and pubic lice that are on inanimate objects are dead or dying.

D. Human lice are not transmitted by animals; they live and breed only on humans.

E. Lice cannot jump or fly from one person to another.

F. Head lice are transmitted by direct contact with an infested person's hair or by contact with hats, brushes, combs, or bedding. Head lice can crawl from one place to another.

G. Head lice do not normally live on the hair shafts of blacks.

H. Head lice will leave the body if the host temperature rises due to fever or drops due to death. (Ova cannot hatch at temperatures below 22°C.)

I. Eggs are laid close to the scalp. Since hair grows approximately a quarter inch each month, any eggs found a greater distance from the scalp are probably empty shells.

J. Do not borrow combs, barrettes, ribbons, hats, helmets, scarves, or pillows.

K. Do not stack or hang coat or hat so it is touching other persons' clothing.

L. Nits must be removed with a fine-tooth comb or manually.

M. Body lice are transmitted by direct contact or by contact with infected clothing or bedding.

N. Lice usually cling to clothing, particularly in the seams, and are least prevalent in areas where personal and general hygiene are good.

O. Pubic lice are transmitted through close personal contact and through clothing, bedding, and, less commonly, toilet seats.

P. Pubic lice are particularly common among persons aged 15–25, probably because of close physical contact, especially sexual intercourse.

Q. Do not use lice spray on a person or a pet.

R. Laundry.

1. Use hot water and detergent.
2. Use hot dryer.
3. Use hot iron.
4. Change all clothing and bed linen daily.

S. Woolens.

1. Dry clean.
2. Press with hot iron, paying particular attention to seams of clothing if infestation with body lice.
3. If expense of dry cleaning is prohibitive, place articles in sealed plastic bag for 35 days (ova generally hatch in 8–9 days but may remain dormant for up to 35 days, and newly hatched nymphs must feed within 24 hours to survive).

T. Furniture.

1. Vacuum.
2. Use R&C Spray® (lice control insecticide) on upholstered furniture.
   or
3. Use hot iron on upholstered furniture.
4. Damp dust or wash other furniture.

U. Kwell

1. Avoid unnecessary skin contact. If treating more than one child, use rubber gloves for applying.
2. Do not use on open cuts or extensive excoriations.
3. It has no residual effects, therefore it should not be used for prevention.
4. Kwell requires a prescription.

V. Notify school nurse. Most schools have a "no nit" policy.

W. Examine all contacts.

IX. Follow-up

Recheck in 3–5 days if child presents with secondary infection.

X. Complications

A. Secondary bacterial infection.

B. Concomitant sexually transmitted diseases seen with pediculosis pubis.

XI. Consultation/referral

A. Concomitant sexually transmitted disease such as gonorrhea, syphilis, *Trichomonas, Chlamydia.*

NOTES

NOTES

PINWORMS

Infestation by intestinal parasite; generally benign; characterized by anal pruritus, especially at night.

I. Etiology

Enterobius vermicularis, a 4-mm worm, inhabits rectum or colon and emerges to lay eggs in the skin folds of the anus. Ingested eggs hatch in the duodenum, mature in the small intestine, and reproduce in the cecum. The worms then migrate to the rectum and eventually to the perianal skin where eggs are laid. The eggs become infectious within 2 to 4 hours. The entire cycle from ingestion of eggs to egg laying phase takes 4 to 6 weeks.

II. Incidence

The most common parasitic infestation in children in the United States. All ages are susceptible, autoinfection is common, and humans are the only host.

III. Incubation period

3–6 weeks following ingestion of eggs.

IV. Communicability

Transmissible through fecal-oral route as long as viable worms are present.

V. Subjective data

- **A.** Perianal pruritus, especially at night.
- **B.** Restlessness during sleep.
- **C.** Females may complain of pain or itching of genitals.
- **D.** If anus is inspected during the night, ova or white, threadlike worms, approximately 0.5–1.0 cm in length, may be seen.

VI. Objective data

- **A.** Rectal excoriation may be present.
- **B.** Inflammation of vulva may be present.
- **C.** Pinworms and/or ova almost never observed in the office.

VII. Assessment

Diagnosis is made by microscopic identification of ova on transparent Scotch tape that has been applied to the perianal area and placed on a glass slide. Prior to microscopic examination, place a drop of toluene between tape and slide.

VIII. Plan

- **A.** Vermox chewable tablets: 100 mg PO, one time, for all ages over 2 years.
- **B.** Treat all family members simultaneously except pregnant women and children under 2 years of age.
- **C.** Sitz baths for rectal or vulva irritation.
- **D.** Desitin to perianal area if irritated from scratching.

IX. Education

- **A.** Teach parent how to prepare slide.
  1. Use *clear* Scotch tape wrapped around finger, sticky side out.
  2. Spread buttocks and tap firmly around perianal area during the night or in the early morning—preferably before child gets up, but at least before toileting.
  3. Apply tape, sticky side down, to clear glass slide.

Note: Slides for diagnosis may be purchased, but above method is less expensive and works just as well.

B. Communicability is high.

C. Transmitted directly by autoinfection: child scratches his anus, gets the eggs under his fingernails, and then puts his fingers in his mouth.

D. Pinworms are contracted through human contact only; they are not worms from dogs or cats.

E. Eggs remain viable in humid environment for several days.

F. Stress personal hygiene to avoid autoinfection.

1. Bathe daily.
2. Wash hands after toileting and before eating.
3. Keep fingernails short and clean.
4. Wear tight cotton underpants.
5. Change underpants twice a day, in the early morning and at bedtime.
6. Change bedding nightly.
7. Laundry should be washed in hot water and dried in a hot dryer. Avoid shaking bedding and clothing prior to laundering.

G. Perianal itching is caused by gravid worm crawling out of anus and laying eggs.

H. Vermox

1. Side effects are abdominal pain and diarrhea.
2. Tablet may be chewed, swallowed, or crushed and mixed with food.
3. Vermox has a 95% cure rate.

I. Recurrences are common, particularly in large families and dormitories.

J. Reassure that course is benign and infestation is easily treated. Pinworm infestation can be very upsetting to parents, and they may go to extremes in environmental control.

X. Follow-up

A. Not generally indicated.

B. Call or return to office in 3 weeks if symptomatic.

C. Treatment with Vermox may need to be repeated.

XI. Complications

A. Vulvovaginitis from migration of worms to vagina.

B. Secondary bacterial infection from excessive scratching.

C. Occasionally, symptoms of appendicitis.

XII. Consultation/referral

A. Pregnant women.

B. Children under 2 years of age.

NOTES

PITYRIASIS ROSEA

An acute, self-limited disease characterized by a superficial scaling eruption. Seen classically on the trunk in a "Christmas tree" configuration.

I. Etiology

Unknown, although presumed to be viral in origin. There is no evidence of contagion.

II. Incidence

Seen frequently in children, adolescents, and young adults. Rare in infants. Occurs most often in spring and fall.

III. Subjective data

- **A.** May be asymptomatic until rash appears.
- **B.** Initially a single scaling, erythematous maculopapular patch with central clearing; generally found on the trunk.
- **C.** Mild prodromal symptoms occasionally: headache, malaise, sore throat, swollen glands.
- **D.** Rash appears 3–10 days after initial lesion.
- **E.** Pruritus of varying degrees.

IV. Objective data

- **A.** Herald patch, or "mother spot."
  - **1.** Initial lesion.
  - **2.** Scaly with central clearing; salmon colored.
  - **3.** Round or oval plaque 3–6 cm in diameter.
  - **4.** Spreads peripherally.
  - **5.** Border erythematous.
- **B.** Rash.
  - **1.** Salmon-colored, oval lesions.
  - **2.** Lesions smaller than herald patch; vary in size.
  - **3.** Lesions scaly, generally macular and papular. Vesicular lesions may be present.
  - **4.** Generally seen on normally clothed areas, i.e., trunk. Occasionally a "reverse" distribution is seen with prominent involvement of the face and proximal extremities.
  - **5.** In typical case, axes of lesions are along cleavage lines, parallel to the ribs, and a Christmas tree configuration can be seen on the back.
- **C.** Mild regional lymphadenopathy.

V. Assessment

- **A.** Diagnosis.Usually readily diagnosed by appearance and distribution of rash.
- **B.** Differential diagnosis
  - **1.** Tinea corporis: primary lesion or "herald" patch is very similar in appearance; usually child is not seen with primary lesion alone.
  - **2.** Seborrheic dermatitis: lesions may appear similar but do not have characteristic distribution.
  - **3.** Secondary syphilis: generalized rashes of secondary syphilis and pityriasis are strikingly similar; a serologic test is often indicated to rule out syphilis in patients who are sexually active.

VI. Plan

Symptomatic treatment.

- **A.** Cool compresses.
- **B.** Calamine lotion.
- **C.** Benadryl or Atarax for marked pruritus.
- **D.** Exposure to sunlight will relieve itching and enhance resolution of rash.

VII. Education

- **A.** No need to isolate; low communicability.
- **B.** Typically, the rash develops over a 2-week period, persists for 2 weeks and then fades over another 2 weeks. The duration of the rash, however, can be as long as 3–4 months.
- **C.** Rash disappears in the reverse order in which it appears.
- **D.** Recurrences are uncommon.
- **E.** Antihistamine may cause drowsiness.
- **F.** Prognosis is excellent; disease is self-limited.

VIII. Follow-up

None indicated as a rule. However, with a severe inflammatory reaction, it is advisable to keep in contact by telephone.

IX. Complications

Lesions excoriated from scratching may be secondarily infected.

X. Consultation/referral

Children with extensive rash and severe pruritus.

NOTES

ROSEOLA (EXANTHEM SUBITUM)

An acute disease of infants and young children characterized by a high fever of 3 to 4 day duration and the appearance of a faintly erythematous maculopapular rash after defervescence.

I. **Etiology**
Confirmation not available, but evidence suggests a virus as the causative agent.

II. **Incidence**
Most commonly seen in the spring and fall, although it does occur year round. Infants and preschoolers are the most susceptible, with 95% of the cases seen between 6 months and 3 years of life. The peak incidence is seen in the second year of life.

III. **Incubation period**
Estimated to be 7–17 days; average 10 days.

IV. **Communicability**
Probably for duration of illness.

V. **Subjective data**

A. Abrupt onset of high fever (up to 103–105°F) for 3–4 days.

B. Irritability.

C. May present with a febrile convulsion.

D. Generally, symptoms are minimal.

VI. **Objective data**

A. Child appears nontoxic.

B. Slight edema of eyelids.

C. Mild pharyngitis.

D. Occipital and cervical lymphadenopathy may be present.

E. Typical clinical course

1. Spiking high fever and irritability for 3–4 days.
2. Fever falls by crisis to normal or subnormal.
3. Exanthem appears just before or shortly after temperature returns to normal. It is a faintly erythematous macular or maculopapular eruption, first appearing at the nape of the neck and behind the earlobes. Spreads mainly to the trunk, rarely on the face, and disappears within 24 hours.

F. Physical exam findings are generally unremarkable.

G. Laboratory findings.

1. Progressive leukopenia to 3000–5000 WBCs on the third to fourth day of illness with a relative lymphocytosis of up to 90%.
2. Urinalysis and culture should be done to rule out urinary tract infection.

VII. **Assessment**

A. Diagnosis is based mainly on clinical findings, particularly if other cases are present in the community.

B. Differential diagnosis

1. Rubella: prodromal period of mild catarrhal symptoms and low-grade fever. Rash concurrent with fever.
2. Rubeola: prodromal period with variable fever, which elevates to 103–

104°F with appearance of rash and remains elevated. Also, cough, coryza, and conjunctivitis are present during prodrome, and Koplik's spots appear on second to fourth day of prodromal period.

3. Meningococcemia: fever, chills, headache, nuchal rigidity, nausea, vomiting, and petechial rash are present. In children over 2 years of age, Brudzinski's and Kernig's signs are positive. Lumbar puncture is positive.
4. Urinary tract infection (prior to onset of rash): do urine culture.
5. Other acute febrile illnesses.

VIII. Plan

A. Treatment is symptomatic.

B. Acetaminophen or PediaProfen for elevated temperature (see Drug Index for dosage and administration).

C. Tepid baths.

D. Encourage fluids.

IX. Education

A. Do not overdress child.

B. Try to keep environment calm and quiet.

C. Use tepid water for bath; allow to air dry, or rub skin briskly to increase skin capillary circulation, facilitating heat loss.

D. Bathe every 2 hours as necessary.

E. Keep child well hydrated—encourage liquids; do not worry about decreased appetite for solids.

F. Give small amounts of liquids frequently; try Popsicles, Jell-O, juice, sherbet.

G. Do not expose to other children until well.

H. One attack probably confers permanent immunity.

I. Disease is self-limited.

X. Follow-up

Maintain daily contact with parents until diagnosis is confirmed.

XI. Complications

Febrile convulsions.

XII. Consultation/referral

A. Prolonged high fever (after rash appears).

B. Febrile convulsions.

C. Signs of meningeal irritation.

NOTES

NOTES

SCABIES

A skin infestation of a mite that causes an intractable pruritus.

I. Etiology

Female mite *Sarcoptes scabiei* burrows into stratum corneum to lay eggs. Larvae hatch within 2–4 days and move to the surface of the skin. After 14–17 days the process is repeated by the now mature larvae.

Sensitization to the ova and feces of the mite occurs about 1 month after the initial infestation, producing the symptom of intense pruritus.

II. Incidence

Pandemic. Cyclical in nature and believed to occur in 30-year cycles, an epidemic lasting 15 years. Scabies affects all ages and both sexes without regard to socioeconomic status, but it is most common in urban areas where crowded conditions enhance the spread of the mite. It also occurs as a nosocomial outbreak.

III. Incubation period

Usually 1–3 weeks, but can be as long as 2 months.

IV. Communicability

Highly communicable. Spread by skin to skin contact.

V. Subjective data

- **A.** Rash.
- **B.** Itching—most intense at night.
- **C.** Restlessness; poor sleep.
- **D.** History of similar rash in other family members or other exposure to similar rash.
- **E.** Symptoms noted 3–4 weeks after infestation.

VI. Objective data

- **A.** Characteristic lesions
  - **1.** Linear, threadlike, grayish burrows 1–10 mm long; burrows may end in a vesicle or papule.
  - **2.** Most predominant in finger webs, flexor surface of wrists, and antecubital fossae.
- **B.** Other lesions
  - **1.** Vesicles, papules (pale pink, pinpoint size), excoriations.
  - **2.** Pustules present with secondary infection.
  - **3.** Bullous lesions are often present on face, palms, and soles of infants and small children.
- **C.** Distribution
  - **1.** Generally below the neck, but palms, soles, head, and neck may be involved in infants and children.
  - **2.** Most common sites of lesions.
    - **a.** Finger webs.
    - **b.** Wrists.
    - **c.** Extensor surfaces of elbows and knees.
    - **d.** Lateral aspect of feet.
    - **e.** Axillae.

f. Buttocks.
g. Intergluteal folds.
h. Waist.
i. Penis and scrotum in males.
j. Nipples in females.

D. Many lesions are secondarily infected.

VII. Assessment

A. Diagnosis. Scrapings of the burrow or papules using a surgical blade may reveal the mite, eggs, or a black speck of feces when viewed under the microscope. These scrapings are best obtained from interdigital areas or the flexor surface of the wrists. Scrapings are often negative, so scabies must then be diagnosed by the clinical signs and symptoms as well as by the epidemiologic data.

B. Differential diagnosis. Impetigo: secondary bacterial infection often occurs and obscures the lesions of scabies. There is a high index of suspicion, however, with widespread impetiginous lesions involving the most frequent sites of involvement of scabies; a history of intense pruritus, especially on retiring; or a positive history of exposure.

VIII. Plan

A. Follow selected treatment plan; do not overtreat. Chemical irritation from medication or a hypersensitivity reaction to the mite may result in persistent itching, which may be seen as a treatment failure. Order only enough medication for treatment schedule.

B. Children under 2 years
1. Bathe thoroughly with soap and warm water using a rough washcloth. Towel dry.
2. Apply Eurax (Crotamiton) Cream—order 60 gm—to entire body from chin down. Apply to facial and scalp lesions, if present.
3. Repeat application in 24 hours. (Child may shower after 24 hours before reapplication.)
4. Bathe 48 hours after last application.
5. Use clean clothing, sheets, and towels after each application and at completion of therapy.

C. Children and adults
1. Kwell lotion:
   a. Bathe thoroughly with soap and hot water using rough washcloth or scrub brush. Towel dry.
   b. Apply Kwell Lotion from chin down. Apply to facial and scalp lesions, if present.
   c. Leave lotion on for 12 hours; then bathe thoroughly again.
   d. Use clean clothing, sheets, and towels after application and after bathing.
   e. Repeat application in 1 week (scabicides are not ovicidal, so a repeat application is needed to kill newly hatched larvae).
2. Elimite (permethrin 5%)—order 30 gms for average adult.
   a. Safe and effective in children aged 2 months and older.
   b. Thoroughly massage into skin from head to soles of feet.

c. Wash off after 8 to 14 hours.

d. One application is curative.

D. Alternative treatment, all ages. Precipitated sulfur (6–10%) applied every 24 hours for 3 days. It is effective but less commonly used because it is messy and smells like sulfur.

E. Secondary bacterial infections

1. Neosporin or bacitracin ointment 3–4 times a day 24 hours after treatment with Kwell or following treatment regimen with Eurax for one or two infected lesions.

2. If infection extensive, penicillin G for 10 days.

F. Pruritus

1. 1% Hydrocortisone cream.

2. Benadryl 5 mg/kg/day in 4 divided doses as needed, if intense.

G. It is reasonable to treat all close contacts (family members and sexual contacts) prophylactically to prevent reinfection.

1. Order:

a. 2 oz of Kwell (maximum) per adult, 1 oz per child.

b. 60 gm of Eurax (maximum) per person.

2. Do not give refills.

3. Eurax is the primary alternative therapy. It is an antipruritic as well as a scabicide, although its cure rates are lower than those of Kwell.

IX. Education

A. Recognize that infestation by scabies can be a traumatic emotional experience for many persons. Support, education, and reassurance are vital to assist them in coping with and eradicating the parasite.

B. Scabies are acquired by close personal contact. They may also be transmitted through clothing or linens.

C. Treat close family and personal contacts if indicated.

D. Female mite can survive for 2–3 days without human contact.

E. Lack of cleanliness does not cause scabies, but scrupulous hygiene can help eradicate and prevent reinfestation.

F. Low economic classes are not the only victims; scabies affects all socioeconomic groups and all ages.

G. Transmission is unlikely 24 hours after treatment is instituted.

H. Symptoms may persist for several weeks after the mites have been killed. Symptoms may be due to persistent infestation, sensitivity to the scabicide, or hypersensitivity to the mite. Patient should call back for an evaluation.

I. Notify school so nurse can be alert for symptoms of infestation in contacts.

J. Laundry.

1. Use hot water and detergent.

2. Use hot dryer.

3. Use hot iron.

4. Change all clothing daily.

K. Woolens.

1. Dry clean.

2. Press with hot iron.
3. If expense of dry cleaning is prohibitive, place woolens in plastic bag and seal for 2 weeks.

L. Furniture.
1. Use R&C spray for upholstered furniture.
2. Damp dust or wash other furniture.

M. Teach parent the signs and symptoms of secondary bacterial infection.

N. Scabicide.
1. Reapply to hands after washing.
2. Do not use on face or scalp unless lesions are present there.
3. Do not get in eyes or on mucous membrane.
4. Be sure to cover all areas of the body, paying special attention to interdigital areas. If any areas are missed, treatment may not be successful.
5. Poisonous if ingested.
6. Side effects: eczematous eruptions.
7. Do not apply to acutely inflamed skin or raw, weeping surfaces.

X. Follow-up

A. Check babies and small children in 7–10 days.
B. Recheck in 3–5 days if child presented with secondary infection of lesions.
C. If persistent pruritus after 2 weeks, repeat scraping of lesion to determine presence of mites.

XI. Complications

A. Secondary bacterial infection.
B. Reaction to scabicide.

XII. Consultation/referral

A. Infants under 2 months and pregnant women.
B. Failure to respond to therapy.
C. Secondary bacterial infection.

NOTES

SCARLET FEVER

A streptococcal infection characterized by fever, pharyngitis, and rash.

I. **Etiology**
Erythrogenic strain of group A beta-hemolytic streptococci.

II. **Incubation period**
Average 1–3 days.

III. **Communicability**
Weeks or months without treatment; generally noninfectious within 24 hours after therapy is started.

IV. **Subjective data**

- A. Acute onset of sore throat.
- B. Fever: 102–104°F (39–40°C).
- C. Listlessness.
- D. Abdominal pain.
- E. Vomiting.
- F. Rash.
- G. Child appears toxic.
- H. History of exposure to streptococcal pharyngitis.

V. **Objective data**

- A. Elevated temperature.
- B. Toxic child.
- C. Circumoral pallor.
- D. Strawberry tongue—protruding red papillae showing on coated surface, which then desquamates.
- E. Tonsils and pharynx intensely erythematous and edematous; purulent yellowish exudate on tonsils.
- F. Palatal petechiae.
- G. Anterior cervical nodes enlarged and tender.
- H. Exanthem.
  1. Appears 12–48 hours after onset of illness.
  2. Bright red, punctate rash with a sandpaper feel, which begins in skin creases and rapidly spreads to involve the trunk, extremities, and face. Rash blanches with pressure.
  3. Lasts 3–6 days, after which desquamation occurs (particularly on fingertips and deep creases).
- I. Pastia's lines—linear streaks of rash in antecubital fossa that do not blanch with pressure.
- J. Objective findings are similar in all respects to strep pharyngitis except for the exanthem and the "strawberry tongue."

VI. **Assessment**

- A. Diagnosis
  1. Throat culture: positive for group A beta-hemolytic streptococcus.
  2. White blood count: usually elevated (12,000–15,000).

B. Differential diagnosis
   1. Rubeola: Koplik's spots; characteristic rash; prodrome of cough, coryza, conjunctivitis; epidemiology.
   2. Rubella: postauricular adenopathy; mild illness; epidemiology.
   3. Fifth disease: "slapped cheek" rash; no pharyngeal signs or symptoms.
   4. Roseola: fever of 3 days; child is not toxic; rash appears after temperature drops.
   5. Enterovirus: gastrointestinal symptoms; negative throat culture; epidemic locally.
   6. Kawasaki syndrome: engorged conjunctival vessels; hands and feet erythematous and edematous; prolonged fever—5 or more days (fever starts high and remains high).

VII. Plan

A. Penicillin G 200,000–400,000 U 4 times a day, for 10 days.

B. If child is allergic to penicillin, give erythromycin 40/mg/kg/day in 4 divided doses for 10 days.

C. Acetaminophen for elevated temperature and discomfort (see Drug Index).

D. Warm saline gargles.

Note: Buffered penicillin G is less expensive, but consider treating with penicillin V, which can be given with meals, if it would enhance compliance. Treat contacts at risk (e.g., child who has had rheumatic fever).

VIII. Education

A. Medication.
   1. Antibiotic must be given 4 times a day for 10 days without fail. Continue drug even if child seems better.
   2. Give penicillin G 1 hour before or 2 hours after meals.
   3. Side effects of medication include nausea, vomiting, diarrhea, and rashes (maculopapular to urticarial).

B. Isolation is unnecessary after 24 hours of antibiotic therapy.

C. Do not send child back to school until temperature has been normal for 24 hours. Child may then resume normal activities.

D. Encourage fluids.
   1. Try Popsicles, sherbet, Jell-O, apple juice.
   2. Avoid orange juice and carbonated beverages; they may be difficult for child to swallow.

E. Sucking hard candies may help relieve discomfort of sore throat.

F. Expect child to improve within 48 hours once on medication.

G. Second attacks are rare.

H. Generally transmitted by direct contact.

IX. Follow-up

A. Call immediately if any symptoms of adverse reaction to penicillin.

B. Call immediately if child unable to retain medication; return to office for IM penicillin.

C. Call immediately if family members complain of sore throat. Cultures should be done on those with symptoms.

D. Call if no improvement within 48 hours, sooner if child seems worse.

E. Call if child improves and then 7–14 days later complains of malaise, headache, fever, anorexia, abdominal pain, edema, dark urine, decreased urinary output, or migratory joint pains.

F. Ideally, child should return for throat culture and urinalysis after completion of penicillin therapy. Follow-up at this time should include a careful cardiac examination.

X. Complications

Complications and sequelae are less likely to occur if treatment is instituted early. However, they may occur despite early, vigorous treatment.

A. Otitis media.

B. Pyoderma.

C. Cervical adenitis.

D. Rheumatic fever.

E. Acute glomerulonephritis.

XI. Consultation/referral

A. Prolonged course or no improvement once on medication for 48 hours.

B. Any signs of complications.

NOTES

SEBORRHEA OF THE SCALP (CRADLE CAP)

Inflammatory, scaling eruption of the scalp.

I. **Etiology**
Presumed to be accelerated epidermal growth. Although it occurs in an area with large numbers of sebaceous glands, there is no documented proof that it is caused by increased sebum production.

II. **Incidence**
Occurs predominantly in newborns and adolescents.

III. **Subjective data**

A. Pruritus.

B. Scaling of the scalp.

C. Dandruff.

D. Often no presenting complaints; nurse practitioner may find it on routine physical examination.

IV. **Objective data**

A. Scalp is primary site.

1. Slight to severe erythema.
2. Yellowish, greasy scales.
3. Excoriations from scratching.

B. Check entire body, since seborrhea may progress to other areas.

1. Face: erythema and scaling may progress to forehead, eyebrows, eyelashes(marginal blepharitis), and cheeks.
2. Ears: dryness, scaling, erythema, and cracking in postauricular areas.
3. Back of neck, groin, umbilicus, and gluteal crease may also have erythema and fine, dry scaling.
4. Secondary infection may occur.

V. **Assessment: Differential diagnosis**

A. Tinea capitis: lesions are round; broken hair stumps in lesions.

B. Tinea corporis: erythematous, circinate or oval scaling patches.

C. Psoriasis: erythematous macules or papules covered with dry, silvery scales.

VI. **Plan**

A. Infants—cradle cap

1. Rub petroleum jelly into scalp to soften crusts 20–30 minutes prior to shampoo.
2. Shampoo daily with baby shampoo, using a soft brush.
3. If lesions are inflammatory or extensive, use corticosteroid lotion (Valisone lotion) daily for scalp only.

B. Toddlers or adolescents—seborrhea of the scalp

1. Antiseborrheic shampoo (Selsun or Sebulex) every other day.
2. If lesions are inflammatory or extensive, use topical corticosteroid lotion (Valisone) daily.

C. Seborrheic blepharitis. See Marginal Blepharitis.

D. Lesions on areas other than scalp. 1% Hydrocortisone cream 2–3 times a day.

VII. Education

A. Stress prevention.
B. Teach mothers of newborns how to shampoo and rinse hair.
C. Reassure that it is all right to wash over "soft spot."
D. Daily shampooing is recommended.
E. Keep shampoo out of eyes.
F. Do not use prescription shampoos if child is not cooperative or any sensitivity results.
G. Continue treatment for several days after lesions disappear.
H. Shampoo at least weekly once resolved.
I. If lesions have spread to forehead and eyebrows, vigorous successful treatment of scalp will generally result in clearing of the face.

VIII. Follow-up

Telephone call in 5–6 days to report progress; return to office if no improvement.

IX. Consultation/referral

A. Secondary impetigo.
B. No response to treatment in 10–14 days.

NOTES

SEROUS OTITIS MEDIA

An accumulation of fluid in the middle ear characterized by decreased or absent mobility of the tympanic membrane and varying degrees of hearing loss.

I. Etiology

A. Eustachian tube obstruction or dysfunction resulting in decreased pressure in the middle ear. The causes of eustachian tube obstruction include allergic rhinitis, upper respiratory infection, enlarged adenoids, cleft palate.

B. Also seen as sequela of otitis media when fluid becomes sterile but does not resolve.

C. May be caused by increased secretions of mucosa of middle ear.

II. Incidence

The most frequent cause of air conduction hearing loss in school-age children; seen most often in 5–7-year-olds.

III. Subjective data

A. Complaints of

1. Ears popping.
2. Ears feeling plugged or full.
3. Voice sounding strange or hollow to child when he talks.

B. Subjective hearing loss.

1. Child may say he does not hear well.
2. Parents may notice diminished hearing.
3. Child does not respond well.
4. Child "never listens."
5. Child sits close to television.
6. School grades go down.
7. Hearing loss may be noted on school audiologic examination.

C. May have history of otitis media, upper respiratory infection, or allergic rhinitis.

D. Condition may be asymptomatic and found on routine well child visit.

IV. Objective data

A. Tympanic membrane.

1. Dull.
2. Opaque.
3. Color varies from white to bluish to orange-blue.
4. Fluid level may be visualized behind tympanic membrane.
5. Air bubbles may be visualized (suggesting intermittent eustachian tube function).
6. Mobility absent or diminished (does not move inward with positive pressure but may move outward with negative pressure).

B. Rinne test reveals bone conduction greater than air conduction.

C. Other positive objective findings would be those associated with causes of eustachian tube obstruction.

1. Mouth breathing.
2. Thin, watery nasal discharge.
3. Nasal turbinates pale and boggy.

D. Audiogram generally shows a 15- to 30-dB air conduction loss with normal bone conduction.

V. Assessment

Diagnosis is made by pneumatic otoscopy which reveals decreased mobility or immobility of the tympanic membrane in the absence of acute inflammation. Tympanometry and examination by acoustic otoscope confirm diagnosis by demonstrating decreased compliance of tympanic membrane.

VI. Plan

A. Antimicrobials: indicated if child has not had a recent course of therapy because of the possibility of an unrecognized infection. Recent studies have indicated that middle ear effusion is not a sterile process. Antibiotic intervention may be used for 2–4 weeks.

1. Amoxicillin: 40 mg/kg/day in 3 divided doses for 10 days.

   or, if child is allergic to penicillin and is over 2 years of age.

2. Trimethoprim (TMP)-sulfamethoxazole (SMX): 8 mg TMP and 40 mg SMX/kg/day in 2 divided doses (every 12 hours) for 10 days.
3. Follow-up in 10 days as for acute otitis media.

B. Oral decongestants: indicated if child has concurrent allergic rhinitis or upper respiratory infection. They are not specific as treatment for serous otitis.

1. Actifed 3 times a day for 2 weeks (see Drug Index for dosage and administration).

   or

2. Dimetapp 3 times a day for 2 weeks.

C. Eustachian tube autoinflation: purpose is to build up positive pressure in nasopharynx.

1. Have child blow up a balloon while mother holds his nose.
2. Have child hold his nose, keep his lips closed, puff his cheeks out, and swallow.
3. Have child chew gum.

D. Corticosteroids have not yet been proven to be effective in the treatment of middle ear effusion.

VII. Education

A. Do not feed infant supine or give bottle in bed.
B. Explain that it is a temporary hearing loss and common in children; normal hearing will return.
C. Speech development may be affected.
D. Speak slowly and distinctly to child when you have his full attention, preferably face-to-face.
E. Do not punish for assumed inattentiveness, but be aware that manipulation may occur.
F. Habit of asking "what?" may be formed.
G. Notify school of problem if child of school age.
H. It may take 2–4 months for problem to resolve.

I. Serous otitis may recur as sequela to otitis media or seasonally in an allergic child.

J. With frequent recurrences in an allergic child, allergic rhinitis should be treated.

K. Recommend that child chew sugarless gum for eustachian tube autoinflation.

VIII. Follow-up

There has been much controversy over the surgical treatment of serous otitis over the past several years, and treatment has changed from aggressive therapy to a more conservative watch-and-wait approach. A child can be followed for 4 months or longer with a unilateral serous otitis. Referral for a myringotomy may need to be made after 1 month of observation if child has bilateral serous otitis, especially if it is interfering with speech development or school progress.

Follow-up, therefore, must be individualized for each patient, and psychosocial factors and development, as well as tympanic membrane mobility and audiogram, must be assessed at each visit. General guidelines:

A. Recheck in 2 weeks. Discontinue antibiotics if tympanic membrane mobility and audiogram are normal. If exam is not within normal limits, continue treatment and recheck in another 2 weeks.

B. Recheck in 2 weeks. (The presence of air bubbles behind the tympanic membrane indicates intermittent functioning of the eustachian tubes.) If child is not handicapped by his hearing loss, continue to recheck at 2 to 4 week intervals.

C. Rechecks should include audiometric evaluation in addition to otoscopic examination.

D. Refer for evaluation for myringotomy with tube insertion if:

1. Persistent effusion between episodes of acute otitis media.
2. Consistent hearing loss of >15dB longer than 3 months.

Note: Tube insertion will decrease scarring of tympanic membrane and middle ear space as well as diminish cholesteatoma formation and chronic conductive hearing loss in these children.

IX. Complications

A. Delayed speech development.

B. Poor school progress.

C. Problems with social adjustment.

X. Consultation/referral

A. Bilateral hearing loss (30–50 dB) interfering with speech development and school progress.

B. No improvement after 2 months.

C. No resolution after 3 months.

D. For evaluation for respiratory allergy, obstructive adenoidal hypertrophy, immunodeficiency, submucous cleft palate.

NOTES

STREPTOCOCCAL PHARYNGITIS

An acute pharyngitis seen in approximately 10% of all children who present with a sore throat.

I. **Etiology**
Group A beta-hemolytic streptococcus *(Streptococcus pyogenes)*.

II. **Incubation period**
1–3 days.

III. **Communicability**
Weeks or months without treatment; generally noninfectious within 24 hours once treatment has started.

IV. **Subjective data**
- A. Acute onset of sore throat.
- B. Fever: 102–104°F (39–40°C).
- C. Vomiting; abdominal pain.
- D. Listlessness.
- E. Dysphagia.
- F. Voice thick or muffled, not hoarse.
- G. Anorexia.
- H. History of exposure to streptococcal pharyngitis.
- I. May have few presenting symptoms.

V. **Objective data**
- A. Typical clinical findings.
  1. Elevated temperature.
  2. Tonsils and pharynx intensely erythematous.
  3. Purulent, yellowish exudate on tonsils.
  4. Palatal petechiae.
  5. Edematous, "beefy" red uvula.
  6. Anterior cervical nodes enlarged and tender.
  7. Infant may present with excoriated nares.
- B. May not present with typical picture; therefore, a throat culture should be done to confirm or deny diagnosis of group A beta-hemolytic streptococcus in any child with pharyngitis.

VI. **Assessment**
- A. Diagnosis. Throat culture positive for group A beta-hemolytic streptococcus.

  Note: Current data on rapid strep tests suggests that the specificity exceeds 90% and the sensitivity ranges from 85–95%. When in doubt, recommendations are to use in conjunction with a conventional throat culture.
- B. Differential diagnosis
  1. Viral pharyngitis: negative rapid strep and/or negative throat culture.
  2. Infectious mononucleosis: positive heterophil antibody or Monospot test; more generalized adenopathy.

VII. **Plan**
- A. Penicillin G, 200,000–400,000 U 4 times a day, for 10 days.

  or

B. If child is allergic to penicillin, give erythromycin 40 mg/kg/day in 4 divided doses.

C. Acetaminophen or ibuprofen for elevated temperature, headache, and general discomfort (see Drug Index).

D. Warm saline gargles.

Note: Although buffered penicillin G is less expensive, consider treating with penicillin V, which can be given with meals, if this treatment schedule would enhance compliance. Treat contacts at risk (e.g., child who has had rheumatic fever).

VIII. Education

A. Medication

1. Antibiotic must be given 4 times a day for 10 consecutive days without fail.
2. Give penicillin G 1 hour before or 2 hours after meals.
3. Continue antibiotic even if child seems better.
4. Side effects of medication include nausea, vomiting, diarrhea, and rashes (maculopapular to urticarial).

B. Isolation is unnecessary after 24 hours of antibiotic therapy.

C. Clinical improvement is generally noted within 24 hours after initiating treatment.

D. Do not send child back to school until temperature has been normal for 24 hours. Child may then resume normal activities.

E. Force fluids.

1. Try popsicles, sherbet, Jell-O, apple juice.
2. Avoid orange juice and carbonated beverages; they may be difficult for child to swallow.
3. Do not be concerned about solid foods.

F. Sucking hard candies may help to relieve discomfort of sore throat.

G. Expect child to improve within 48 hours once on medication.

H. Immunity is not conferred, but some resistance is built up.

I. Streptococcal pharyngitis is transmitted by direct or close contact.

IX. Follow-up

A. Call immediately if any symptoms of adverse reaction to medication.

B. Call immediately if child unable to retain medication; return to office for IM medication.

C. Call back if child is not improved within 48 hours.

D. Call immediately if other family members complain of sore throat. Those with symptoms should have a throat culture.

E. Call if after 7–14 days child complains of malaise, headache, fever, anorexia, abdominal pain, edema, dark urine, decreased urinary output, or migratory joint pains.

F. Ideally, child should return for throat culture and urinalysis after completion of antibiotic therapy. Follow-up should include a careful cardiac examination.

G. Follow-up throat culture and eradication of carrier state indicated when:

1. When family has a history of rheumatic fever.
2. When "ping-pong" spread of GABHS has occurred within a family.

3. When outbreaks occur in closed or semi-closed communities.
4. When tonsillectomy is considered because of chronic GABHS.
5. When family is inordinately anxious about GABHS.
6. Treatment for eradicating carrier state:
   a. Rifampin 20 mg/kg every 24 hours for 4 doses during the last 4 days of penicillin therapy.
   b. Oral clindamycin 20mg/kg/day in 3 divided doses for 10 days.

X. Complications

Complications and sequelae are less likely to occur if treatment is instituted early. However, they may occur despite early, vigorous treatment.

A. Otitis media.
B. Pyoderma.
C. Cervical adenitis.
D. Rheumatic fever. (Risk approximately 0.3%.)
E. Acute glomerulonephritis. (Risk is 10–15% if infecting strain is nephritogenic.)

XI. Consultation/referral

A. Prolonged course.
B. Any signs of peritonsillar abscess (e.g., asymmetrical swelling of tonsils, uvula shifted to one side, edema of palate).
C. Any signs or symptoms of acute glomerulonephritis or rheumatic fever.

NOTES

SUICIDE PREVENTION*

Suicide is the act of taking one's own life. Suicide attempts are acts of life-threatening behavior that fall short of completion. Suicidal ideas are thoughts or plans about self-destruction. Death by suicide is by nature secretive.

Because suicide is such a strong social taboo, many health care workers are reluctant to even ask patients about it. Many persons feel that suicide is a sign of craziness, weakness, lack of courage, "possession by the devil," or moral inadequacy. Health care workers often miss opportunities to interview or help persons considering suicide.

I. Etiology

The causes of suicide are many; the most prevalent is the turmoil of adolescence, that critical period during which a person is establishing his identity, learning to be independent, growing physically and intellectually, choosing a career, and developing love relationships. For some persons adolescence is a time of great unhappiness, rebellion, confusion, and disturbance.

II. Incidence

Because of family instability and mobility, children may be deprived of the nurturing and love they need to withstand the pressures of growing up. It uscd to be that suicide affected primarily adolescents, but in recent years there has been an increase of 150% in the incidence of suicide among persons aged 10–24. Ten percent of deaths of adolescents and young children are by suicide. Many suicides are now occurring in clusters of high school students, often three or four in one class in one week (a recent phenomenon). Suicide attempts in the United States are estimated to number 300,000–500,000 per year, and an estimated 12,000 suicides occur annually in the United States among children aged 14 years or younger. Ninety percent of suicides in adolescent girls are by ingestion of drugs, and 90% of suicides in adolescent boys are by hanging.

III. Reasons

A. To get even ("You'll be sorry when I'm gone").

B. Way out of conflicts with parents; lack of close relationships.

C. Desire to be with someone who died.

D. Impulsiveness.

IV. Personality characteristics

A. Children at risk

1. Impulsive, acting-out.
2. Depressed.
3. Angry.
4. Loner; lacks social skills, has few friends, is withdrawn.
5. In crisis owing to loss of parent through divorce or death of loved one.
6. Lacks ability to communicate; suicide attempt is cry for help.

B. Suicide completers

1. Often very bright intellectually.

---

*This section was written by Rose Boynton.

2. May go to highly competitive schools.
3. Does not solve problems well.
4. Exceedingly demanding of himself.
5. Sees things as right or wrong.
6. Achiever and hard worker.
7. Does not respond to therapist in diagnostic interview.
8. Loner or socially withdrawn.
9. *Most importantly,* displays termination behaviors: gives important things away and disengages from usual activities.

V. Warning signs and symptoms

A. Previous attempts, 8 of 10 successful suicides are carried out by persons who have attempted the act before.

B. Threat of suicide.

C. Depression: extreme sadness; feelings of helplessness, hopelessness, and worthlessness; low self-esteem.

D. Changes in school behavior that last for more than 2–3 weeks: emotional outbursts, failing grades, falling asleep in class, inability to communicate, problems with drugs or alcohol.

E. Changes in appetite, usually decreasing but sometimes increasing.

F. Changes in sleep patterns; too much or too little sleep may be indicative of depression.

G. Increase in substance abuse (drugs or alcohol).

H. Changes in peer group or peer relationships.

I. Stresses.

1. Parent-child conflict.
2. Physical/sexual abuse by parents.
3. Dysfunctional family unit (due to recent divorce, death, substance abuse, etc.).
4. Rejection or neglect by others; feeling that "nobody cares."

VI. Management

A. Immediate response and rapid intervention are critical.

B. Reassure child he does have someone to turn to.

C. *Don't lecture.* Point out all the reasons a person has to live, but listen and reassure child that he can be treated; take him seriously, show you care. Do not show shock or disapproval.

D. If a child is depressed, do not be afraid to ask "Do you feel like killing or harming yourself?"

E. Assess safety of child; get him to agree not to act on suicidal impulses, and refer him to mental health professional.

F. Be ready to intervene against any suicide attempt.

G. Individual psychotherapy should include family (in group therapy as well as initial interview), school personnel, and peers. Child may be hospitalized to provide protective, comprehensive therapeutic setting.

H. Record in writing all events, information given, and plan of referral.

NOTES

THRUSH

Oral candidiasis characterized by white plaques on inflamed oral mucosa. It is often associated with cutaneous candidiasis in the diaper or intertriginous areas.

I. Etiology

Candida albicans.

II. Incidence

Seen primarily in newborns and infants up to 6 months of age. They have less immunity than older children to *C. albicans.*

III. Incubation period

Highly variable.

IV. Subjective data

- **A.** Fussy, irritable infant.
- **B.** Difficulty feeding or refusal to nurse.
- **C.** "White spots" on tongue and inside of mouth.
- **D.** Mother may have history of vaginal candidiasis.
- **E.** Nursing mother may have concomitant infection of nipples and areola.
- **F.** Infant may have history of concurrent or previous antibiotic therapy.

V. Objective data

- **A.** White, curdlike plaques on inflamed oral mucosa.
- **B.** Located on tongue, buccal mucosa, gingivae, and throat.
- **C.** Plaques cannot be easily removed. If they are wiped away, bleeding occurs.
- **D.** Early lesions start as pinpoint in size and grow larger.
- **E.** Cracks or fissures may appear in corners of mouth.
- **F.** Lesions may extend to esophagus.
- **G.** Inspect skin for concomitant candidiasis of diaper area and/or intertriginous areas.

VI. Assessment

- **A.** Diagnosis is readily made by the clinical picture.
- **B.** Differential diagnosis. Milk deposits: may resemble thrush but are easily removed by wiping with a gauze pad.

VII. Plan

- **A.** Mycostatin Oral Suspension
    1. Infants: 1 ml in each side of mouth 4 times a day.
    2. Premature or low-birth-weight infants: 0.5 ml in each side of mouth 4 times a day.
    3. Continue for 48 hours after symptoms disappear.
- **B.** Candidiasis in diaper area: see Candidiasis—Diaper Rash.

VIII. Education

- **A.** Give infant small amount of water before medication to rinse inside of mouth.
- **B.** Try to remove large plaques with cotton swab moistened with water.
- **C.** Call immediately if infant refuses liquids.

D. Try infant feeder if infant refuses bottle or breast.

E. Diaper rash may occur concomitantly. Leave diaper area exposed as much as possible to help eliminate the warmth and moisture that *C. albicans* thrives on. (See Candidiasis—Diaper Rash.)

F. Sterilize nipples and/or pacifiers.

G. Wash toys well to prevent reinfection.

H. If breast-feeding, wash nipples well with warm water before and after feeding. Allow to air dry.

I. Observe careful hand-washing technique.

J. Notify office if infant does not improve or seems worse.

K. If mother has any symptoms of vaginal candidiasis, she should be referred for treatment.

L. Newborns can be infected during passage through the vagina of a mother with *Candida Albicans.*

M. Infants can contract it from mothers with breast infection.

IX. Follow-up

Telephone contact in 3–4 days to assess progress. If no improvement noted by mother, return visit is indicated.

X. Complications

A. Persistent or recurrent thrush.

B. Systemic candidiasis in debilitated infants or those on immunosuppressive therapy.

XI. Consultation/referral

A. Persistent or recurrent thrush for evaluation of immunologic status.

B. No improvement in 5 days.

C. Mother with vaginal candidiasis.

NOTES

TINEA CORPORIS

Ringworm of the body—a superficial fungal infection of the nonhairy skin.

I. **Etiology**
Trichophyton and *Microsporum* dermatophyte fungi.

II. **Incidence**
Most prevalent in hot, humid climates. Children are the most susceptible.

III. **Incubation period**
4–10 days

IV. **Subjective data**

- A. Pruritic or asymptomatic lesions.
- B. Complaint of rash, round sores, or ringworm.
- C. History of exposure to infected person or animal.

V. **Objective data**

- A. Lesions.
  1. Flat, erythematous papules.
  2. Spread peripherally.
  3. Clear centrally.
  4. Develop into circinate or oval lesions with scaling papular or vesicular advancing borders.
- B. Distribution: most commonly seen on face, neck, arms, but may affect any part of the body.
- C. Check feet and scalp for tinea pedis (interdigital scaling, maceration, and fissures) and tinea capitis (patchy hair loss with broken stumps in oval or circinate lesions with central clearing).

VI. **Assessment**

- A. Diagnosis.
  1. Scrapings from borders of lesions in potassium hydroxide fungal preparation demonstrate hyphae.
  2. History and physical findings may be adequate for diagnosis .
- B. Differential diagnosis.
  1. Pityriasis rosea: herald patch may resemble tinea corporis.
  2. Candidiasis: lesions more inflamed; no central clearing; satellite lesions present.
  3. Psoriasis: lesions erythematous, circumscribed, and covered with silvery scales.

VII. **Plan**

- A. Use one of the following topical creams:
  1. Nizoral (ketoconazole) 2% Cream: apply once daily for 2 weeks.
  2. Oxistat Cream 1%: apply once daily for two weeks.
  3. Lotrimin (Clotrimazole): apply 3 times a day for 2 weeks.
- B. Systemic treatment for severe or unresponsive cases:
  1. Grifulvin V
     a. Weight 30 to 50 pounds: 125–250 mg daily.

b. Weight over 50 pounds: 250–500 mg daily. c. Continue treatment for 2–4 weeks.

VIII. Education

A. Transmitted by direct and indirect contact.
B. Communicable as long as lesions are present.
C. Observe for involvement of other family members or sexual contacts.
D. Ringworm lives on humans and animals; avoid contact with pets.
E. Check dog or cat for *M. Canis.*
F. Do not lend or borrow clothing.
G. Bathe or shower daily.
H. Use talcum or antifungal powder (Caldesene, Tinactin) in intertriginous areas.
I. Keep skin dry; ringworm thrives in moist areas.
J. Do not wear tight, constricting clothing; absorbent cotton is preferable.
K. Launder clothing and linens in hot water.
L. May see no improvement for 5–6 days; generally takes 1–3 weeks for effective cure.
M. Continue treatment for 1 week after disappearance of symptoms.
N. Use of corticosteroids will exacerbate lesions.

IX. Follow-up

A. Telephone call in 4–5 days to report progress.
B. Recheck in 7–9 days if no significant improvement.
C. Return sooner if lesions appear worse or become inflamed.

X. Complications

A. Secondary bacterial infection.
B. Sensitivity to topical antifungal cream.

XI. Consultation/referral

A. If severe or extensive, may require treatment with griscofulvin.
B. If tinea capitis is present.

NOTES

TINEA CRURIS

Ringworm of the groin, or "jock itch"—a superficial fungal infection of the groin.

I. Etiology

Epidermophyton floccosum and *Trichophyton* dermatophyte fungi.

II. Incidence

Seen most often in athletes and obese children. Incidence increases in hot, humid weather.

III. Subjective data

A. Groin and upper inner thighs are red, raw, and sore.

B. Pruritic when healing.

C. Hurts with activity.

D. Complaint of "jock itch."

E. History of exposure to tinea cruris.

V. Objective data

A. Symmetric rash with butterfly appearance on groin and inner aspects of thighs; scrotum, gluteal folds, and buttocks may also be involved.

B. Rash erythematous with a sharp, raised border with tiny vesicles, central clearing, and peripheral spreading.

C. Check entire body.

1. Tinea pedis is often present.
2. Intertriginous areas are susceptible to infection.

V. Assessment

A. Diagnosis. Scrapings from lesions in potassium hydroxide fungal preparation reveal hyphae and spores. Diagnosis may also be made from history and typical appearance of rash.

B. Differential diagnosis.

1. Intertrigo: rash is erythematous with oozing, exudation, and crusting; borders not sharply defined; no central clearing.
2. Seborrheic dermatitis: lesions are semiconfluent, yellow, and thick with greasy scaling.
3. Candidiasis: lesions moist and intensely erythematous with sharply defined borders and satellite lesions.
4. Contact dermatitis: distribution and configuration are the distinguishing features; rash is erythematous with vesicles, oozing, erosion, and eventually ulceration.

VI. Plan

A. For lesions with erythema and pruritus, order one of the following:

1. Nizoral (Ketoconazole) 2% Cream once daily (also effective against *Candida albicans*).
2. MicaTin cream *or* Lotrimin cream 3 times daily (also effective against *Candida albicans*).
3. Tinactin cream 3 times daily (over-the-counter preparation; ineffective against *C. albicans*).

B. For acute inflammatory lesions, order the following:
   1. Domeboro solution compresses: 30 minutes 3 times daily for 3 days. Dissolve 1 powder packet in 1 pt of warm water.
   2. Antifungal cream as above.

VII. Education

A. Expect gradual improvement once treatment is instituted.

B. Continue treatment for 1 week after lesions have cleared.

C. Domeboro solution becomes concentrated on exposure to air; keep in covered container.

D. Use a soft cloth for soaks.

E. Eliminate sources of heat and friction.

F. Hygiene.
   1. Bathe daily; dry thoroughly after bathing.
   2. Use cotton underwear.
   3. Change clothing daily.
   4. Use clean athletic supporter daily.
   5. Use fresh towels daily.
   6. Launder linens and clothing in hot water.

G. Tinea is highly communicable and is transmitted by both direct and indirect contact.

H. Check siblings carefully for signs of infection.

I. Alert child and parents to signs and symptoms of secondary infection.

Note: Prevention is of primary importance. Athletes in particular should be educated about the need for clean, dry clothing and the importance of avoiding direct contact with someone who has jock itch. Athletic supporters, shorts, and socks should not be loaned or borrowed. Daily showers should be encouraged, as well as the prophylactic use of antifungal powders such as Caldesene or Tinactin daily or twice daily.

VIII. Follow-up

A. Telephone call in 3–4 days.

B. If severe, with oozing, consider rechecking in 5 days.

IX. Complications

A. Secondary infection.

B. Chronic infection (80% of patients acquire immunity; 20% may develop chronic infection).

C. Allergic response to topical antifungal cream (erythema, stinging, blistering, peeling, pruritus).

X. Consultation/referral

No clinical improvement after 2 weeks. Griseofulvin may be indicated.

NOTES

TINEA PEDIS

Ringworm of the foot, or "athlete's foot"—a superficial fungal infection of the foot.

I. Etiology

Trichophyton mentagrophytes and *T. rubrum,* dermatophyte fungi, invade the skin following trauma.

II. Incidence

Occurs most frequently in adolescents and adults but is found with increasing frequency in preadolescent children, probably because of the use of occlusive footwear.

III. Subjective data

A. One or both feet may be involved.

B. Pruritus.

C. Cracks between toes.

D. Scaling of feet.

E. Blisters on soles.

F. Pain with deep fissures.

G. History of exposure to predisposing factors (e.g., communal showers, prolonged use of sneakers). Often seen following trauma or in conjunction with atopic dermatitis.

IV. Objective data

A. Interdigital fissures.

B. Widespread fine scaling; extension onto sides of foot and heel is frequent.

C. Maceration.

D. Vesicular eruption on plantar surface.

E. Secondary infection may be present.

F. Regional adenopathy.

G. Involvement of nails may occur.

H. Vesicular eruption of the hands—an "id" reaction—may occur.

I. Unilateral tinea pedis is common.

V. Assessment

A. Diagnosis.

1. Scrapings from lesions in potassium hydroxide fungal preparation reveal hyphae and spores.
2. Unilateral involvement is a significant positive clinical finding.

B. Differential diagnosis.

1. Interdigital candidiasis: interdigital lesions are moist and erythematous, with well-defined borders and satellite lesions.
2. Hyperhidrosis: macerated, tender, peeling, and erythematous. Diagnosis is made by history and appearance.
3. Contact dermatitis: reaction to shoes, sneakers, dye, soap, nylon socks. Diagnosis is generally arrived at by history, distribution of rash, and appearance of rash, which is erythematous, vesicular, and oozing.

VI. Plan

A. Domeboro soaks 4 times daily for acute lesions with blistering and oozing—1 tablet or powder packet to 1 pint of water.

B. Antifungal creams—use one of the following:

1. Oxistat cream 1%, once daily for 4 weeks.
2. Lotrimin cream *or* Halotex cream 3 times daily for 4 weeks (also effective against *Candida albicans).*
   or
3. Tinactin cream 3 times daily (over-the-counter preparation; ineffective against *C. albicans).*

C. For severe or unresponsive cases in children over 50 lb: Grifulvin V, 250–500 mg daily for 4 to 8 weeks.

VII. Education

A. Expect gradual improvement once treatment is instituted.

B. Continue treatment for several days after lesions have cleared.

C. Soak feet 2–4 times a day; use a small basin.

D. Domeboro solution concentrates when left exposed; store in covered container.

E. Hygiene.

1. Dry interdigital areas thoroughly after bathing.
2. Use white cotton socks; no colored tights or nylons.
3. Change socks at least daily.
4. Use sandals if possible.
5. Avoid sneakers and plastic footwear.

F. Communicable as long as lesions are present.

G. Causative organisms are long lived, surviving more than 5 months.

H. Transmitted to traumatized skin by both direct and indirect contact.

I. Alert child and parents to signs and symptoms of secondary infection.

J. Prevention.

1. Use Tinactin or Caldesene powder daily.
2. Use clogs for showers.
3. Do not lend or borrow shoes.

VIII. Follow-up

A. Telephone call in 3–4 days.

B. If tinea pedis is severe, with deep fissures and oozing, recheck in 5 days; recheck sooner if no improvement is noted.

IX. Complications

A. Secondary infection.

B. Allergic response to topical antifungal cream (erythema, stinging, blistering, peeling, pruritus).

C. Untreated or improperly treated tinea presents with scaling and erythema of the sides and dorsum of the foot as well as interdigital areas and plantar surface. The tinea may be distributed in a shoe or sneaker pattern.

X. Consultation/referral

A. No clinical improvement after 2 weeks.

B. Severe involvement or secondary infection.

NOTES

TINEA VERSICOLOR

A chronic, superficial fungal infection characterized by fine scaling and decreased or increased pigmentation, mainly on the trunk.

I. Etiology

A superficial fungal infection caused by *Malassezia furfur,* a yeastlike fungus.

II. Incidence

Seen most often in young adults in temperate zones. Uncommon prior to puberty.

III. Subjective data

A. Slightly pruritic or asymptomatic.

B. Chief complaint is cosmetic; patient complains of white, pink, or tan spots on normal skin.

C. Often no complaints but found on routine physical examination.

IV. Objective data

A. Lesions.

1. Circinate macules with fine scales that can be demonstrated by light scratching.
2. Characteristically tan or reddish brown but may vary from white to brown.
3. On skin exposed to the sun, lesions appear hypopigmented, since they do not tan. Lesions may be darker than surrounding skin in winter and lighter than surrounding skin in summer.
4. Areas may coalesce.

B. Distribution.

1. Primarily on the trunk.
2. Less commonly on the neck and face.

V. Assessment

A. Diagnosis.

1. Microscopic examination of scales in potassium hydroxide fungal preparation reveals hyphae and budding yeasts.
2. Examination by Wood's light: lesions may show gold to orange fluorescence.

B. Differential diagnosis in tanned patients.

1. Vitiligo: by family history; lesions pure white.
2. Postinflammatory or posttraumatic hypopigmentation: by history.

VI. Plan

A. Nizoral (ketoconazole) 2% Cream: once daily for 2 weeks.

B. Exelderm Cream or Solution 1%: apply gently once daily for 3 weeks.

C. Selenium sulfide (Selsun Lotion) 2%, order 8 oz.

1. Daily for 7 days:
   a. Bathe.
   b. Rub lesions with a coarse towel.
   c. Apply Selsun to entire trunk and other affected areas.
   d. Lather with a small amount of water.

e. Leave on skin for 10–20 minutes.
f. Rinse thoroughly.

D. Frequent recurrences:
1. Nizoral 200 mg PO daily for 2 weeks.

VII. Education

A. Rub lesions with a coarse towel before applying medication.
B. Launder clothing, towels, and sheets in hot water.
C. Scaling should disappear within several days.
D. Continue treatment for several weeks.
E. Pigment changes resolve slowly. On sun-exposed skin, lesions will not appear normal until they acquire a tan or until existing tan fades; this may take 6 months.
F. Recurrence is common.
G. Selsun may irritate skin.
H. Do not use Selsun on genitalia.
I. Nizoral is for adolescents and adults.

VIII. Follow-up

A. Recheck in 2 weeks; scaling should not be present, but pigment changes will still be evident.
B. Recurrences should be retreated. If resistant to treatment, use Nizoral by mouth for one week.

IX. Complications

None; of cosmetic significance only.

X. Consultation/referral

No improvement after skin color has had an opportunity to return to normal. Repigmentation may take 3–6 months.

NOTES

UMBILICAL CORD CARE

Cord care begins in the newborn nursery and is continued until the stump falls off and the area is totally healed. Complete healing may take several weeks.

I. Subjective data

A. Cord clamped; drying begins within hours.

B. Clamp removed on first or second day of life.

C. Black, hard stump remains attached for approximately 6–12 days.

II. Objective data

A. Stump clean and dry.

B. No inflammation surrounding umbilicus.

C. No bleeding, discharge, or odor.

III. Assessment

Normal healing of umbilical cord.

IV. Plan

A. Wash with soap and water and dry thoroughly twice a day.

B. Apply antibiotic ointment (neosporin) to umbilicus 2–3 times a day.

or

C. Clean with alcohol once a day.

D. Clean depression with a cotton swab after stump falls off.

V. Education

A. Keep diapers folded below umbilicus.

B. With disposable diapers, fold plastic to the outside.

C. Keep rubber pants below umbilicus.

D. Watch for oozing, odor, bleeding, or inflammation.

E. A small amount of discharge is normal for 1–2 days after the cord drops off.

F. Keep depression clean and dry. It can become a site for the collection of dead skin, powder, etc., leading to infection.

VI. Follow-up

None necessary unless bleeding, discharge, odor, swelling, or inflammation occurs.

VII. Complications

Infection.

VIII. Consultation/referral

A. Bleeding.

B. Discharge.

C. Foul odor.

D. Edema.

E. Inflammation.

F. Moistness at base of cord (may be urachus).

NOTES

UMBILICAL GRANULOMA

A small, pink lesion that forms at the base of the umbilical cord.

I. Etiology

Believed to be the result of a mild infection.

II. Subjective data

A. Umbilicus moist, oozing.

B. Pink mass on umbilicus.

C. Foul odor may be present.

D. History of mild infection with mucopurulent drainage or delayed drying of cord.

III. Objective data

A. Soft, pink granulation tissue on umbilicus.

B. Seropurulent discharge.

C. Examine for bleeding, erythema, purulent discharge, edema of stump.

IV. Assessment

A. Diagnosis is made by typical appearance of granulation tissue.

B. Differential diagnosis

1. Umbilical polyp: larger (7–10 mm), firmer mass.
2. Patent urachus: fistula between bladder and umbilicus that discharges urine when infant voids.

V. Plan

A. Cauterize with silver nitrate stick. Do not touch surrounding skin with silver nitrate.

B. Wash umbilicus 3–5 minutes after cauterizing.

VI. Education

A. Keep diapers and rubber pants below umbilicus.

B. Clean with alcohol sponge at least 3 times a day.

C. Watch for oozing, odor, bleeding.

VII. Follow-up

Recheck in 5–7 days to check healing. Repeat cauterization if granuloma is still present.

VIII. Complications

Secondary infection.

IX. Consultation/referral

Persistence of granuloma after repeat treatment with silver nitrate.

NOTES

URINARY TRACT INFECTION

A bacterial infection of any portion of the urinary tract. It may be limited to asymptomatic bacteriuria or may progress to involve the renal pelvis and parenchyma, causing pyelonephritis.

I. Etiology

Escherichia coli is the most common causative organism. Other organisms include Klebsiella, Proteus, Pseudomonas, Enterobacteriaceae, and less commonly, *Staphylococcus aureus.*

II. Incidence

A. Most commonly seen between 2 months and 2 years of age; more frequent in girls than in boys. The recurrence rate after the first infection is estimated at about 40%.

B. Often related to sexual activity in adolescent females.

III. Subjective data

A. Classic signs.
   1. Elevated temperature—may be as high as 104.5°F.
   2. Chills.
   3. Anorexia.
   4. Urinary frequency and urgency.
   5. Dysuria.
   6. Incontinence.
   7. Enuresis—nocturnal and diurnal.
   8. Costovertebral angle tenderness (flank pain).
   9. Suprapubic pain.
   10. Back pain.

B. Typical symptoms.
   1. Infants
      a. Failure to thrive.
      b. Fever of unknown origin.
      c. Irritability.
      d. Strong odor to urine.
   2. Preschool-age children
      a. Abdominal pain.
      b. Vomiting.
      c. Fever.
      d. Strong-smelling urine.
      e. Enuresis.
      f. Urinary frequency and urgency.
      g. Dysuria.
   3. School-age and older children
      a. Symptoms as for preschool children.
      b. Costovertebral angle tenderness.

C. Pertinent subjective data to obtain.

1. Character of urinary stream.

2. History of previous urinary tract infection or symptoms.

3. History of possible causes of urethral irritation.

a. Use of bubble bath or feminine sprays.

b. Vaginitis.

c. Pinworms.

d. Masturbation.

e. Sexual activity.

4. Personal hygiene practices.

5. Change in urinary habits.

6. History of constipation.

Note: Urinary tract infection should be suspected in all children who present with failure to thrive, fever of unknown origin, or recurrent abdominal pain.

IV. Objective data

A. Obtain accurate weight and blood pressure.

B. Poor growth rate.

C. Fever of up to 104.5°F.

D. Abdominal examination may reveal suprapubic and/or costovertebral angle tenderness.

E. Child may appear toxic with acute infection.

F. Laboratory tests: urinalysis and urine culture.

1. Since infection may be completely asymptomatic, routine urinalysis should be done yearly on all children to detect asymptomatic bacteriuria. Approximately 2% of females screened are found to have significant bacteriuria.

2. Proteinuria may be present.

3. Criteria for diagnosis by urine culture in a symptomatic child:

a. >10 WBCs per high-power field (HPF) in centrifuged sediment.

b. >100,000 bacteria/ml (of the same type of microorganism) in a culture of a clean-voided specimen. Growth of more than one organism is usually indicative of contamination, not infection.

c. Any pathogens in a suprapubic aspirate or from a catheter specimen (if first 10 ml is excluded) indicate infection.

4. Order sensitivity studies as well as urine culture if specimen is to be taken to the laboratory (results will take 24–48 hours).

5. Ideally, two or more urine cultures should be done unless the specimen is obtained by suprapubic aspiration (by physician) or sterile catheterization.

6. If child is not toxic or does not have severe symptoms, postpone treatment and request a first-morning clean-voided specimen the next day.

7. Repeat any culture with a count between 10,000 and 100,000/ml.

V. Assessment

A. Diagnosis is established by positive urine culture.

B. Differential diagnosis

1. Vaginitis: pyuria of >10 WBCs/HPF; urine culture nonspecific. Symptoms may be those of "cystitis": frequency, burning, urgency.

2. Urethritis: normal urine culture. Symptoms may be those of cystitis: frequency, burning, urgency.
3. Gonococcal urethritis: urethral culture positive; urine culture negative.

VI. Plan

A. Pharmacologic therapy:
   1. Bactrim or Septra (Trimethoprim-sulfamethoxazole). Dosage: 8 mg/kg trimethoprim and 40 mg/kg sulfamethoxazole in 24 hours in two divided doses.
      or
   2. Sulfisoxazole (Gantrisin), 150 mg/kg/24 hours in 4 divided doses. Start with initial loading dose of one-half of the 24 hour dose. Treat for 2 weeks.
      or
   3. Amoxicillin, 40 mg/kg/24 hours in 3 divided doses. Treat for 2 weeks.
   4. Acetaminophen for fever and discomfort (see Drug Index).

B. Repeat urine culture in 48 hours.

C. Encourage fluids.

D. Plan should include attempts to determine mechanism causing infection; consult with physician for referral for urologic evaluation.

E. Indications for IVP and VCUG:
   1. Child under 6 years.
   2. Toxicity
   3. First infection in male.
   4. Second infection in female.

F. Ultrasonography with suspicion of upper UTI.

VII. Education

A. Urine collection
   1. Do not force fluids before collecting specimen.
   2. Collection of clean-voided, midstream specimen
      a. Use sterile container; boil thoroughly washed jar and cover for 10 minutes.
      b. Female. Clean labia from front to back, using a fresh, soft, clean cloth or gauze sponge for each wipe. Cleanse each side with lightly soaped sponges; then spread labia and cleanse from clitoris to anus. Use fresh sponges to rinse.
      c. Male. Retract foreskin and cleanse glans, first with a lightly soaped cloth or sponge, then with water.
      d. Have child initiate voiding and then stop. Obtain specimen when child commences voiding again.
      e. Take specimen to the office immediately; if a delay of more than a few minutes is expected, refrigerate specimen at 4°C.
   3. U-bag collection. It is very difficult to obtain a specimen free of contamination using this method.
      a. Female
         (1) Clean genitalia as above.
         (2) Dry genitalia thoroughly.

(3) Remove protective covering from bag; apply first to perineum, pressing firmly to assure adherence; then apply pressure from perineum forward. Be sure seal is tight.

b. Male

(1) Clean external genitalia.

(2) Dry thoroughly.

(3) Apply bag with firm pressure to ensure a tight seal.

c. Seal edges of bag once infant has voided and take to the office or laboratory immediately.

B. Force fluids during treatment.

C. Try to give medication every 6 hours. Give all medication.

D. Call back immediately if child develops a rash or has nausea, vomiting, diarrhea, or headache.

E. Expect child to improve within 24–48 hours.

F. Teach parent and child to be alert to signs and symptoms of urinary tract infection.

G. Do not use bubble baths or feminine sprays.

H. Use showers instead of baths if child is old enough.

I. Do not use deep water for baths.

J. Stress perineal hygiene—wiping from front to back after toileting.

K. Encourage child to void at regular intervals and not to stall voiding.

L. For sexually active adolescent, encourage voiding after intercourse.

M. Minimize constipation. (See protocol, p. 235).

VIII. Follow-up

A. Repeat urine culture in 48 hours.

B. Repeat urine culture 48 hours after treatment is discontinued and every month for 3 months, then every 3 months for 1 year.

IX. Complications

A. Recurrent urinary tract infection.

B. Pyelonephritis.

C. Failure to thrive in undiagnosed or untreated cases.

X. Consultation/referral

A. Infants—for urologic evaluation.

B. All males with first urinary tract infection—will require urologic evaluation.

C. All females with second urinary tract infection—will require urologic evaluation.

D. If patient is symptomatic 2–3 days after initiation of therapy.

NOTES

VARICELLA (CHICKENPOX)

A benign, highly contagious viral disease characterized by a mild constitutional prodrome followed by a pruritic rash consisting of macules, papules, vesicles, and crusted lesions, which appear in crops and rapidly progress through various stages.

I. Etiology

Varicella-zoster virus. (Primary infection.)

II. Incidence

Peak incidence is 2–8 years of age. Epidemics are seen in 3 to 4 year cycles, mainly from January to May.

III. Incubation period

Can vary from 10–21 days; average period is 14–16 days.

IV. Communicability

One day prior to appearance of rash to 6 days after. Transmitted by droplet infection and by direct contact. Dried crusts are not infectious. Chickenpox can be contracted from patients with herpes zoster.

Note: Licensure of live varicella vaccine (VZV) is anticipated in the near future in the United States. The VZV vaccine was developed in Japan where it is licensed for administration. In Japan, nearly all vaccinees seroconverted in one month and were seropositive 5 years later. The protective effect was about 83% and those that had the disease had a mild clinical course with few lesions. Similarly, the VZV vaccine is currently undergoing clinical trials in the United States.

V. Subjective data

- **A.** History of exposure about 2 weeks prior to appearance of lesions or a history of chickenpox in the community.
- **B.** Lesions appear in crops.
- **C.** Lesions in various stages of development at one time.
- **D.** Prodrome: child may have low-grade temperature, upper respiratory infection, anorexia, headache, and malaise for 24–48 hours prior to appearance of lesions, or constitutional symptoms may appear simultaneously with exanthem. Prodrome may be recognized in retrospect only.
- **E.** Lesions: few spots on trunk or face initially; then a 3- to 4-day period during which successive crops erupt on trunk, face, scalp, extremities, and mucous membranes. Lesions are seen in greatest concentration centrally and on proximal portions of the extremities. They tend to be more abundant on clothed areas and in areas of local inflammation (e.g., diaper area in a child with diaper rash). Lesions are found on the scalp, the mucous membranes, and the conjunctiva.

VI. Objective data

- **A.** Skin
  1. Lesions appear as small red macules and rapidly progress to papules to clear vesicles on an erythematous base to umbilicated to cloudy vesicles to crusted lesions. (Drying occurs in the center of the vesicle, producing an umbilicated appearance prior to crusting.)
  2. Lesions are seen in various stages in one area. (They progress through the stages in 6–8 hours, with crusts forming in 2–4 days.)
  3. Total number of lesions is generally 200 to 400.

B. Mucous membranes
  1. Vesicles rupture rapidly, so are most commonly seen as shallow white ulcers 2–3 mm in diameter.
  2. Lesions may be present on genital mucosa, palpebral conjunctiva, ear canals, and mouth.

C. Lymphadenopathy. May be generalized.

D. Severity
  1. Varies from mild cases with a few lesions and no systemic symptoms to severe toxicity with hundreds of lesions and elevated temperature (104°F).
  2. Systemic manifestations subside after the first 3 days as new crops of lesions cease to appear.

VII. Assessment

A. Diagnosis is usually made by history of contact and development of an exanthem that rapidly progresses through stages (macule to papule to vesicle to crusting) and is found in various stages in one area.

B. Differential diagnosis
  1. Smallpox: severe prodrome; lesions are seen in the same stage, are more prominent peripherally, and progress more slowly (5–6 days) through stages.

     Note: Variola has virtually been eradicated throughout the world and is not a diagnostic consideration in the United States at this time.
  2. Impetigo: lesions to not appear in crops, differ in appearance and distribution, and do not involve mucous membranes of the mouth. There are no constitutional symptoms.
  3. Insect bites: lesions do not have vesicular appearance and are not present on mucous membranes. Constitutional symptoms are not present.
  4. Scabies: lesions do not have characteristic appearance, are not present on mucous membranes, but are characteristically present in the interdigital spaces.
  5. Herpes zoster: lesions are painful and usually confined to dermatome.

VIII. Plan

A. Symptomatic treatment to alleviate itching
  1. Baking soda or Aveeno oatmeal baths.
  2. Calamine lotion as needed to skin.
  3. Antihistamines for pruritus.
     a. Benadryl

        or

     b. Atarax (see Drug Index).

B. Acetaminophen as indicated for temperature elevation (see Drug Index).

C. Oral lesions. Warm saline or hydrogen peroxide mouth rinses.

D. Genital lesions. Warm saline or hydrogen peroxide compresses.

E. Infected lesions
  1. One or two lesions: wash lesions well and apply the following:
     a. Neosporin ointment 4 times daily.

        or

     b. Bacitracin ointment 4 times daily.
  2. Many lesions: see Impetigo.

F. Zovirax (acyclovir): Infectious disease experts do not recommend routine use of acyclovir in varicella. There are instances, however, where administration may be indicated since, if given within 24 hours of onset of rash, it results in a milder illness.. The indications for uses should be defined and included in guidelines for individual health centers.

IX. Education

A. Transmitted by direct contact or inhalation from nose and throat secretions.

B. Communicable from 24–48 hours prior to first lesion and until all lesions have crusted.

C. Crusts do not contain active virus.

D. Second attacks are rare. Lifelong immunity is generally conferred.

E. In mild cases, crusting occurs within 5 days. In severe cases, crusting occurs in 10 days.

F. Keep child home from school until all vesicles are crusted; this generally takes 7 days.

G. Do not expose to pregnant women or infants.

H. Do not expose to children with eczema or malignancies or those on immunosuppressive therapy.

I. Call immediately if cough, dyspnea, or chest pain occurs within 2–5 days of onset of exanthem.

J. Call immediately if child develops high fever, stiff neck, headache, listlessness, or hyperirritability.

K. Keep nails trimmed. Put gloves on child if scratching is a problem.

L. Use careful hygiene to prevent superimposed infection; keep nails clean, bathe child daily, and change clothing daily.

M. Encourage fluids.

N. If genital lesions cause dysuria, encourage child to void in tub.

O. Crusts fall off in 5–20 days.

P. When scabs fall off, a shallow pink depression remains. This eventually becomes white, and repigmentation occurs later.

Q. Scarring is caused by premature removal of scabs or secondarily infected lesions.

R. Do not use aspirin.

S. Aveeno baths: mix 1 cup Aveeno with 2 cups cold water. Shake until well mixed, then pour in tub of tepid water.

X. Follow-up

A. Generally not indicated in uncomplicated cases.

B. Return to office if there is

1. Any question of secondary infection.
2. Cough, dyspnea, or chest pain.
3. Persistent vomiting, abdominal pain.
4. Headache, fever, stiff neck, lethargy, or irritability.
5. Fever over 104°F, or any fever after one week.
6. Lesions continue to develop after one week.

XI. Complications

A. Most common: secondary bacterial infection.

B. Rare: encephalitis, pneumonia, Guillain-Barré syndrome, hemorrhagic varicella, Reye's syndrome.

C. Disseminated varicella.

XII. Consultation/referral

A. Suspected complications.

B. Infants and children with debilitating conditions for prophylaxis if exposed to, or for antiviral therapy if infected by, varicella.

1. Varicella-zoster immune globulin (VZIG) should be given within 96 hours of exposure to:
    a. Newborns whose mothers had varicella less than 5 days prior to delivery or 48 hours after delivery.
    b. Premature infants.
    c. Children with cancer or collagen-vascular disease.
    d. Organ or bone marrow transplant recipients.
    e. Children being treated with steroids, cytotoxic chemotherapy, or radiation.
    f. Immunodeficient children.
    g. Children with severe burns or eczema.
    h. Pregnant women.
2. Zovirax is given to the VZV susceptible "high risk" child if he is beyond the fourth day post exposure when there would be no beneficial effect of passive immunization with VZIG. It is generally given IV to:
    a. Children with an immunodeficiency syndrome.
    b. Children with cancer undergoing chemotherapy.

NOTES

VIRAL CROUP

Laryngotracheobronchitis characterized by inspiratory stridor. Inflammation of the respiratory mucosa of all airways is generally present. The classic symptoms are caused by inflammation and edema in the larynx and subglottic area.

I. **Etiology**

Generally caused by the parainfluenza virus. Less commonly caused by the respiratory syncytial virus, influenza virus, and adenoviruses.

II. **Incidence**

Most common age range is 3 months to 3 years. Generally occurs in late fall or early winter.

III. **Subjective data**

A. History of gradual onset.
B. Symptoms of upper respiratory infection for several days prior to onset.
C. Fever—low-grade or moderate.
D. Harsh, barking cough.
E. Wheezing—with lower respiratory tract involvement.
F. Hoarseness.
G. "High-pitched sound" on inspiration; often occurs at night.
H. Child does not appear toxic.
I. Important questions to ask in history to rule out epiglottitis:
   1. Acute onset?
   2. Dysphagia?
   3. Drooling?
   4. Apprehension and air hunger?

   If answer is affirmative for any of the above or child appears toxic, do not attempt to examine child but refer to physician immediately.

IV. **Objective data**

A. Elevated temperature.
B. Slight hyperemia and edema of nasopharynx.
C. Inspiratory stridor—usually of abrupt onset.
D. Harsh, barking cough.
E. Hoarseness.
F. Dyspnea.
G. Wheezing—with lower respiratory tract involvement.
H. Prolonged expiratory phase.
I. With increased obstruction, breath sounds decrease and anxiety increases.
J. Laboratory test: WBCs normal or low.
K. Lateral neck x-ray to rule out epiglottitis.

V. **Assessment: differential diagnosis**

A. Bacterial croup (epiglottitis): toxic, drooling, dysphagic, acute onset, anxious. Age range generally 3–7 years.

B. Foreign body: fever absent; dysphagia, visualization of foreign body, sudden onset of coughing and wheezing; careful history may reveal episode of choking just prior to onset of wheezing.

C. Congenital laryngeal stridor: stridor present from birth.

D. Bronchiolitis, pneumonia, bronchitis: see following table, Differential Diagnosis of Viral Croup, Bronchiolitis, Pneumonia, and Bronchitis.

VI. Plan

A. Home management if child
   1. Is well hydrated and pink.
   2. Has little or no retraction.
   3. Has normal air exchange on auscultation.
   4. Has respirations and pulse within normal range.
   5. Has absence of stridor at rest.

B. Cool-mist vaporizer: use continuously.

C. Force fluids, especially clear liquids.

D. Monitor respiratory rate.

VII. Education

A. Cool-mist vaporizers are preferred over steam vaporizers. Warm steam may have a partial drying effect and may raise the temperature of a febrile child. Also, steam vaporizers are more dangerous to use around small children.

B. Fluids—especially clear liquids—are important in the acute phase. They help keep secretions thin.

C. Croup is generally self-limited.

D. Inspiratory obstruction at a maximum for the first 24–48 hours. Respiratory symptoms persist for 1 week.

E. Recurrences are common until 5–6 years of age.

F. Do not use antihistamines; they tend to cause inspissation of laryngeal and tracheal secretions.

G. Restlessness and anxiety are indications of hypoxemia.

H. Monitor respiratory rate; teach parent how to count respirations.

I. Symptoms generally increase at night.

J. For immediate relief of acute symptoms, take child into bathroom and turn on hot water. Symptoms also improve when child is taken outside. If no improvement after 5 minutes, take child to hospital.

K. Signs and symptoms of airway obstruction are tachypnea, cyanosis, increased retractions, and increased anxiety or restlessness. Should any of these occur, call physician immediately.

VIII. Follow-up

A. Call immediately if child becomes restless or anxious.

B. Call immediately if respiratory rate or retractions increase.

IX. Complications

Principal complication is asphyxia secondary to laryngeal obstruction.

X. Consultation/referral

A. Any child with an acute onset of inspiratory stridor, tachypnea, retractions, or diminished breath sounds.

B. Any child with cyanosis, restlessness, anxiety, and/or flaring of the alae nasi.

Differential Diagnosis of Viral Croup, Bronchiolitis, Pneumonia, and Bronchitis

Criteria	Viral Croup (Laryngotracheobronchitis)	Bronchiolitis	Pneumonia	Bronchitis
Etiology	Viral Parainfluenza viruses (most common) Influenza viruses Adenoviruses Rhinoviruses Respiratory syncytial virus	Viral Respiratory syncytial virus (most common) Parainfluenza viruses Adenoviruses Influenza viruses Allergy Inflammation of small and terminal bronchioles Occasionally, secondary bacterial infection	Bacterial Pneumococci Hemolytic streptococci *Hemophilus influenzae* Staphylococci Viral Respiratory syncytial virus Parainfluenza viruses Adenoviruses Influenza viruses Mycoplasmal	Viral, bacterial (including mycoplasmal and fungal)
Incidence	Most common ages: 3 months–3 years Generally seen during late fall or early winter	Most commonly seen under 2 years; spans ages 3 months–3 years Most common in winter	All age groups Most common in winter	Uncommon in childhood as an isolated entity
Subjective findings	History of upper respiratory infection Low-grade or moderate fever Gradual onset of cough and dyspnea Sudden onset of stridor, usually at night	Mild rhinitis for 1–2 days Low-grade or no fever Abrupt onset of dyspnea Wheezing Cough	History of upper respiratory infection Abrupt rise in temperature Cough Tachypnea Chills Chest pain or abdominal pain Bacterial pneumonia presents with acute onset Viral pneumonia presents with insidious onset	Low-grade fever Dry, hacking, nonproductive cough for 4–6 days Productive cough after 4–6 days Chest pain with coughing

(Cont'd)

Differential Diagnosis of Viral Croup, Bronchiolitis, Pneumonia, and Bronchitis (cont'd)

Criteria	Viral Croup (Laryngotracheobronchitis)	Bronchiolitis	Pneumonia	Bronchitis
Objective findings	Variable fever Harsh, barking cough Nasopharynx slightly hyperemic with mild edema Inspiratory stridor Supracluvicular and intercostal retractions Diminished breath sounds	Marked respiratory distress Rapid, shallow respirations Flaring of alae nasi Intermittent cyanosis Rales (diffuse) Expiratory wheezes/grunts Decreased breath sounds Prolonged expiratory phase Displacement of liver edge below costal margin (hyperinflation of lungs leads to depression of the diaphragm, resulting in liver displacement) Tachycardia Hyperresonance on percussion Bilateral involvement	Elevated temperature: 39.5–40.5°C (103.1–104.9°F) Respiratory distress varies from mild to marked Tachypnea Decreased breath sounds Inspiratory rales, rales may not be heard until infection is resolving Retractions Hyporesonance over areas of consolidation Unilateral or bilateral involvement	Fever mild or absent Coarse inspiratory rhonchi, which disappear with coughing
Laboratory	WBCs normal or low	WBCs normal Eosinophilia (nasal and peripheral) in allergic infants	WBCs elevated to 18,000–40,000/mm^3 (mainly polys)	WBCs normal or slightly elevated
X-ray		Hyperinflation Increased bronchovascular markings Mild infiltrates	Patchy infiltrates Increased bronchovascular markings Lobar consolidation	Normal or increased bronchovascular markings

Duration of illness	5–7 days	Acute symptoms 2–7 days Total resolution 7–10 days	7–10 days	7–14 days
Diagnosis	Generally apparent from inspiratory stridor and harsh, barking cough	Generally made by history of abrupt onset of dyspnea and wheezing in infant; hyperinflation of lungs and retractions support the diagnosis	Usually made by x-ray studies and physical signs of consolidation; etiology established by culture and clinical features Mycoplasmal (school-age children and adolescents) Insidious onset Nonproductive cough Fever Staphylococcal (children under 3 years) High fever Abdominal distention Respiratory distress Toxic Unilateral involvement Viral Upper respiratory infection often precedes pneumonia Insidious onset WBCs slightly elevated *H. Influenzae* (infants and young children) Symptoms similar to any of above Failure to respond to penicillin therapy	Diagnosis made by signs and symptoms

(Cont'd)

Differential Diagnosis of Viral Croup, Bronchiolitis, Pneumonia, and Bronchitis (cont'd)

Criteria	Viral Croup (Laryngotracheobronchitis)	Bronchiolitis	Pneumonia	Bronchitis
Treatment	Outpatient management Cool-mist vaporizer Parents to monitor respirations and to watch for tachypnea, cyanosis, retractions, anxiety Increase liquid intake Refer for physician management children with an acute onset of inspiratory stridor; respiratory distress; signs of acute epiglottitis (sudden onset, elevated temperature, toxic, drooling, anxious)	Refer to physician for airway maintenance and oxygenation; probable hospitalization Cool humidified oxygen Increase liquid intake Antibiotics indicated only with secondary bacterial infection	Penicillin G Streptococcal Staphylococcal Pneumococcal Ampicillin *H. influenzae* Erythromycin Mycoplasma Viral Antibiotic therapy only if secondary bacterial infection is suspected Cool-mist vaporizer Increase liquid intake	Symptomatic Postural drainage Chest percussion Avoid inhalants Cool-mist vaporizer Antibiotic therapywith elevated WBCs or production of purulent sputum; amoxicillin is generally the drug of choice

NOTES

VIRAL GASTROENTERITIS

An acute, generally self-limited inflammation of the gastrointestinal tract, manifested by a sudden onset of vomiting and diarrhea.

I. Etiology

Reovirus, echovirus, Coxsackie virus, adenoviruses, polioviruses, and parvovirus are the common causative agents.

II. Incidence

Seen sporadically in day care, schools and communities in epidemic proportions. Common in all age groups, and seen most frequently in winter.

III. Incubation period

24–48 hours.

IV. Communicability

Transmissible during acute stage via fecal–oral route.

V. Subjective data

A. Vomiting. Assess duration, frequency, character, amount.

B. Diarrhea. Assess duration, frequency, consistency of stools, presence of blood or mucus. Stools are loose with unpleasant odor. Blood or mucus is rarely present.

C. Pertinent subjective data to obtain

1. History of exposure to others with similar symptoms.
2. History of illness in the community.
3. Urinary output: frequency and amount.
4. Elevated temperature.
5. Abdominal pain.
6. Weight loss.
7. Type and amount of feedings prior to and since onset.

D. Pertinent subjective data to rule out other causes

1. Exposure to turtles.
2. Exposure to food source outside of home.
3. Ingestion of drugs or toxic substances: if history is positive, refer immediately to physician.
4. Exposure to stressful situation.
5. Ingestion of home-canned foods: if history is positive, refer immediately to physician.

VI. Objective data

A. Physical examination should include other systems to rule out other infections.

1. Ears.
2. Throat.
3. Adenopathy.
4. Chest.
5. CNS for signs of meningeal irritation.
   a. Nuchal rigidity.
   b. Fontanelle.

c. Kernig's sign.
d. Brudzinski's signs.
e. Irritability, especially paradoxical.
f. Level of sensorium.

6. Abdomen for distention, visible peristalsis, bowel sounds, tenderness, spasm, organomegaly, masses.
7. Assess state of hydration (see Appendix D, Clinical Signs of Dehydration).
8. Weight, pulse, blood pressure, temperature.

B. Laboratory tests
1. Urinalysis, include specific gravity to assess state of dehydration.
2. Stool culture.
a. It is not necessary to culture stools of all children seen with acute gastroenteritis.
b. Indications for culture.
(1) Diarrhea persisting over 4 days.
(2) Infants.
(3) Blood in stools.

VII. Assessment

A. Diagnosis is made by history of exposure, clinical course, and clinical picture. It is generally a diagnosis of exclusion if the history is not suggestive of other bacterial or parasitic etiologies and if done, a negative stool culture and the absence of leukocytes on stool exam.

B. Differential diagnosis
1. *Escherichia coli* gastroenteritis: commonly seen in children under 2 years of age. Gradual onset of diarrheal stools, which are loose, slimy, green, and foul smelling; vomiting and fever are not usually prominent symptoms.
2. Salmonella gastroenteritis (including food poisoning): incubation period usually 12–24 hours but can range from 6–72 hours. Severe abdominal cramps and loose, slimy, green stools with odor of rotten eggs are characteristic; vomiting is common. Diagnosis is confirmed by stool culture.
3. Staphylococcal food poisoning: explosive onset 2–6 hours after ingestion of food contaminated with staphylococci; other persons who ingested the same food have a similar illness. Not transmitted from person to person.

VIII. Plan

A. If concurrent infection is found in addition to gastroenteritis (e.g., pneumonia, otitis media, pharyngitis), treat according to protocol. Initially antibiotics may have to be given parenterally.

B. Dietary management is directed primarily toward fluid and electrolyte management.
1. First 24 hours
a. Pedialyte or Ricelyte: 1–2 oz every 30–60 minutes.
or
b. Clear liquids (water, cola, ginger ale, Gatorade): 1–2 oz every 30–60 minutes.
c. To control vomiting, begin with 1 tsp every 5–10 minutes.
d. When tolerated, increase to 1–2 oz every 30–60 minutes. Gradually increase the amount and decrease the frequency as vomiting subsides.

If vomiting recurs, resume giving 1 tsp every 5 minutes and again gradually increase amounts.

2. Second day
   a. If diarrhea has not improved, continue clear liquids (water, cola, ginger ale, weak tea, apple juice, Gatorade, Popsicles), 1–2 oz every 30–60 minutes.
   b. If diarrhea has improved, add the following bland solids in small amounts:
      (1) Infant rice cereal mixed with water.
      (2) Banana flakes or mashed ripe banana.
      (3) Saltines.
      (4) Dry cereal.
      (5) Toast with jelly.
      (6) Jell-O.
   c. At this point in treatment, skim milk diluted with equal parts water, or half-strength ProSobee or Isomil, may be added in amounts adequate to ensure hydration.
3. Third day
   a. If bland solids have not been added, start with small amounts of the foods listed in 2.b above.
   b. If bland solids have been started and diarrhea has improved, continue as above and add baked potato and chicken. Progress to full-strength skim milk, ProSobee, or Isomil. Regular formula may be added if diarrhea has stopped.
   c. Gradually return to normal diet, avoiding whole milk, juices, and foods with roughage until diarrhea has completely subsided.

IX. Education

A. Explain that the disease is self-limited. The usual duration of illness is 5 to 7 days. Medications such as paregoric, Kaopectate, and Lomotil are not indicated.

B. Aim of treatment is to keep child well hydrated.
   1. Clear liquids should be at room temperature. Cola or ginger ale is preferable if "flat."
   2. Do not give large amounts. Set timer and adhere to 5- to 10-minute intervals initially.
   3. If large amounts of cola are used, the caffeine may cause stimulation and increase the severity of the diarrhea.
   4. Do not give whole milk for at least 48 hours.
   5. Do not use boiled skim milk; it has a high solute load.

C. Once vomiting is under control, increase amount of clear liquids and decrease frequency to avoid too frequent stimulation of the gastrocolic reflex, which might aggravate the diarrhea.

D. Stress the importance of strict adherence to the dietary regime in order not to prolong the course of the illness.

E. If clear liquids only are given for more than 48 hours, reactive loose stools may occur.

F. Starvation stools—scanty, mucousy, loose, green-brown—may mistakenly be construed to be diarrheal stools.

G. Monitor temperature and urinary output.

H. Use petroleum jelly on perianal area to prevent excoriation.

I. Support and encourage parent; treatment is time-consuming.

J. Gastroenteritis may occur in the entire family. It is highly communicable by the fecal-oral or fecal-respiratory route.

1. Careful hand-washing technique must be followed to control spread.
2. Do not let other children drink from the sick child's glass or use the same utensils.

X. Follow-up

A. Close telephone follow-up every 2 hours if vomiting and diarrhea are frequent.

B. Daily weight measurement until weight is stabilized.

C. Daily or twice daily telephone contact until all gastrointestinal symptoms have stopped.

XI. Complications

The most important complication is dehydration.

XII. Consultation/referral

A. Infants under 3 months of age.

B. Vomiting persisting over 12 hours.

C. Diarrhea persisting over 3 days.

D. Any signs or symptoms of dehydration.

E. Abdominal pain or tenderness on examination.

NOTES

VOMITING—ACUTE

The forceful ejection of stomach contents through the esophagus and mouth; a common symptom throughout infancy and childhood.

I. Etiology

Associated with a variety of illnesses, infections, and emotional stress. It is often indicative of an abnormality or infection of the gastrointestinal tract, urinary tract, or central nervous system. The etiology varies according to age group.

II. Incidence

One of the most common symptoms throughout infancy and childhood.

III. Subjective data

Pertinent subjective data to obtain:

A. Is nausea associated with vomiting?
B. Does child appear ill?
C. Duration of vomiting—acute or chronic.
D. Frequency of vomiting.
E. Character of vomitus—undigested food, bile, fecal material, blood.
F. Relation to intake.
G. Projectile vomiting or "spitting up?"
H. Associated temperature elevation.
I. Diarrhea or constipation.
J. Exposure to similar illness.
K. Any weight loss or last accurate weight.
L. Decrease in urinary output.
M. Detailed dietary history.
N. Ingestion of drugs or other substances.
O. Stress or changes—family, school.
P. Associated symptoms.
   1. Pulling at ears or complaints of ear pain.
   2. Sore throat or distress when swallowing.
   3. Stiff neck.
   4. Cough.
   5. Abdominal pain.
   6. Headache.
   7. Changes in vision.
   8. High-pitched cry.
   9. Convulsions.
Q. History of injury (e.g., fall on head).

IV. Objective data

A. Physical examination should encompass other systems to rule out other infectious processes.
   1. Ears.
   2. Throat.
   3. Adenopathy.

4. Chest.
5. CNS for signs of meningeal irritation:
   a. Nuchal rigidity.
   b. Fontanelle.
   c. Kernig's sign.
   d. Brudzinski's sign.
   e. Irritability, especially paradoxical.
   f. Level of sensorium.
6. Abdomen for distention, visible peristalsis, bowel sounds, tenderness, spasm, organomegaly, masses.
7. Assess state of hydration (see Appendix D, Clinical Signs of Dehydration).
8. Weight, head circumference, pulse, blood pressure, temperature.

B. Laboratory test. Urinalysis; include specific gravity to assess state of hydration.

V. Assessment

A. Type of vomiting
1. Projectile
   a. Etiology: upper gastrointestinal tract or increased intracranial pressure.
   b. Refer to physician.
2. Vomiting without nausea
   a. Etiology: probable increased intracranial pressure.
   b. Refer to physician.
3. Vomiting with nausea.
   a. Etiology: infection or toxicity.

B. Vomiting in infants (neonates to toddlers 2 years of age).
1. Most acute vomiting in this age group is in conjunction with infection. The following causes must also be considered:
   a. Overfeeding.
   b. Poor feeding techniques (e.g., failure to burp baby, propping of bottle).
   c. Congenital anomalies.
      (1) Gastrointestinal lesions.
         (a) Pyloric stenosis: onset of vomiting at 2–3 weeks of age; progresses to projectile vomiting.
         (b) Chalasia: vomiting or regurgitation after feedings.
         (c) Intussusception: currant jelly stools, distention, visible peristalsis, bile-stained vomitus.
         (d) Volvulus.
      (2) Hydrocephalus: increased head circumference, bulging fontanelle.
2. Infections: almost any disease with fever at onset.
   a. Gastroenteritis.
   b. Urinary tract infection.
   c. Meningitis.
   d. Pneumonia.
   e. Otitis media.
3. Poisoning.

C. Vomiting in children (2 years of age and older). Infection is also the most common etiology in acute vomiting in children over the age of 2 years, but ingestion of toxic substances becomes of increasing importance in this age group. The following are important causes to be considered in this age group:

1. Acute infection.
    a. Gastroenteritis.
    b. Urinary tract infection.
    c. Meningitis.
    d. Pneumonia.
    e. Pharyngitis.
    f. Otitis media.
    g. Acute glomerulonephritis.
    h. Hepatitis.
2. Appendicitis.
3. Central nervous system.
    a. Increased intracranial pressure due to brain tumor, hydrocephalus.
    b. Migraine headaches.
4. Poisoning.
    a. Lead.
    b. Medications, drugs, salicylates.
    c. Poisons.

VI. Plan

A. Acute vomiting due to infectious cause

1. First 24 hours
    a. Clear liquids—tea, cola, ginger ale, water, Gatorade: 1 tsp every 5 minutes
    or
    b. Oral rehydration solution (Lytren or Pedialyte): 1 tsp every 5 minutes.
    c. After cessation of vomiting, increase amounts and decrease frequency to avoid overstimulating gastrocolic reflex and causing diarrhea. Give 1–2 oz every 30–60 minutes.
    d. If vomiting recurs, resume 1 tsp every 5 minutes until tolerated, and again gradually increase amounts.
2. Second day.
    a. Add infant rice cereal mixed with water, banana, saltines, toast with jelly, Jell-O.
3. Third day.
    a. Gradually resume regular diet, avoiding strong-flavored foods and fried foods until child is completely well.

B. Treatment for concurrent infectious processes must be instituted. Initially antibiotics may have to be given parenterally.

VII. Education

A. Set timer and give 1 tsp of clear liquids every 5 minutes.

1. Cola or ginger ale is tolerated better if flat and at room temperature.
2. Cola contains caffeine, so large amounts may stimulate child.
3. Some children will not take Pedialyte readily.

B. Monitor temperature, intake, and output.

C. Support and encourage parent; this treatment is time-consuming but is the most effective way to treat vomiting and prevent dehydration.

D. Give parent specific dietary instructions—written if possible—and stress importance of strict adherence to regimen.

E. If clear liquids are used for more than 48 hours, child may have reactive loose stools or starvation stools.

F. Stress hygiene and proper hand-washing technique to prevent spread if vomiting due to infectious process.

G. Use tepid baths for temperature control if indicated.

VIII. Follow-up

A. Telephone contact at least every 3–4 hours while child is vomiting. Call immediately if any symptoms of dehydration.

B. Check weight in 24 hours.

C. Follow-up for other infectious process per protocol.

IX. Complications

The most important complication of acute vomiting due to infection is dehydration.

X. Consultation/referral

A. Infant under 6 months of age.

B. Child of any age who appears toxic.

C. Any signs or symptoms of dehydration.

D. Child with projectile vomiting.

E. Blood, fecal material, or bile in vomitus.

F. Vomiting persisting over 12 hours.

G. Child with any positive findings on abdominal examination.

NOTES

VULVOVAGINITIS IN THE PREPUBERTAL CHILD

Inflammation of the vulva and vaginal introitus characterized by dysuria, pruritus, and vaginal discharge.

I. **Etiology**

Often a contact reaction to irritants such as bath soaps, bubble bath, laundry products, deodorants, perfumed powders, nylon underpants, panty hose, or tights. Anal scratching (secondary to pinworm infestation), poor perineal hygiene, and masturbation may cause contamination of the vaginal area. The lack of estrogen makes the immature vaginal mucosa susceptible to infection.

II. **Incidence**

Common in prepubertal females.

III. **Subjective data**

- **A.** Vaginal discharge.
- **B.** Dysuria.
- **C.** Pruritus.
- **D.** Inflammation.
- **E.** Pertinent subjective data to obtain
  1. Use of bubble bath.
  2. Use of harsh soaps.
  3. Recent change in laundry products.
  4. Use of nylon underpants, tights, tight jeans.
  5. Improper toileting hygiene. (Have child demonstrate toileting technique.)
  6. Symptoms of pinworm infestation (see Pinworms).
  7. Exposure to infection (e.g., streptococcal upper respiratory infection).
  8. Recent infection (e.g., group A beta-hemolytic streptococcus).
  9. Recent course of antibiotics.
  10. Determine duration, amount, and type of discharge—bloody, purulent, mucoid.
  11. Masturbation.
  12. Detailed history to determine any question of sexual abuse. Include any behavioral changes which may suggest a possibility of abuse.

IV. **Objective data**

- **A.** Vaginal discharge—thin and mucoid, but may be copious and purulent.
- **B.** Erythema of vulva and vaginal introitus.
- **C.** Check hymenal opening. (A minute high hymenal opening can impair vaginal drainage.)
- **D.** If symptoms are severe, examine vagina with child in the knee-chest position using an otoscope with a nasal speculum or veterinary otoscope.
- **E.** Check for anal excoriation.
- **F.** Rectal exam—to detect foreign body or mass.
- **G.** Laboratory tests
  1. Urinalysis—to rule out UTI and diabetes.
  2. Hematocrit—to rule out anemia.

3. Culture of purulent discharge—both aerobically and on Thayer-Martin medium.

V. Assessment

A. Diagnosis. Eighty percent of cases in prepubertal children are nonspecific vulvovaginitis.

B. Differential diagnosis

1. Physiologic leukorrhea.
2. Foreign body: foreign body visualized; foul-smelling drainage.
3. Gonorrhea: culture positive for *Neisseria gonorrhoeae.*
4. Herpes simplex: vesicular eruptions; may be ulcerations; painful. Herpes simplex type 1 can cause simultaneous lesions in the mouth and vulva of young girls.
5. Monilia: vulvar and vaginal erythema; white, cheesy vaginal discharge; presence of Candida in potassium hydroxide wet preparation.
6. Trichomonas vaginitis: vaginal erythema; profuse frothy discharge that is gray or green in color and malodorous. Trichomonas is seen as motile, pearshaped, flagellated protozoa on microscopic examination of wet preparation. Trichomonas may also be detected by Pap smear.
7. Pinworms: pinworm eggs visualized microscopically on Scotch tape slide.
8. Sexual abuse. Rule out by careful history. If high index of suspicion and history negative, refer to mental health worker with expertise in the field.

VI. Plan

A. Sitz baths 3 times a day.

B. Proper perineal hygiene.

C. White cotton underpants.

D. Use mild soap—Lowila, castile, Dove.

E. Scotch tape slide for pinworms if infestation suspected.

F. Neosporin ointment or 1% hydrocortisone cream applied locally 3–4 times a day.

G. Antibiotics as indicated by culture:

1. Group A beta-hemolytic streptococcus or pneumococcus:
   a. Penicillin 125–250 mg qid for 10 days.

   or

   b. Erythromycin 50 mg/kg/day in 4 divided doses for 10 days.
2. *Hemophilus influenzae:* amoxicillin 40 mg/kg/day in 3 divided doses for 10 days.
3. *Neisseria gonorrhoeae:* consult with physician for parenteral penicillin; order serology for syphilis.

VII. Education

A. Teach careful perineal hygiene.

1. Use cool, wet tissue, cotton balls, or Tucks (witch hazel pads).
2. Wipe from front to back.

B. Sitz baths.

1. Warm water.
2. May add baking soda.
3. Duration of 15–20 minutes.

4. Pat dry or air dry after bathing (do not rub). May use hair dryer on cool setting.

C. Avoid shampooing hair in bathtub.

D. Do not use bubble bath.

E. Use Dove or other bland soap in bath.

F. Change underpants frequently. White cotton underpants should be used; they are more absorbent than synthetic materials and free of dyes.

G. Use Ivory Snow for laundry.

H. Discontinue use of bleach and fabric softeners.

I. Avoid perfumed powders.

J. Avoid nylon underpants, tight jeans or slacks, panty hose, and tights; they lead to maceration of the vulva.

K. Encourage child to void in tub if dysuria is a problem.

L. Wash all new items of clothing before child wears them.

M. Avoid long periods of time in wet bathing suits or spandex.

N. Overweight girls are particularly prone to recurrences.

VII. Follow-up

A. Mild symptoms. Have parent call back in 5 days.

B. Moderate to severe symptoms

1. Have parent call back in 24–48 hours.
2. If pruritus is still a problem, use
   a. 1% Hydrocortisone cream 3 times daily on vulva.
   or
   b. Benadryl PO, 5 mg/kg/day in 4 doses.

C. Most cases of nonspecific vulvovaginitis improve within 2 weeks. If symptoms have not improved, vaginal examination and cultures must be done. If no specific causative organism is found, give amoxicillin 3 times daily (dosage according to age and weight) and Vagitrol or Sultrin cream locally.

IX. Consultation/referral

A. Any question of sexual abuse.

B. No improvement within 2 weeks using plan outlined above.

C. Culture positive for *N. gonorrhoeae.*

NOTES

WARTS—COMMON AND PLANTAR

Benign intraepidermal tumors of the skin.

I. Etiology

A papovavirus that grows within the nucleus of the epithelial cells causing hyperplasia.

II. Incidence

Worldwide in occurrence. Plantar and common warts are most frequently seen in children from 12–16 years of age. Both are more common in females.

III. Subjective data

A. Common warts—Verruca vulgaris
   1. Complaints of warts that started as small papules and grew over a period of weeks or months.
   2. There may be no presenting complaints, but warts may be found on physical examination.
   3. Complaint is generally prompted by cosmetic appearance; however, some large warts in certain areas may be irritated by pressure (e.g., use of a pencil may cause pain in wart on finger).

B. Plantar warts—Verruca plantaris
   1. Pain on the sole of the foot on weight bearing or walking.
   2. Corn or callus on the sole of the foot.
   3. Complaint of plantar wart.
   4. May be history of trauma.

IV. Objective data

A. Common warts
   1. Lesions begin as tiny, translucent papules and progress to sharply circumscribed, circinate, firm lesions. Surface is roughened and pitted with papillary protuberances. Black pinpoint spots are often seen on the surface (thrombosed capillaries). Color of lesions ranges from skin-colored to gray-brown.
   2. Found most often in multiple distribution on the hands, but may occur anywhere on epidermis, usually on sites subjected to trauma.

B. Plantar warts
   1. Lesions are flat (because of weight bearing) or slightly elevated.
   2. Resemble a callus with pinpoint depressions on the surface.
   3. Capillary dots may be seen.
   4. Interrupt natural skin lines (calluses do not).
   5. May be a single wart or a multiple distribution.

V. Assessment

A. Diagnosis is usually made by appearance.

B. Differential diagnosis
   1. Molluscum contagiosum: umbilicated waxy papules; molluscum body can be expressed.
   2. Foreign body reaction: by history and surrounding erythema.
   3. Callus: does not interrupt skin lines as does a plantar wart.

VI. Plan

There are many treatments available for warts. Vigorous treatment, which may cause pain and scarring, is not generally recommended. Treatment is not always successful, the rate of recurrence is high, and many times the warts resolve spontaneously (66% within 2 years). The treatment modality selected must be individualized according to the child and the location of the wart.

A. Common warts

1. Occlusive therapy.

a. Completely occlude wart with adhesive tape.

b. Leave tape undisturbed for 1 week.

c. After 1 week, soak wart thoroughly in warm water.

d. Scrape surface of wart with emery board.

e. Reapply adhesive tape, and repeat process.

f. May take several weeks for wart to disappear.

Note: Periungual and subungual warts, which tend to be painful, may well respond to the above occlusive therapy.

2. Duofilm (salicylic and lactic acid in collodion).

a. Soak wart for 10 minutes.

b. Scrape surface with emery board.

c. Apply Duofilm to wart only, using a toothpick.

d. Allow to dry.

e. Repeat every 24 hours.

3. Trans-ver-sal patch (salicylic acid 15%)—6 mm or 12 mm size.

a. Cut patch to size of wart.

b. Clean skin and smooth wart surface with emery file.

c. Moisten wart with drop of water.

d. Apply patch and secure with tape.

e. Apply at bed time and remove in A.M., about 8 hours later.

f. Use nightly until wart is gone.

B. Plantar warts

1. Duofilm.

a. Soak foot in warm water for 10 minutes.

b. Scrape surface of wart with emery board.

c. Apply Duofilm to wart with a toothpick; allow to dry and apply more if necessary to cover wart.

d. Apply adhesive tape to wart once Duofilm is dry, and leave on for 24 hours.

e. Repeat process daily.

2. Trans-plantar patch (salicylic acid 21%)—20 mm size.

a. Follow directions as for Trans-ver-sal patch.

3. Hyperthermia.

a. Hot water (113°F) immersion 1/2–3/4 hour 2–3 times a week for 10 treatments.

b. Wart virus is thermolabile.

VII. Education

A. Warts are a virus.

B. Warts generally occur following trauma to the skin.

C. Warts are transmitted by direct contact, but plantar warts can be transmitted by fomites and floors.

D. Virus concentration is greatest in warts of 6–12 months' duration.

E. Most warts eventually disappear without treatment. Approximately 66% resolve spontaneously within 2 years.

F. Recurrences occur in 20–30% of all cases.

G. Duofilm.

1. Do not use applicator with Duofilm; drops are large and apt to get on surrounding skin.
2. Do not apply to surrounding skin; causes desquamation and tissue destruction.
3. Keep Duofilm bottle tightly closed.
4. With erythema or tenderness, discontinue treatment until inflammation subsides.
5. Do not use on infected or recently treated areas.
6. Overtreatment will cause scarring.

H. Trans--plantar or Trans-ver-sal.

1. Do not apply to surrounding skin.
2. Do not use on any other lesions. Use only on warts that have been diagnosed as such.
3. Patient directions and emery file are included in package.

I. Wear correctly fitting shoes to avoid pressure and trauma to the feet.

J. Treatment may require several weeks.

K. With occlusive therapy, if skin is sensitive to tape, use Micropore or Dermicel.

L. Visible clinical improvement should be noted in 2–4 weeks. Complete resolution may take 6–12 weeks.

VIII. Follow-up

A. Return in 1 week if using Duofilm.

B. Phone in 2 weeks with occlusive therapy.

C. Recheck periungual or subungual warts treated with occlusive therapy every 10–14 days.

IX. Complications

A. Secondary infection.

B. Trauma to surrounding skin.

X. Consultation/referral

A. For more vigorous treatment: electrodesiccation for common warts or laser surgery for plantar warts.

B. Diabetics.

C. Venereal warts (condyloma acuminatum): soft, friable, vegetative clusters on the foreskin, penis, labia, vaginal mucosa, or perianal area.

NOTES

BIBLIOGRAPHY

Adolescents, AIDS and HIV. Compiled by Christina Biddle. Center for Population Options, Washington, DC, July 1991.

Adolescents and Condoms. Compiled by Elizabeth Armstrong. Center for Population Options, Washington, DC, September 1991.

American Academy of Pediatrics, Committee on Infectious Diseases. Parvovirus, erythema infectiosum, and pregnancy. *Pediatrics* 85:1, January 1990.

American Academy of Pediatrics, Committee on School Health. School attendance of children and adolescents: HTLV-III/LAV infection. *Pediatrics* 77:430–432, March 1986.

Ammann, A. J., and Shannon, K. Recognition of acquired immune deficiency syndrome (AIDS) in children. *Pediatrics in Review* 7:4, October 1986.

Barkin, R. M., and Rosen, P. (Eds.). *Emergency Pediatrics* (3rd ed.). St. Louis: C. V. Mosby, 1989.

Behrman, Richard E., and Kliegman, Robert. *Nelson Essentials of Pediatrics.* Philadelphia: W. B. Saunders, 1990.

Behrman, Richard E., and Kliegman, Robert. *Nelson Textbook of Pediatrics* (14th ed.). Philadelphia: W. B. Saunders, 1992.

Berkowitz, Carol D. Child sexual abuse. *Pediatrics in Review* 13:12, December 1992.

Bogdasarian, Ronald S. Q & A on tympanostomy tubes. *Contemporary Pediatrics* 8:5, May 1991.

Ceftriaxone-Associated Biliary Complications of Treatment of Suspected Disseminated Lyme Disease—New Jersey, 1990–992. *Morbidity and Mortality Weekly Report,* 42:2, January 1993.

Chetham, Michele M., and Roberts, Kenneth B. Infectious mononucleosis in adolescents. *Pediatric Annals* 20:4, April 1991.

Coping with AIDS: Psychological and Social Considerations in Helping People with HTLV-III Infection. Rockville, MD: National Institute of Mental Health, 1986.

Connor, Edward. Pediatric HIV infection: What you can do. *The Journal of Respiratory Diseases* 14:1, January 1993.

Craft, Joe C., and Steere, Allen C. Lyme disease. *Mediguide to Infectious Diseases* 6:4. Lawrence Della Corte Publications, Inc., New York, NY, Miles Pharmaceuticals, 1986.

Cranston, Kevin. *Notes from the VIII International Conference on AIDS.* Amsterdam, July 1992.

Eigen, Howard. Asthma diagnosis: Getting back to the basics. *The Journal of Respiratory Diseases* 13:10 Supplement, October 1992.

Emans, S. J., and Goldstein, D. P. *Pediatric and Adolescent Gynecology* (3rd ed.). Boston: Little, Brown, 1990.

Fairbanks, K.D., Lockhart, B., and Sharp, V. AIDS update. *Clinician Reviews* 2:9, October 1992.

Fischbach, Frances. *A Manual of Laboratory & Diagnostic Tests* (4th ed.). Philadelphia: J. B. Lippincott, 1992.

Fitzpatrick, T. B., Polano, M. K., and Suurmond, D. *Color Atlas and Synopsis of Clinical Dermatology* (7th ed.). New York: McGraw-Hill, 1988.

Fiumara, Nicholas J. *Pictorial Guide to Sexually Transmitted Diseases.* New York: Cahners, 1989.

Gentry, Stokes. Allergic rhinitis: Always in season. *Contemporary Pediatrics* 8:4, April, 1991.

Gerber, Michael, and Markowitz, Milton. Streptococcal pharyngitis: Clearing up the controversies. *Contemporary Pediatrics* 9:10, October 1992.

Governor's Task Force on AIDS: Policies and Recommendations, rev. ed. Boston: Massachusetts Department of Public Health, 1986.

Guidelines for the Diagnosis and Management of Asthma. Bethesda, MD: National Asthma Education Program, U.S. Department of Health and Human Services, August 1991.

Harrrison, Christopher J., and Belhorn, Thomas H. Antibiotic treatment failures in acute otitis media. *Pediatric Annals* 20:11, November 1991.

Healy, Gerald B. Consultation with the specialist: Otitis media. *Pediatrics in Review* 13:1, January 1992.

HIV/AIDS Surveillance. Atlanta, GA: U.S. Department of Health and Human Services, October 1992.

HIV/HBV in Health Care Settings. AIDS Newsletter. Boston: Massachusetts Department of Public Health, December 1992.

Hoole, A. J., Greenberg, R. A., and Pickard, C. G., Jr. *Patient Care Guidelines for Nurse Practitioners* (3rd ed.). Boston: Little, Brown, 1988.

Hoth, D. F., Jr., Myers, M. W., and Stein, D. S. Current status of HIV therapy: Antiretroviral agents. *Hospital Practice* 27:9, September 1992.

Konig, Peter. A step-wise approach to the changing drug therapy of Asthma. *Pediatric Annals* 21:9, September 1992.

Kruks, Gabe. Gay and lesbian homeless/street youth: Special issues and concerns. *Journal of Adolescent Health* 12:7, November 1991.

Le, Chinh T. Choosing an antibiotic: Efficacy, side effects—and cost. *Contemporary Pediatrics* 8:6, June 1991.

Leads from the MMWR: Recommendations for prevention of HIV transmission in health-care settings. *Journal of the American Medical Association* 258:10, September 1987.

Lichenstein, R., King, J. C., Jr., and Tunnessen, W. W., Jr. If the shoe doesn't fit, don't wear it! *Contemporary Pediatrics* 9:4, April, 1992.

Mandel, E. M., Rockette, H. E., Bluestone, C. D., Paradise, J. L., and Nozza, R. J. Efficacy of amoxicillin with and without decongestant—Antihistamine for otitis media with effusion in children. *New England Journal of Medicine* 316 (8):432–437, 1987.

Mansfield, M.J., and Eliot, A.O. *Eating Disorders: Obesity, Anorexia and Bulimia Nervosa.* Syllabus Postgraduate Course Adolescent Medicine, Children's Hospital, Boston, May 1992.

McFadden, E. R., Jr. Exercise and asthma. *New England Journal of Medicine* 317 (8):502–504, August 1987.

Meyers, Burt R. *Antimicrobial Therapy Guide.* Newtown, PA: Antimicrobial Prescribing, 1992.

Mofenson, Lynne. *Update on Fifth Disease (Erythema Infectiosum).* Boston: Massachusetts Department of Public Health, Center for Disease Control, March 1989.

Moffitt, John E., and Feldman, Sandor. Chickenpox: New dangers, new therapies. *Contemporary Pediatrics* 8:11, November 1991.

Oski, Frank A. *Principles and Practice of Pediatrics* (2nd ed.). Philadelphia: J. B. Lippincott, 1994.

The Pediatrician's Compendium of Drug and Patient Information. New York: Biomedical Information Corporation, 1986.

The Pediatric Spectrum of HIV Disease in Massachusetts. AIDS Newsletter. Boston: Massachusetts Department of Public Health, January 1993.

Physician's Compendium of Drug Therapy. Secaucus, NJ: Compendium Publications, 1993.

Platts-Mills, Thomas A.E. Controlling indoor allergens in patients with asthma. *The Journal of Respiratory Diseases* 13:10 Supplement, October 1992.

Rachelefsky, Gary S. Guidelines for effective long-term use of theophylline. *The Journal of Respiratory Diseases* 13:10 Supplement, October 1992.

Reese, Richard E., and Betts. Robert, F. *A Practical Approach to Infectious Diseases* (3rd ed.). Boston: Little, Brown, 1990.

Report of the Committee on Infectious Diseases (22nd ed.). Elk Grove Village, IL.: American Academy of Pediatrics, 1991.

Richards, Warren. Asthma, Allergies, and School. *Pediatric Annals* 21:9, September 1992.

Santosham, M., Brown, K. H., and Sack, R. B. Oral rehydration therapy and dietary therapy for acute childhood diarrhea. *Pediatrics in Review* 8(9):273–278, March 1987.

Saryan, John A. and O'Loughlin, John M. Anaphylaxis in Children. *Pediatric Annals* 21:9, September 1992.

Schmitt, Barton D. Overcoming bed-wetting in the teen years. *Contemporary Pediatrics* 9:9, September 1992.

Schotte, D. E., and Stunkard, A. J. Bulimia vs. bulimic behaviors on a college campus *Journal of the American Medical Association* 258:9, September 1987.

Schuster, C. S., and Ashburn, S. S. *The Process of Human Development* (3rd ed.). Philadelphia: J. B. Lippincott, 1992.

Shadick, Nancy A., and Liang, Matthew H. Management of Lyme disease. *Brigham and Women's Hospital Medical Update* 5:1, January 1993.

Shapiro, Eugene D. Bacterial respiratory infections and otitis media. *Pediatric Annals* 20:8, August 1991.

Shapiro, Gail G. Childhood asthma: Update. *Pediatrics in Review* 13:11, November 1992.

Sheffer, Albert L. Where beta$_2$-adrenergics fit into step care for asthma. *The Journal of Respiratory Diseases* 13:10 Supplement, October 1992.

Some Things Don't Change—Others Do. Research Triangle Park, NC: Burroughs Wellcome, November 1980.

Sonnenblick, Howard C. Abstract: Erythema infectiosum. *Pediatrics in Review* 13:6, June 1992.

Strasburger, Victor C., and Brown, Robert T. *Adolescent Medicine* (1st ed.). Boston: Little, Brown, 1991.

Survival with AIDS in Massachusetts. AIDS Newsletter, Massachusetts Deparment of Public Health, November 1992.

Teele, David W. Strategies to control recurrent acute otitis media. *Pediatric Annals* 20:11, November 1991.

Washington, William L. When to expect and how to detect Lyme disease. *The Journal of Musculoskeletal Medicine,* March 1988.

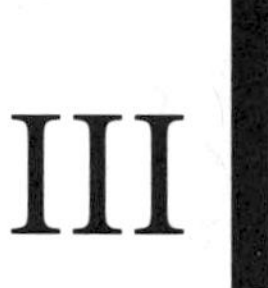

Drug Index

Rose W. Boynton

The Drug Index provides a quick reference to help medical professionals confirm their knowledge of medications. It contains a list of many drugs generally used in ambulatory pediatric practices. This part of the manual provides a comprehensive outline of each medication, incorporating the generic name and composition, pediatric dosage, action of the drug, and the facts parents should know about the drug.

ACLOVATE

I. **Generic name.** Alclometasone dipropionate (synthetic corticosteroid).

II. **Composition.** Alclometosone diproprionate cream, 0.05%; ointment, 0.05%.

III. **Route.** Topical cream or ointment.

IV. **How supplied.** (Glaxo dermatologic) 15-gm, 45-gm, or 60-gm tubes (both cream and ointment).

V. **Uses.** Used for symptoms of inflammatory and pruritic rashes when corticosteroid activity is required.

VI. **Dosage.** Apply a small amount of either cream or ointment to the affected area 2 or 3 times a day, massage gently into skin until cream or ointment is absorbed. Or 3–4 days occlusive dressing may be more beneficial in the treatment of psoriasis or lichen simplex chronicus.

Directions for occlusive dressing:

1. Cover lesion with medication and light gauze dressing and then cover the area with pliable plastic film.
2. Seal the edges with tape.
3. Leave dressing in place for 1–4 days.

VII. **Side effects.** Burning, itching, dryness, hypopigmentation, allergic contact dermatitis.

VIII. **Contraindications.** Any individual who are hypersensitive to any ingredients in these preparations or to other corticosteroids.

IX. **Precautions.**

A. Pediatric patients may show a greater sensitivity to topical corticosteroid-induced HPA axis suppression and Cushing's syndrome than do older people, because of a larger skin surface to body weight ratio. Manifestations of adrenal suppression in children include mental retardation, retardation of linear growth, poor weight gain, low plasma cortisol levels, absence of ACTH stimulation, bulging tentanules, headaches, and bilateral papilledema.

B. Limit medication to the least amount compatible with effective therapeutic regimen.

C. Do not use over extended period of time in pediatric patients.

D. Not suggested for use on pregnant patients.

E. Medication is excreted in breast milk, use with caution for nursing woman.

X. **Education.**

A. Keep all medication out of children's reach.

B. Children may absorb proportionately more of topical corticosteroids and therefore be more susceptable to toxicity.

C. If irritation or side effects or infections develop, discontinue use immediately and call the office.

D. Do not use medication near or in the eyes.

E. Do not use medication over a prolonged period of time or over large surface areas.

F. Do not bandage or cover skin area unless advised to do so by medical provider.

G. Store medication at 36°–86°F.

ACTIFED (ANTIHISTAMINE–DECONGESTANT)

I. **Composition.**
   A. Syrup—Triprolidine hydrochloride 1.25 mg/5 ml and pseudoephedrine hydrochloride 30 mg/ml.
   B. Tablets—Triprolidine hydrochloride 2.5 mg and pseudoephedrine hydrochloride 60 mg.

II. **How supplied.** (Burroughs-Wellcome)
   A. Syrup—40-oz and 1-pt bottles
   B. Tablets—bottles of 100 and 1000; boxes of 12, 24, and 48.

III. **Route.** PO.

IV. **Dosage.**
   A. Adults and children age 12 and over—2 teaspoonsful every 4–6 hours.
   B. Children age 6–12—1 teaspoonful every 4–6 hours.
   C. Do not give medication to children under age 6 unless recommended by a physician.

V. **Action and uses.** Used as an antihistamine and decongestant in cases of seasonal and perennial rhinitis, allergic rhinitis, mild upper respiratory symptoms and sinus congestion.

VI. **Contraindications.** Contraindicated in people with high blood pressure, heart disease, diabetes, thyroid disease, asthma, and glaucoma.

VII. **Precautions.** Medication reacts to monooxidase inhibitors and tricyclic antidepressants.

VIII. **Education.**
   A. May cause excitability in some children.
   B. Do not give Actifed syrup to children under the age of 6 unless directed by physician.
   C. Medication may cause drowsiness.
   D. Do not exceed 4 doses in 24 hours.
   E. Store syrup at controlled temperature 59°–77°F and protect from light.
   F. Keep this and all drugs out of the reach of children.

ADRENALIN CHLORIDE SOLUTION (EPINEPHRINE HYDROCHLORIDE)

I. **Composition.** Sterile solution contains 1 mg of adrenaline (epinephrine as a hydrochloride in each 1-ml ampoule (1:1000).

II. **How supplied.** (Parke-Davis)
   A. Ampoules—Packages of 10.
   B. Solution—30-ml vial.

III. **Route.** SC or IM.

IV. **Dosage.**
   A. 0.2–1 ml (mg) SC. Use small dose to start; increase if required.
   B. Pediatric dose. 0.01 mg/kg to a maximum of 0.5 mg SC q4h.

V. **Action.** Epinephrine is a sympathomimetic drug. It stimulates an adrenergic receptive mechanism on effector cells and imitates all actions of the sympathetic nervous system except those on the arteries of the face and on the sweat glands.

VI. **Uses.** Epinephrine is most commonly used to relieve respiratory distress due to bronchospasm, especially bronchial asthmatic paroxysms. It also is used to relieve hypersensitivity to drugs and other allergens and to control rhinitis, urticaria, and acute sinusitis.

VII. **Side effects.** Anxiety, headache, fever, palpitations.

VIII. **Contraindications**

A. Patients with congestive glaucoma or organic brain disease.
B. Patients receiving local anesthesia of certain areas (e.g., toes or fingers); it may cause vasoconstriction and sloughing of tissue.
C. Patients receiving digitalis, mercurial diuretics, or other drugs that sensitize the heart to arrhythmias.

IX. **Education.**

A. Keep medication out of children's reach.
B. Protect from exposure to light.
C. Do not remove from carton until ready to use.
D. Do not use if medication is brown in color or a precipitant is evident.
E. The action of epinephrine may be affected by tricyclic antidepressants and certain antihistamines.
F. Repeated local injections of epinephrine may result in necrosis at injection sites.
G. Epinephrine-fastness can occur with prolonged use.
H. Use in pregnancy is recommended only if the benefit outweighs the risk to the fetus.
I. Use with caution in patients with long-standing bronchial asthma and emphysema who have developed degenerative heart disease.
J. Use with caution in persons with cardiovascular disease, hypertension, diabetes, or hyperthyroidism, and in psychoneurotic persons.
K. Overdose or inadvertent intravenous injection of epinephrine may cause cerebrovascular hemorrhage due to the sudden increase in blood pressure.
L. Epinephrine may cause pulmonary edema due to peripheral constriction and cardiac stimulation.
M. Rapid-acting vasodilators such as nitrates or alpha-blocking agents may counteract the marked pressure effects of epinephrine.

AMOXICILLIN (SYNTHETIC ANTIBIOTIC)

I. **Generic name.** Amoxicillin.

II. **Composition.**

A. Pediatric drops—50 mg/ml.
B. Oral suspension—125 mg/ml and 250 mg/5 ml.
C. Chewables—250 mg (Amoxil).
D. Capsules—250 mg and 500 mg.

III. **Route.** PO.

IV. **Dosage**

A. For infections other than of lower respiratory tract, 20 mg/kg/day in divided doses q8h.
   1. Under 13 lbs—0.75 of pediatric drops q8h.
   2. 13–18 lbs—1 ml of pediatric drops q8h.
   3. 18 lb and over—125 mg or 250 mg q8h.
   4. 20 kg and over—250 mg q8h.

B. For infections of lower respiratory tract, 40 mg/kg/day in divided doses q8h.
   1. Under 13 lbs—1.25 ml of pediatric drops q8h.
   2. 13–18 lbs—2 ml of pediatric drops q8h.
   3. 18 lbs and over—125 mg or 250 mg q8h.
   4. 20 kg and over—500 mg q8h.

C. Oral prophylaxis prior to dental surgery or dental procedures.
   1. 3.0 gm PO 1 hour before procedure then 1.5 gm 6 hours after treatment.

V. **Action and uses.** Used for treatment of both upper and lower respiratory tract infections caused by gram-negative and gram-positive organisms. Effective in infections of the ears, nose, throat, soft tissues, skin, and genitourinary tract. Amoxicillin is also being used prior to oral surgical procedures.

VI. **Side effects.** Nausea, vomiting, diarrhea, urticaria, maculopapular rash.

VII. **Contraindications.**

A. Patients with allergy to penicillin.
B. Patients with renal or hepatic malfunction.

VIII. **Precautions.** Safety of use in pregnancy has not been established.

IX. **Education.**

A. Keep all medication out of children's reach.
B. Take medication for 10 full days even though symptoms disappear.
C. Medication may be given with meals.
D. Suspension may be placed directly in mouth for swallowing or may be mixed with juice, formula, or soft drinks.
E. Shake both oral suspension and pediatric drops well before using.
F. Keep bottle tightly capped.
G. Discard unused portion of medication after 14 days.
H. Refrigeration preferred but not required.
I. Diabetics using Clinitest will get false high sugar reading.
J. If side effects occur discontinue use and call the office.

AMPICILLIN (ANTIBIOTIC)

I. **Generic name.** Ampicillin trihydrate.

II. **Composition.**

A. Oral suspension—125 mg/5 ml and 250 mg/5 ml.
B. Capsules—250 mg and 500 mg.

III. Route. PO, IM, and IV.

IV. Dosage.

A. 25–50 mg/kg/day in divided doses q8h.

B. For septicemia and bacterial meningitis—50–200 mg/kg/day in divided doses q4h.

C. 11–22 lbs—125 mg q6h PO.

D. Over 25 lbs—250 mg q6h PO.

V. Action. Inhibition of cell wall synthesis.

VI. Uses. Broad-spectrum activity against gram-negative and gram-positive bacteria. Used for treatment of genitourinary, respiratory, and gastrointestinal infections caused by *Escherichia coli, Hemophilus influenzae, Neisseria gonorrhoeae,* salmonellae, shigellae, *Proteus mirabilis,* septicemia, and bacterial meningitis. Also effective against gram-positive pneumococcal staphylococci, groups A and B beta-hemolytic streptococci, and *Bacillus anthracis.*

VII. Side effects. Nausea, vomiting, stomatitis, diarrhea, urticaria, rash (maculopapular or erythema multiforme), and black, hairy tongue. Hematologic side effects (e.g., anemia, thrombocytopenia, purpura, eosinophilia, agranulocytosis).

VIII. Contraindications. Patients with a history of hypersensitivity to any penicillins.

IX. Precautions.

A. Not suggested for, or to be used with caution in, children with asthma, severe hayfever, or allergies.

B. Treatment may cause overgrowth of nonsusceptible organisms.

C. Smaller dosages are suggested for premature infants and neonates; use with caution in this age group because of poor renal clearance.

X. Education.

A. Keep all medication out of children's reach.

B. Discontinue drug if signs of allergy appear and call the office.

C. Take medication on an empty stomach 1 hour before or 2 hours after eating.

D. Shake liquid well before using.

E. Take for 10 full days as instructed.

F. Store liquid form in refrigerator.

ANAPROX

I. Generic name. Naproxen sodium.

II. Composition. 275 mg of naproxen sodium equivalent of 250 mg ; 250 mg of naproxen sodium with 25 mg (1 mEq) sodium.

III. How supplied. Bottles of 100 film-coated tablets, or in carton of 100 individually blister-packed tablets.

V. Route. PO.

V. Dosage.

A. Mild to moderate pain in primary dysmenorrhea, acute tendonitis and bursitis. Starting dose 2 tabs (550 mg) followed by 1 tablet (275 mg) 6–8 hours. Total daily dose not to exceed 1,375 mg.

B. Children age 2 and older with juvenile arthritis. Single dose of 2.5–5 mg/kg. Total dose not to exceed 15 mg/kg/day. Anaprox 275-mg tablet is not well suited for younger children; use Naprosyn 250-mg scored tablet or 125-mg/5 ml suspension in cases of juvenile arthritis in younger children.

C. Adult rheumatoid arthritis, osteoarthritis, and ankylosing spondylitis. Dose: 1 tablet of 275 or 500 mg twice daily, lower dose may suffice. For long-term administration, do not treat more than twice daily.

VI. **Action.** Recommended for use in mild to moderate pain associated with primary dysmenorrhea, acute tendinitis, bursitis, or juvenile arthritis, rheumatoid arthritis osteoarthritis, and ankylosing spondylithis and acute gout.

VII. **Side effects.** Gastrointestinal discomfort, drowsiness, dizziness, vertigo, or depression. Serious side effect of gastrointestinal bleeding may require hospitalization or might be fatal.

VIII. **Contraindications.**

A. In persons with allergy to ingredients of medication or individuals with sensitivity to aspirin or other nonsteroidal/antiinflammatory medications that induce asthma, rhinitis or nasal polyps, or hypertension.

B. Not indicated for use in persons with known history of peptic ulcer disease, or alcoholism; or history of GI bleeding disorders or renal dysfunction, hypertension, and heart disease.

IX. **Precautions.**

A. Do not use concomitantly with the drug Naprosyn.

B. Long-term use of Anaprox can result in acute interstitial nephritis with hematuria, proteinuria, and occasionally nephrotic syndrome.

C. Not recommended for use by nursing mothers or during pregnancy.

X. **Education.**

A. Keep all medication out of children's reach.

B. If side effect occurs, discontinue use and call the medical office.

C. If overdose occurs, call the office immediately.

D. Safety in use in children under age 2 is not established.

E. Do not use if pregnant or a nursing mother.

F. Do not exceed daily recommended dose of medication. Do not use medication longer than is necessary.

G. Single daily dose is recommended in children with juvenile arthritis.

H. When treating for primary dysmenorrhea prescribe only 8 tablets of medication at a time. Do not treat longer than 3 days, call the office regarding effectiveness after next menstral period. Reevaluate patient every 3–4 months with follow-up visit at the office.

ARISTOCORT A (TOPICAL CREAM)

I. **Generic name.** Triamcinolone acetonide. Topical cream with aguatin hydrohilic case.

II. **Composition.** Each gram of 0.025% topical cream contains 0.25 mg of the highly active steroid triamcinolone acetonide. Each gram of 1% topical cream contains 0.1 mg of triamcinolone acetonide.

III. **How supplied.** 15-gm and 60-gm tubes.

IV. **Route.** Topical.

V. **Dosage and administration.** Apply a light film sparingly to the affected area three times daily.

VI. **Action and uses.** Indicated for the relief of inflammatory and pruritic rashes, minor skin irritations and allergic contact dermatitis.

VII. **Contraindications.**

A. Anyone sensitive to the ingredients of the medication.

B. Safety during pregnancy has not been established, it is not suggested for use by nursing mothers.

VIII. **Precautions.** Children may absorb proportionally larger amounts of topical corticosteroids and therefore more susceptible to systemic toxicity than more mature patients because of larger skin surface area to body weight ratio.

IX. **Education.**

A. Keep all medication out of children's reach.

B. Administration of topical corticosteroids to children should be limited to the lease amount compatible with an effective therapeutic regimen.

C. Chronic corticosteroid therapy may interfere with growth and development in children.

D. If skin does not respond to medication, immediately discontinue use.

E. Do not use in management of extensive area, particularly in small children.

F. Occlusive dressings may be used rarely for the management of psoriasis or recalcitrant conditions. If infection develops, the use of occlusive dressings should be discontinued and appropriate antimicrobial therapy instituted.

G. If favorable response does not occur, the corticosteroid should be discontinued.

H. Medication should be used as directed.

I. Avoid contact with the face and eyes.

J. Do not use medication for any rash other than that described or prescribed.

K. Do not use medication under tight-fitting diapers, or plastic pants in children.

ASPIRIN (ANALGESIC)

I. **Generic name.** Acetylsalicylic acid.

II. **Composition.** Orange-flavored chewable tablets, 1$^1/_4$ grains.

III. **Route.** PO.

IV. **Dosage**

A. 65 mg/kg/day in divided doses q6h.

B. Administer q4h, not more than 5 times a day.

1. 2–4 years—2 tablets.
2. 4–6 years—3 tablets.
3. 6–9 years—4 tablets.
4. 9–11 years—5 tablets.

V. **Action.** Antipyretic, antiinflammatory, analgesic.

VI. **Uses.** Used for headaches, simple upper respiratory infection, teething discomfort, immunization discomforts, otitis media, and pharyngitis.

VII. Contraindications.

A. Any child sensitive to salicylates.

B. Not recommended for influenza symptoms or chickenpox because risk of Reye's syndrome.

VIII. Precautions. Use cautiously in patients with peptic ulcer or asthma or those on anticoagulant therapy.

IX. Education.

A. Use of aspirin in pregnancy and nursing, usually not advised.

B. Do not use aspirin especially during last three months of pregnancy, it may cause fetal problems or complications during delivery.

C. Do not use over a prolonged period of time.

D. If intense itching and general rash occur, discontinue medication and call the office.

E. Tinnitus is an early sign of toxicity; discontinue use or lower dosage.

F. Prolonged high doses of aspirin can lead to iron-deficiency anemia, especially in young woman.

G. High levels of salicylates can cause gastric irritation and gastric bleeding.

H. *Caution.* Keep all medication out of children's reach. One of the most common causes of poisoning in children is accidental ingestion of aspirin, and this drug is often used in teenage suicides, particularly by females.

ATARAX

I. Generic name. Hydroxyzine hydrochloride.

II. Composition.

A. Syrup—10 mg/5 ml in pint bottles.

B. Tablets—10 mg, 25 mg, 50 mg, and 100 mg.

III. Route. PO.

IV. Dosage.

A. Children under age 6—50 mg daily in qid doses.

B. Children over age 6—50–100 mg daily in qid doses or tid.

V. Action. Suppression of activity in certain regions of subcortical area of central nervous system, i.e., primary skeletal muscle relaxant, bronchodilator activity with antihistamine and analgesic effects. It may also show an antiemetic effect.

VI. Uses.

A. In the management of pruritus due to allergic conditions, i.e., chronic urticaria, atopic and contact dermatitis, and in histamine-medicated pruritus.

B. In cases for symptomatic relief of anxiety and tension.

C. Useful as a sedation in premedication and following general anesthesia—*Atarax potentiate Demeral and barbiturates. So their use in preanesthetic adjunctive therapy should be modified. Atropine and other belladonna alkaloids are not affected.*

Digitalis may be used with Atarax successfully.

VII. Side effects. Dry mouth, drowsiness, rare instances of trauma and convulsions.

VIII. Contraindications.

A. Safety during pregnancy has not been established.

B. People who have shown a previous hypersensitivity to Atarax.

C. Not suggested in use by nursing mothers. It is not known whether this drug is excreted in human milk.

IX. Precautions. Potentiating action of hydroxyzine must be considered when drug is used in conjunction with central nervous system depressants.

X. Education.

A. Keep all medication out of children's reach.

B. Atarax patients should be advised against the simultaneous use of CNS depressants and caution that the effect of alcohol may be increased.

C. Overdose of Atarax causes hypersedation.

D. If overdose occurs, call the office immediately.

E. There is no specific antidote. If vomiting has not occurred spontaneously—it should be induced immediately; gastric lavage is also recommended.

F. Effectiveness of Atarax as an antianxiety agent (more than 4 months) has not been established by clinical studies.

AUGMENTIN (ORAL ANTIBIOTIC)

I. Composition. Amoxicillin/clavulanate potassium.

II. How supplied. (Beecham Laboratories).

A. 250-mg and 500-mg white coated tablets.

B. 125-mg and 250-mg chewable tablets.

C. 125-mg and 250-mg orange-flavored or banana-flavored suspension.

III. Route. PO.

IV. Dosage.

A. 20 mg/kg/day; based on amoxicillin component.

B. 18 lbs and over—125 mg or 250 mg q8h.

C. 40 kg and over—500 mg q8h.

V. Action and uses. Used for treatment of lower respiratory tract infections (especially beta-lactamase-producing strains of *Hemophilus influenzae)*, otitis media, sinusitis, skin and skin structure infections, and urinary tract infectionscaused by *Escherichia coli, Klebsiella,* and *Enterobacter* species.

VI. Side effects. Loose stools or diarrhea, vomiting, skin rash, urticaria, vaginitis, flatulence, headache, and abdominal discomfort.

VII. Contraindications.

A. Patients with allergy to penicillin.

B. Nursing mother (Augmentin is secreted in breast milk).

VIII. Education.

A. Keep all medication out of children's reach.

B. Take medication for 10 full days even though symptoms disappear.

C. Shake oral suspension well before using.

D. Suspension must be refrigerated.

E. Discard medication after 10 days.

F. Augmentin may be administered with meals.

G. Discontinue drug if signs of allergy appear.

H. Augmentin 250-mg and 500-mg tablets contain the same amount of clavulanic acid; two Augmentin 250-mg tablets are not equivalent to one Augmentin 500-mg tablet. Do not substitute two Augmentin 250-mg tablets for one Augmentin 500-mg tablet for treatment of severe infections.

AURALGAN OTIC SOLUTION (TOPICAL OTIC ANALGESIC)

I. **Generic name and composition.** Antipyrine, benzocaine, dehydrated glycerin.

II. **How supplied.** (Ayerst Laboratories) 1/2-oz bottles.

III. **Route.** External canal of the ear.

IV. **Dosage and administration.** Instill drops until ear canal is filled. Do not touch ear with dropper. Insert a wick of cotton into the meatus; moisten cotton with Auralgan. Repeat procedure every 1–2 hours until pain is relieved.

V. **Action and uses.** Topical analgesic to reduce inflammation and pain associated with acute otitis media.

VI. **Contraindications.**

A. Any individuals who show hypersensitivity to any of the components or substances related to them.

B. Safety to fetus unknown; not recommended in pregnancy or by nursing mothers.

IX. **Education.**

A. Keep all medication out of children's reach.

B. Warm bottle by holding in palm of hand; do not heat in hot water.

C. Keep bottle tightly closed.

D. Do not rinse dropper after use; water reduces strength of medication.

E. Discard remaining medication after treatment has been completed.

F. Protect solution from light and heat.

G. Do not use solution if brown or it contains precipitate.

H. *Discard product six months after dropper is first placed in drug solution.*

BACTRIM OR SEPTRA (SYNTHETIC ANTIBACTERIAL)

I. **Composition.**

A. Cherry-flavored suspension. Trimethoprim 40 mg/5 ml and sulfamethoxazole 200 mg/5 ml.

B. Tablets—Trimethoprim 80 mg and sulfamethoxazole 400 mg.

C. Double-strength tablets—Trimethoprim 160 mg and sulfamethoxazole 800 mg.

II. **Route.** PO.

III. **Dosage.** Administer twice daily for 10 days.

Weight	Suspension		Tablets
22 lbs	1 tsp (5 ml)	or	1/2 tablet
44 lbs	2 tsp (10 ml)	or	1 tablet
66 lbs	3 tsp (15 ml)	or	1 1/2 tablets
88 lbs	4 tsp (20 ml)	or	2 tablets or 1 double-strength tablet

IV. **Action and uses.** Treatment of urinary tract infection, otitis media, and *Pneumocystis carinii* pneumonitis. The organisms most affected in urinary tract infections are *Escherichia coli, Klebsiella-Enterobacter, Proteus mirabilis, P. vulgaris,* and *P. morganii.* Also traveler's diarrhea in adults.

V. **Side effects.**

A. Blood dyscrasia, allergic manifestations (e.g., urticaria, erythema multiforme, pruritus, periorbital edema, photosensitivity, gastrointestinal complaints, nausea, vomiting, diarrhea, headaches, tinnitus, vertigo, and insomnia.)

B. Minor side effects: mild fluid retention, itching of skin, ringing of ears.

VI. **Contraindications.**

A. Patients with known sensitivity to sulfonamides.

B. Infants less than 2 months of age.

C. Patients with renal insufficiency.

D. Patients with severe allergy or asthma.

E. In pregnancy and nursing mothers (drug passes the placenta barrier and is excreted in breast milk).

VII. **Precautions.**

A. Not to be used in treatment of streptococcal pharyngitis.

B. Not to be used by AIDS patients—they may not tolerate or respond to Bactrim in the same manner as non-AIDS patients.

C. Not indicated for prophylactic or prolonged treatment in otitis media at any age.

D. Bactrim should be discontinued at the first appearance of skin rash or any adverse reaction.

Warning: Fatalities associated with administration of sulfonamides have occurred due to severe adverse reactions (i.e., Stevens-Johnson syndrome, toxic epidermal necrolysis, agranulocytosis, aplastic anemia, fulminant hepatic necrosis.

VIII. **Education.**

A. Keep all medication out of children's reach.

B. Increase fluid intake by several glasses of water a day.

C. Discontinue drug if any signs of allergy occur and call the office immediately.

D. Take medication for 10 full days as directed.

BACTROBAN 2% OINTMENT (FOR DERMATOLOGIC USE)

I. **Generic name.** Mupirocin.

II. **Composition.** Each gram contains 20-mg mupirocin in a bland, water-miscible ointment base.

III. **Route.** Topical ointment. *Not for ophthalmic use.*

IV. **Dosage.**

A. Apply a small amount of Bactroban ointment to the affected area tid for 3–5 days.

B. Supplied in 1-gm single unit packages and in 15-gm and 30-gm tubes.

V. **Action and uses.** Bactroban is effective in topically treating impetigo due to streptococcus pyogenes, staphylococcus aureus and beta-hemolytic streptococcus.

VI. **Side effects.** Itching, burning, stinging, rash, nausea, dry skin, tenderness, swelling, increased exudate.

VII. **Contraindications.** In individuals with a history of sensitivity reactions to any components of the drug.

VIII. **Precautions.**

A. Safety of use in pregnancy has not been established.

B. If a reaction suggesting sensitivity or chemical irritation should occur, treatment should be discontinued.

C. Nursing mothers: Nursing should be temporarily discontinued while using Bactroban. It is not known whether Bactroban is present in breast milk.

IX. **Education.**

A. Keep all medication out of children's reach.

B. Patients not showing a clinical response within 3–5 days should be reevaluated.

C. Store medication between 15° and 30°C (59° and 86°F) controlled room temperature.

D. The area treated may be covered with a gauze dressing if desired.

E. Prolonged use may result in overgrowth of nonsusceptible organisms including fungi.

F. Due to the mode of action, Bactroban shows no cross resistance with chloramphenicol, erythromycin, fusidic acid, gentamicin, lincomycin, methicillin, neomycin, novobiocin, penicillin, streptomycin and tetracycline (mupirocin inhibits bacterial protein synthesis by reversibly and specifically binding to bacterial isoleucyl transfer-RNA synthetase).

BROMFED–DM (COUGH SYRUP)

I. **Composition.**

A. Each teaspoon contains:
2 mg brompheniramine maleate
30 mg pseudoephedrine hydrochloride
10 mg dextromethorphan hydrobromide

B. Tablets—4 mg brompheniramine maleate; 60 mg pseudoephedrine hydrochloride

C. Capsules—6 mg brompheniramine maleate; 60 mg pseudoephedrine hydrochloride.

II. **How supplied.** (Muro Pharmaceutical, Inc.) 16-fluid oz bottles, capsules, or tablets.

III. **Route.** PO.

IV. **Dosage.**

A. Syrup: Children age 6–12—1 tsp q4–6h
Children age 12 years and older—2 tsp q4–6h
Adults—2 tsp q4–6h

B. Bromfed–PD
Capsules: Children age 6–12—1 capsule q12h
Children age 12 years and older —1–2 capsules q12h
Adults—1–2 capsules q12h
Tablets: Children age 6–12—1/2tablet q4h *(not to exceed 6 doses in 24 hours).*
Children 12 years and older—1 tablet q4h *(not to exceed 6 doses in 24 hours).*
Adults—1 tablet q4h *(not to exceed 6 doses in 24 hours).*

V. **Action and uses.** For relief of seasonal and allergic rhinitis, vascular rhinitis, and nasal congestion.

VI. **Contraindications.** Any individual who shows hypersensitivity to any of the ingredients and individuals who have severe hypertension, coronary disease, patients on MAO inhibitor therapy, patients with narrow-angle glaucoma, urinary retention, peptic ulcer, or anyone during an asthmatic attack. Caution in patients with diabetes, hyperthyroidism, and mitral ocular pressure.

VII. **Precautions.** Safety of use of this medication in pregnancy has not been established. Do not use in nursing mothers.

VIII. **Adverse reaction.** Drowsiness, nausea, dry mouth, blurred vision, cardiac palpitations, flushing, increased irritability or excitement especially in children.

IX. **Education.**

A. Antihistamines may cause irritability and excitability in children, and at dosages higher than recommended, dizziness, sleeplessness and nervousness may occur.

B. Do not give medication to children under age 6, except under the advise of a physician.

C. Keep all medication out of the reach of children.

D. Pseudoephedrine is excreted in breast milk; use by nursing mothers is not recommended.

E. Keep capsules and tablets in an air tight container.

F. Store at controlled temperature 59–86°F.

G. Dispense in child resistant container.

CECLOR (CEFACLOR)

I. **Composition.** Semisynthetic cephalosporin antibiotic.

II. **How supplied.** (Eli Lilly & Co.)

A. Oral suspension—125 mg/5 cc, 187 mg/5 cc, 250 mg/5 cc, and 375 mg/5 cc.

B. Pulvules—250 mg and 500 mg.

III. **Route.** PO.

IV. **Dosage.**

A. Children—usual recommended daily dose is 20/mg/kg/day in divided doses in 8 hours.

B. In serious infections 40 mg/kg/day with maximum dosage 1 gm/day.

Child's Weight	125 mg/5 ml	250 mg/5 ml
9 kg	1/2 tsp tid	1/2 tsp tid
18 kg	1 tsp tid	—

Ceclor suspension 40 mg/kg/day.

Child's Weight	125 mg/5 ml	250 mg/5 ml
9 kg	1 tsp tid	1/2 tsp tid
18 kg		— 1 tsp tid

(bid option—For the treatment of otitis media and pharyngitis, the total daily dosage may be divided and administered every 12 hours)

V. **Actions and uses.** Used for treatment of clinical infections caused by staphylococci, group A beta-hemolytic streptococci, *Streptococcus pneumoniae, Escherichia coli, Proteusmirabilis, Klebsiella* species, *Hemophilus influenzae,* and some beta-lactamase-producing ampicillin-resistant strains; also used to treat otitis media, urinary tract infections, lower and upper respiratory infections, and skin and skin-structure infections. It is not known whether Ceclor is effective in preventing rheumatic fever.

VI. **Contraindications.**

A. Any persons with known allergy to cephalosporin group.

B. Safety in use of infants age less then 1 month of age is unknown.

C. In penicillin-sensitive children, cephalosporin antibiotics should be administered cautiously. Some laboratory cross-allergenicity of the cephalosporins and penicillin have shown reactions, including anaphylaxis.

D. Caution in administrating to nursing mothers and use in pregnancy only if clearly needed.

VII. **Education.**

A. Keep all medications out of children's reach.

B. Some serum sickness like reactions can occur in children, i.e., erythema multiforme, signs of arthritis, arthralgia with or without fever.

C. Toxic signs may include severe epigastric distress, diarrhea. More severe signs of toxicity include Stevens-Johnson syndrome.

D. Hepatic—elevate SGOT-SGPT and alkaline phosphatase values.

E. If side effects occur, discontinue use and call the office immediately.

COLACE (STOOL SOFTENER)

I. **Generic name.** Docusate sodium.

II. **Composition.**

A. Syrup—20 mg/5 ml (1 tsp).

B. Liquid drops—1% solution 10 mg/ml.

C. Capsules—50 mg and 100 mg.

III. **How supplied.** (Mead Johnson)

A. Syrup—bottles of 8 fl oz and 16 fl oz.

B. Liquid drops—1% solution with calibrated dropper (16 fl oz or 30 fl oz).

C. Capsules 50 mg—bottles of 30, 60, 250, or 1000; or 100 single unit packs.

D. Capsules 100 mg—bottles of 30, 60, 250, or 1000; or 100 single unit packs.

IV. **Route.** PO.

V. **Dosage.**

A. Under 3 years—10–40 mg/day or 10 mg tid (1/2 tsp of syrup tid).

B. 3–6 years—60 mg/day or 20 mg tid (1 tsp of syrup tid).

C. 6–12 years—40–120 mg/day (2 tsp of syrup tid).

D. Older children—50–200 mg/day (one 50-mg capsule tid).

E. Higher doses are suggested for initial therapy.

VI. **Action and uses.** A stool softener, not a laxative; used in persons with chronic constipation and in children with anal fissures.

VII. **Side effects.** Throat irritation, nausea, rash, and bitter taste in mouth.

VIII. **Education.**

A. Keep all medications out of children's reach.

B. There are no contraindications to the use of Colace.

C. During pregnancy and in nursing mothers ask advice of physician before taking Colace.

D. Not habit forming.

E. Given in formula, juice or milk to mask the flavor.

F. Store capsules at room temperature.

G. Medication will take effect in 1–3 days.

H. Adjust dosage to individual.

I. Keep child on medication for 1 week; then call office regarding results.

J. Gradually taper off medication.

DOMEBORO POWDER PACKETS (TOPICAL SOLUTION)

I. **Generic name.** Aluminum sulfate and calcium acetate.

II. **Composition.**

A. 1 packet with 1 pt of water = Burow's solution 1:40 dilution.

B. 2 packets with 1 pt of water = Burow's solution 1:20 dilution.

III. **How supplied.** (Miles Pharmaceuticals) Powder packets, boxes of 12 and 100; each packet contains 2.2 gm.

IV. **Route.** External use topical solution.

V. **Dosage and administration.** Apply wet soaks to skin every 15–30 minutes for 4–8 hours.

VI. **Action and uses.** Used for severe inflammatory dermatitis, poison ivy, insect bites, diaper rash, and athlete's foot.

VII. **Education.**

A. Keep medication out of children's reach.

B. Dissolve 1 or 2 packets in 1 pt of water.

C. Stir until mixture is dissolved.

D. Shake well.

E. Apply as wet dressing.

F. Do not use plastic or rubber pants or occclusive bandages.

G. For external use only.
H. May be stored for 7 days at room temperature.
I. Keep away from eyes.
J. May treat for symptomatic relief for 1 week; if conditions are worse or not relieved in 1 week, discontinue use and seek medical advise.

DONNAGEL (ANTIDIARRHEAL)

I. **Composition.**
   A. Each tablespoon (15 ml) contains 600 mg attapulgite, USP.
   B. Each chewable tablet contains 600 mg attapulgite, USP.
II. **How supplied.** (Robbins)
   A. 4-fl oz and 16-fl oz bottles.
   B. Packages of 18.
III. **Route.** PO.
IV. **Dosage.**
   A. Adults—2 tablespoons or 2 tablets after each loose bowel movement.
   B. Age 12 years or older—2 tablespoons after loose bowel movement.
   C. Age 6–12 years—1 tablespoon after loose bowel movement.
   D. Age 3–6 years—1/2 tablespoon after loose bowel movement.
   E. Do not exceed 7 doses in a 24-hour period.
V. **Actions and uses.** Recommended for symptomatic relief of diarrhea, it relieves cramping, reduces the number of loose stools, and improves the consistency of the stool.
VI. **Contraindications.** In patients with hypersensitivity to any of the ingredients in the medication.
VII. **Education.**
   A. Keep all medications out of children's reach.
   B. Not recommended for use in children age 3 or under unless under care and consultation of a physician.
   C. Not recommended for pregnant women or nursing mothers unless directed by physician.
   D. Tablets are to be chewed well then swallowed.
   E. Shake liquid medication well before using.
   F. Store medication in controlled room temperature (59°–86°F).
   G. Discontinue use of medication and call health provider if any signs of dehydration, i.e., sunken fontanel, dry mouth, decreased urination, or sunken eyes.
   H. Call health provider if symptoms persist beyond 2 days.
   I. Call health provider if temperature is above 100°F or if child is vomiting.
   J. Do not exceed recommended dosage.
   K. Call Poison Control if overdose occurs.

DONNATAL (ANTICHOLINERGIC/ANTISPASMODIC, MILD SEDATION)

I. **Composition.** Each tablet, capsule, or teaspoon contains phenobarbital (1/4 grain) 16.2 mg, hyoscyamine sulfate 0.1037 mg, atropine sulfate 0.0194 mg, and hyoscine hydrobromide 0.0065 mg.

II. **How supplied.**

A. Green citrus-flavored in 4-fl oz bottle.

B. Tablets—bottle of 100 or 1000; or dose package of 100.

C. Capsules—bottle of 100 or 1000.

III. **Route.** PO.

IV. **Dosage.** Children (elixir). May have every 4–6 hours.

Body Weight	q4h	q6h
10 lbs	0.5 ml	0.75 ml
20 lbs	1.0 ml	1.5 ml
30 lbs	1.5 ml	2.0 ml
50 lbs	1/2 tsp	3/4 tsp
75 lbs	1/4 tsp	1 tsp
100 lbs	1 tsp	1 1/2 tsp

Older children and adults—tablets and capsules—1–2 tablets or capsules 3–4 times a day.

V. **Action and uses.** An anticholinergic/antispasmodic with mild sedation used in colic and irritated bowel syndrome.

VI. **Side effects.** Headaches, blurred vision, drowsiness, constipation, suppression of lactation, nervousness, and hyperactivity in some.

Overdose—severe headache, nausea, vomiting, hot and dry skin, dilated pupils, dry mouth, difficulty swallowing, CNS stimulation. Treated by gastric lavage, emetics and activated charcoal.

VII. **Contraindications.** Any child with bleeding disorder, cardiac disease or any question of pyloric stenosis or hepatic dysfunction, during pregnancy and nursing mothers.

VIII. **Education.**

A. Keep all medications out of children's reach.

B. Medication may be habit forming.

C. Do not use in patients with history of drug dependency.

D. Return call in 1 week regarding progress of colic.

E. Use with caution in a very warm climate because of association with increased heat prostration and heat stroke due to increased sweating.

F. Safety in use during pregnancy unknown.

G. It is not known whether drug is excreted in human breast milk, but it does suppress lactation.

H. If overdose call the office immediately.

DORCOL PEDIATRIC COUGH SYRUP

I. **Composition.** Pseudoephedrine hydrochloride 15 mg, guaifenesin 50 mg, dextromethorphan hydrobromide 5 mg in each 5 ml.

II. **How supplied.** Grape-flavored 4-fl oz or 8-fl oz bottle with tamper-proof, child-resistant cap.

III. **Route.** PO.

IV. **Dosage.**

A. 3–12 months—3 gtt/kg/body weight q4h (given by advice of M.D. only).

B. 12–24 months—7 gtt (0.2 ml)/kg/body weight q4h (given by advice of M.D. only).

C. Age 2–6 years—1 tsp q4h.

D. Age 6 –12 years—2 tsp q4h.

E. By weight:

Children 25–45 pounds—1 tsp q4h

Children 46–85 pounds 2 tsp q4h

Do not exceed 4 doses in 24 hours.

V. **Actions and uses.** Temporary relief of common cold. Prompt relief of upper respiratory infection, and aids in excretion of mucus secretions. It contains a decongestant, expectorant and antitussive. Antihistamine-free formula.

VI. **Side effects.** Dizziness, gastrointestinal upset, insomnia, hyperactivity.

VII. **Contraindications.**

A. Children and adults with ongoing chronic cough due to bronchitis, bronchial asthma or emphysema.

B. Do not use in patients with diabetes mellitus, high blood pressure, heart disease, or thyroid disease.

VIII. **Education.**

A. Do not exceed recommended dose.

B. Keep all medications out of the reach of children.

C. If overdose occurs call Poison Control immediately.

D. If cough persists longer than 1 week call back.

E. Return to office or call if rash appears, persistent headache, vomiting, or high fever occurs.

F. Do not give medication if patient is on antidepressants or antihypertensive medications.

DURICEF

I. **Generic name.** Cefadroxil monohydrate, USP.

II. **Composition**

A. Capsules 500 mg, film-coated tablets 1 gm; both in bottles of 50.

B. Oral suspension 125 mg/5 ml, 250 mg/5 ml, or 500 mg/5 ml. Orange and pineapple flavor. All available in 50-ml or 100-ml size or in (strips) of 10 blisters and 4 packs of individually labeled blisters.

III. Route. PO.

IV. Dosage.

Child's Weight

lbs	kg	125 mg/5 ml	250 mg/5 ml	500 mg/5 ml
10	4.5	1 tsp		
20	9.1	2 tsp	1 tsp	—
30	13.6	3 tsp	$1^1/2$ tsp	—
40	18.2	4 tsp	2 tsp	1 tsp
50	22.7	5 tsp	$2^1/2$ tsp	$1^1/4$ tsp
60	27.3	6 tsp	3 tsp	$1^1/2$ tsp
70+	31.8+	—	—	2 tsp

Adult Dose—1–2 gm/day in divided doses or single dose, i.e.:

A. Uncomplicated urinary tract infection 1 gm daily.

B. More severe urinary tract infection is 2 gm daily.

C. Skin and skin structure infections 1 gm daily.

D. Group A beta-hemolytic streptococcus pharyngitis and tonsillitis 1 gm/day in single or divided doses for 10 days.

Warning: Use with caution in penicillin-allergic patients. There is evidence that those individuals may be also cephalosporin allergic. It is safer not to use in known penicillin allergy patients.

V. Actions and uses.

A. Treatment for the previously identified infections—found by culture and sensitivity tests.

B. Urinary tract infections caused by *E. coli, P. mirabilis* and *Klebsiella* species.

C. Skin and suture infections caused by staphylococci and/or streptococci.

D. Pharyngitis and tonsillitis caused by A. beta-hemolytic streptococci. (Penicillin is still the drug of choice in the treatment and prevention of streptococcal infections.)

E. *The efficacy of Duricef in prevention of rheumatic fever is unknown.*

VI. Side effects. Pseudomembranous colitis, diarrhea, rashes, urticaria and angioedema, genital pruritus, genital moniliasis, vaginitis, and neutropenia.

VII. Contraindications.

A. Not known to be safe in pregnancy or nursing mothers.

B. Individuals with known sensitivity to penicillin.

C. Individuals with known impaired renal function.

VIII. Precautions.

A. For prolonged use, it may result in overgrowth of nonsusceptible organisms.

B. Positive Coombs test may be reported while patient is on Duricef.

C. Use with caution in those individuals with gastrointestinal disease, particularly colitis.

IX. Education.

A. Keep all medications out of children's reach.

B. Do not use medication if packaging or seal on the cap is broken.

C. If side effects occur, discontinue medication and call the office immediately.

D. Medication may be given with or without food, but will be more easily tolerated if given with meals.

E. Shake suspension well before administration.
F. Keep cap tightly closed.
G. Keep medication in the refrigerator.
H. Discontinue use of Duricef after 14 days.

ERYCETTE TOPICAL SOLUTION

I. **Generic name.** 2% erythromycin topical solution.

II. **Composition.** 20 mg of erythromycin base in a vehicle of alcohol (66%) and propylene glycol.

III. **Route.** Topical solution supplied in boxes of 60 swabs.

IV. **Dosage.** Apply topically to affected area bid after skin is thoroughly washed and dried.

V. **Actions and uses.** Indicated for topical control of acne vulgaris on face, neck, shoulders, back and chest. Reduces inflammatory acne vulgaris assumed by its antibiotic action.

VI. **Contraindications.** Contraindicated for use in individuals with known sensitivity to its ingredients.

VII. **Side effects.** Tenderness, dryness, erythema, desquamation, pruritus of affected areas.

VIII. **Precautions.** Discontinue use immediately if urticaria or side effects occur.

IX. **Education.**

A. Keep all medication out of children's reach.
B. Store at controlled room temperature 15–30°C (59°–86°F).
C. Not intended for ophthalmic use, or use in mouth or nose.
D. If overgrowth of bacterial organisms occur, discontinue use and call the office.
E. Use one swab (pledget) once—discard after use.
F. Safety of use during pregnancy is unknown.
G. Safety in use in nursing mothers is unknown—use cautiously.

ERYTHROMYCIN (ANTIBIOTIC)

I. **Generic name.** Erythromycin ethylsuccinate.

II. **Composition.**

A. Tablets—125 mg, 250 mg, and 500 mg
B. Base tablets—250-mg film tablets
C. Erye pellets—125 mg and 250-mg capsules.
D. Liquid—200 mg/5 ml and 400 mg/5 ml.
E. Granules—200 mg/5 ml.
F. Chewable tablets—250 mg.
G. Drops—100 mg/2.5 ml 1/2 tsp.

III. Route. PO.

IV. Dosage

A. 30–50 mg/kg/day or 15–25 mg/kg bid.

B. Pertussis—40–50 mg/kg/day for 14 days.

C. *Chlamydia trachomati*—500 mg qid for 7 days.

D. Oral prophylaxis prior to oral surgery or procedure—800 mg or 1 gm PO 2 hours before procedure then 1/2 dose 6 hours after surgery or procedure.

V. Action and uses. A macrolide group of antibiotics used to inhibit protein synthesis without changing the nucleic acid synthesis. Used for upper and lower respiratory tract infections (e.g., bronchitis, pneumonia, pertussis, intestinal infections, for soft tissue and nasal, pharyngitis infections, primary syphilis, Legionnaire's disease; for long term prophylaxis against rheumatic fever, urologic/gynecologic infections due to *Chlamydia trachomatis* and prevention of bacterial endocarditis. As oral prophylaxis used prior to oral surgery and surgical procedures.

VI. Side effects. Nausea, vomiting, abdominal pain.

A. Adverse reactions—symptoms of hepatic dysfunction with or without abnormal liver function.

B. Rashes may appear with pruritus (urticaria, eczema, or bullaes).

C. Severe anaphylaxis can occur and some transient deafness.

VII. Contraindications.

A. Patients with hypersensitivity to the medication.

B. Safety during pregnancy has not been established.

C. The effect during labor and delivery is unknown.

D. Medication (erythromycin) is excreted in breast milk.

E. Effect in use with Seldane—can be toxic.

F. Not recommended in use with Seldane.

G. Children receiving high levels of theophylline may show an increase of serum theophylline and potential theophylline toxicity if erythromycin is taken together with theophylline.

VIII. Education.

A. Prolonged use of this antibiotic may effect an overgrowth of bacteria or a fungal infection. If so, discontinue use.

B. Some organisms are resistant to erythromycin. Whenever possible obtain specimens for culture and sensitivity and when indicated, incision and drainage or other surgical procedure are best done, as well as antibiotic therapy.

C. Ideally, give medication without food. However, suspension and tablets may be given with meals if GI symptoms occur.

D. Mix ERYC pellets with applesauce before administering.

E. Store liquid medication in the refrigerator.

F. Chewable tablets should be chewed or crushed, never swallowed.

G. Suspensions are stable for 14 days at room temperature, but palatability increases if they are kept refrigerated.

H. Order generic form to minimize cost. Best ordered in coated tablets or caplet form to reduce occurrence of side effects.

EURAX (SCABICIDE ANTIPRURITIC)

I. **Generic name.** Crotamiton

II. **How supplied.** (Westwood Squibb) Lotion and cream 60-gm tubes 10% of synthetic crotamiton.

III. **Route.** Topical use only.

IV. **Dosage.** Apply lotion or cream to skin areas from neck down. Massage into skin, leave cream on overnight, wash off in the morning.

V. **Uses.** Antipruritic/antiscabie medication. For eradication of scabies and for symptomatic treatment of pruritus of the skin.

VI. **Contraindications.**

- A. In patients with sensitivity or known allergy to the ingredients.
- B. In pregnant patients and nursing mothers.
- C. Safety in children has not been established.

VII. **Side effects.** Primary irritation of the skin.

VIII. **Education.**

- A. Keep all medication out of children's reach.
- B. Shake medication well before using.
- C. For scabies—After routine bath or shower, pat dry, massage medication into the skin, covering all the areas from the neck down. A second application may be advisable 24 hours later (60-gm tube is sufficient for 2 applications).
  1. Bed linens, clothing, and hands should be washed in hot, soapy water and changed the next morning. Other contaminated clothing dry cleaned.
  2. A cleansing bath is recommended 48 hours after the last treatment.
- D. For pruritus—Apply small amount of medication, massage gently into affected area.
  1. Discontinue all medication if skin becomes severely irritated.
  2. Keep all medications away from eyes and mouth.
- E. If ingested, call Poison Control immediately.
- F. Do not apply to acutely inflamed skin that has open sores, is weeping or severely red.

FEOSOL ELIXIR (NONPRESCRIPTION IRON SUPPLEMENT)

I. **Generic name** Ferrous sulfate.

II. **Composition.** 200 mg/5 ml of ferrous sulfate (44 mg of elemental iron).

III. **How supplied.** Clear orange liquid in 16 oz bottle. Also available in tablets and capsules

IV. **Route.** PO.

V. **Dosage.**

- A. 6 mg/kg/day.
- B. Infants—Begin with 4 gtt, then increase to 1/2 tsp tid x 1 month.
- C. Children—1/2–1 tsp tid × 4 weeks, between meals.
- D. Adults—1–2 tsp tid.

VI. **Actions and uses.**

A. Keep all medication out of the reach of children.

B. If overdose, call Poison Control immediately.

C. Do not take iron supplements within 2 hours of tetracycline due to malabsorption.

D. If gastrointestinal irritation occurs, take iron supplement with meals starting with a lower dose, gradually increasing until recommended dose is obtained.

E. Iron may cause constipation, dark-colored stools, or diarrhea.

F. Liquid may cause temporary staining of teeth—always dilute the Feosol elixir with water or juice and use a straw.

G. Do not mix with milk, milk products, or wine-based materials.

H. Take medication for 3—4 weeks and return for reevaluation.

I. Request tamper-resistant packing. If seal is broken or missing, do not use this product.

J. If overdose occurs, call the office immediately.

ILOTYCIN OPHTHALMIC OINTMENT (ERYTHROMYCIN)

I. **Composition.** Erythromycin in a sterile ophthalmic base.

II. **How supplied.** (Dista) 5 mg/gm in 1/8 oz tamper-resistant tube.

III. **Route.** Topical ophthalmic ointment.

IV. **Dosage.** Apply a ribbon of ointment 1 cm in length to the lower conjunctival sac 1 or more times a day, depending on severity of the infection.

V. **Actions and uses.**

A. Used for the treatment of ocular infections involving conjunctiva or cornea.

B. For prophylaxis of neonatal ophthalmia.

VI. **Contraindications.**

A. Patients with known sensitivity to erythromycin.

B. Safety in use during pregnancy is unknown.

VII. **Education.**

A. Keep all medication out of children's reach.

B. Occasionally an overgrowth of antibiotic organisms occurs; if this happens stop all medications and call the office.

C. Always apply to both eyes.

D. Do not flush ointment from eyes following application.

E. Medication may cause temporary blurring of vision shortly after application.

F. Use a separate tube of medication for each patient.

G. If eyes seem sensitive to medication, stop medication and call physician or nurse practitioner.

KEFLEX (CEPHALOSPORIN ANTIBIOTIC)

I. **Generic name.** Cephalexin (Dista).

II. **Composition.**
   A. Oral suspension—125 mg/5 ml and 250 mg/5 ml.
   B. Pulvule—250 mg or 500 mg.
   C. Pediatric drops—100 mg/ml.

III. **Route.** PO.

IV. **Dosage.**
   A. 25–50 mg/kg/day.
   B. Otitis media—75–100 mg/kg/day.

V. **Action and uses.** For the treatment of bacterial infections.
   A. Respiratory tract infections caused by pneumonia and group A beta-hemolytic streptococci (not rheumatic fever).
   B. Otitis media due to *Streptococcus pneumoniae, Hemophilus influenzae,* streptococci, staphylococci, and *Neisseria catarrhalis.*
   C. Soft tissue infections caused by staphylococci and streptococci.
   D. Bone infections caused by staphylococci or *Proteus mirabilis.*
   E. Genitourinary infections caused by *Escherichia coli, P. mirabilis,* and *Klebsiella.* (Culture is necessary in all urinary tract infections before administration of medication.)

VI. **Side effects.**
   A. Headaches, diarrhea, vomiting, abdominal cramps, dyspepsia; hypersensitivity (i.e., urticaria, rash, angioedema).
   B. Genital and anal pruritus.
   C. Dizziness and fatigue.

VII. **Contraindications.** Children with known allergy to *any* antibiotics, especially penicillin-sensitive patients.
   A. Safety for use in pregnancy unknown.
   B. Caution in use with nursing mothers.
   C. Use with caution in people with a history of colitis.

VIII. **Education**
   A. Keep all medication out of children's reach.
   B. Diabetics will have false high readings on Clinitest.
   C. After mixing the medication, store in the refrigerator.
   D. Mixture may be kept for 14 days.
   E. Shake well before using.
   F. Keep cap tightly closed.
   G. May be given without regard to meals.
   H. Medication is rapidly absorbed.
   I. Require culture sensitivity tests prior and during therapy when indicated.

KWELL LOTION (PARASITIC)

I. **Composition.** Lindane 1%.

II. **How supplied.** (Reed & Carnrick) Bottles of 2 oz, 16 oz, and 1 gallon.

III. **Route.** Topical (skin).

IV. **Dosage.** Apply a thin layer of lotion to the skin from the neck down over all of body after bathing and patting dry; leave the lotion on overnight, washing it off in the morning. One application generally is effective.

V. **Precautions.**

A. Overdose or oral ingestion of Kwell can cause central nervous system reaction.

B. Do not exceed recommended dose.

VI. **Uses.** Used for treatment of scabies.

VII. **Contraindication.**

A. For premature infants.

B. People with known seizure disorder.

C. In people with known sensitivity to any components in Kwell.

D. Known safety of lindane is unknown for use in pregnancy. Pregnant women should not exceed 2 treatments during pregnancy.

E. Lindane is excreted in low concentrations in breast milk.

F. Lindane can cause central nervous system toxicity, especially in the young.

G. Use only as directed.

VIII. **Education.**

A. Do not use on open cuts or abrasions.

B. Some children continue to have pruritus following treatment; this is not a sign of treatment failure.

C. Do not retreat unless live mites are a consideration.

D. Treat sexual contacts.

E. Keep all medication out of children's reach.

F. Do not use near eye area.

KWELL SHAMPOO (PARASITIC)

I. **Composition.** Lindane 1%.

II. **Route.** Topical (head). Shampoo.

III. **Dosage.**

A. 1 oz. Apply shampoo to dry hair and leave it on for 4 minutes; add enough water to provide a good lather; wash; rinse thoroughly with water and towel dry.

B. Remove nits with a nit comb.

IV. **Contraindications.**

A. Premature infants.

B. People known to have seizures.

C. People with known sensitivities to any component in Kwell.

V. **Uses.** For treatment of head lice.

VI. **Education.**

A. Do not use on open cuts of abrasions.

B. Some children continue to have pruritus following treatment; this is not a sign of treatment failure.

C. Keep all medication out of children's reach.
D. Do not retreat unless live mites are a consideration.
E. Never to be used as preventative to possible infestation.
F. Seizures do occur following excessive use or oral ingestion of lindane.
G. Treat household contacts.
H. Lindane is absorbed through the skin and can cause central nervous system toxicity— especially at a young age.
I. Lindane is excreted in low concentrations in breast milk.
J. Use cautiously during pregnancy. Do not exceed 2 treatments during pregnancy.
K. Hair oils may enhance absorption—encourage applying Kwell shampoo onto clean hair.
L. Avoid any contact to eyes.

LOTRIMIN CREAM 1% (ANTIFUNGAL)

I. **Generic name.** Clotrimazole.
II. **Composition.** 10 mg/gm.
III. **How supplied.** (Schering) 12-gm, 24-gm tubes..
IV. **Route.** Topical.
V. **Dosage and administration.** Gently massage into affected area and surrounding skin bid.
VI. **Action.** Broad-spectrum antifungal.
VII. **Uses.** Inhibits growth of pathogenic dermatophytes, yeasts, and *Malassezia furfur.* Tinea pedis, cruris, corporis.
VIII. **Side effects.** Erythema, stinging, blistering, peeling, edema, pruritus, urticaria, generalized irritation of the skin.
IX. **Contraindications.** Persons with hypersensitivity to any components of the medication.
X. **Precautions.**
   A. Use in first trimester of pregnancy only if essential to patient's welfare.
   B. Discontinue use if irritation develops and call the office.
XI. **Education.**
   A. Keep all medication out of children's reach.
   B. Clinical improvements usually occur within the first week of treatment. If no improvement after 1 week, review the diagnosis.
   C. Store between 34° and 86°F.
   D. Not for ophthalmic use.
   E. Lotrimin is not suggested to be used for the nails or scalp.

LURIDE

I. **Generic.** Sodium fluoride.

II. How supplied. (Colgate-Hoyt Laboratories)

A. Drops—Approximately 0.125 mg fluoride per drop in squeeze bottles of 30 ml (peach-flavored).

A. Tablets—1.0-mg, 0.5-mg, or 0.25-mg fluoride bottles of 120.

III. Dosage. Drops and tablets.
Drinking Water: Daily Use

Birth to Age 3	Age 3–5	Age 5–12
<0.3 ppm	2 gtt or	4 gtt or 8 gtt or
1–0.25 tab	0.50-mg tab	1.0-mg tab
0.3–0.7 ppm	1/2 above dosage	
>0.7 ppm		

Fluoride supplement contraindicated.

IV. Actions and uses. For the use of dental caries prevention in children, birth to age 12.

V. Contraindications. Contraindicated if drinking water >0.7 ppm of fluoride.

VI. Precautions. Do not exceed recommended daily dose, excessive fluoride will result in fluorosis.

VII. Education.

A. Keep all medication out of children's reach.

B. If overdose occurs, call immediately.

C. Give only daily recommended dose, preferably at bedtime, after brushing teeth.

D. Medication is poorly absorbed if given with dairy foods.

E. Prolonged daily dose will result in pitting of the teeth, a condition known as fluorosis.

F. Dispense only one 15-ml bottle or 120 tablets at a time.

G. When dispensing tablets recommend chewing tablets before swallowing.

H. Federal law prohibits dispensing without prescription.

I. Always check the amount of fluoride in drinking water before prescribing the correct amount.

MONISTAT 7 VAGINAL CREAM (ANTIFUNGAL)

I. Generic name and composition. Water-miscible white cream containing miconazole nitrate 2%.

II. How supplied. (Ortho Pharmaceutical) 1.66-oz (47-gm) tubes with applicator.

III. Route. Intravaginal.

IV. Dosage and administration. One applicatorful intravaginally once a day hs for 7 days, only in age 12 and older.

V. Action. Exhibits fungicidal activity against species of the genus *Candida.* Mode of action unknown.

VI. Uses. Repeated local treatment of moniliasis (vulvovaginal candidiasis) previously diagnosed by M.D., confirmed by KOH.

VII. Side effects. Vulvovaginal burning, itching, irritation; vaginal burning, pelvic cramps, hives, skin rash, headaches.

VIII. Contraindications. Patients with hypersensitivity to the drug.

IX. Precautions.

A. Discontinue if irritation develops.

B. Do not use in first trimester of pregnancy unless essential to patient's welfare.

C. Do not use tampons while using cream.

X. Education.

A. Keep all medications out of children's reach.

B. Course may be repeated after other pathogens have been ruled out by appropriate smears and cultures.

C. Do not continue use of medication if infection worsens or does not improve in 3 days.

- Fever about 100°F orally
- or lower abdominal pain, back or shoulder pain
- or odoriferous vaginal discharge

D. Condoms or diaphragms are not reliable forms of birth control, or preventative for sexually transmitted diseases, when using Monistat 7 Cream. (Oil from cream weakens the latex in the product.)

E. If ingested call office and Poison Control immediately.

MOTRIN (ANTIRHEUMATIC, ANALGESIC)

I. Generic name. Ibuprofen.

II. Composition. 300-mg, 400-mg, and 600-mg tablets or caplets.

III. How supplied. Bottles of 24, 50, 100, or 165.

IV. Route. PO.

V. Dosage

A. For rheumatoid arthritis and osteoarthritis, the dosage is tailored to each patient. Do not exceed 6 tablets in 24 hours.

B. For menstrual pain, 1 tablet at the start of period or cramping, then 1 tablet q6h for 1–2 days.

VI. Action. This nonsteroidal, antiinflammatory, and antiarthritic agent also has analgesic and antipyretic properties. Mode of action is unknown.

VII. Uses. For relief of signs and symptoms of rheumatoid arthritis and osteoarthritis. For relief of mild to moderate pain (especially helpful for menstrual pain).

VIII. Interactions. Can occur with:

A. Coumadin-type anticoagulants.

B. Aspirin; there is a net decrease in antiinflammatory activity.

IX. Side effects.

A. Most frequent: nausea, epigastric pain, diarrhea, abdominal distress, vomiting, dizziness and headaches, edema, tinnitus, maculopapular rash.

B. Infrequent: gastric or duodenal ulcers, blurred vision, scotomas or changes in color vision, erythema multiforme, leukopenia, circulatory impairment in patients with marginal cardiac function.

X. Contraindications.

A. Children less than 12 years old.

B. Patients with hypersensitivity to this drug.

C. Patients with symptoms of nasal polyps, angioedema, and bronchospastic reactivity to aspirin or other nonsteroidal antiinflammatory agents.

XI. **Precautions.**

A. Not recommended during pregnancy or breastfeeding.

B. Stop if patient experiences blurred or diminished vision, scotomas, and/or changes in color vision.

C. Use with caution in patients with history of cardiac decompensation.

D. Use with caution in patients with intrinsic coagulation defects and those on anticoagulant therapy.

E. Store at room temperature.

F. Motrin can inhibit platelet aggregation and prolong bleeding time.

G. Patients on prolonged corticosteroid therapy should have their therapy tapered slowly rather than discontinued abruptly when Motrin is added.

H. Not recommended for pain more than 10 days or fever more than 3 days.

I. Keep all medication out of the reach of children. If ingested call Poison Control immediately.

XII. **Education.**

A. Smallest dose of Motrin that yields acceptable control should be employed.

B. Stop drug immediately with appearance of black stools, blurred vision, skin rashes, weight gain, edema or fever.

C. If GI disturbances occur, administer Motrin with meals or milk.

D. May cause dizziness; use caution with hazardous mechanical operations.

MYCELEX-G 500 MG (VAGINAL TABLET)

I. **Generic name.** Clotrimazole.

II. **Composition.** 500 mg.

III. **How supplied.** (Miles Pharmaceuticals) Bullet-shaped vaginal tablet with plastic applicator.

IV. **Route.** Intravaginal.

V. **Dosage.** One tablet intravaginally 1 time at bedtime.

VI. **Uses.**

A. For treatment of vulvovaginal candidiasis when one-time therapy is warranted. In cases of severe vulvovaginitis due to candidiasis, longer antimycotic therapy is recommended.

B. Diagnosis should be confirmed by KOH smears and cultures.

VII. **Side effects.** Vaginal irritation.

VIII. **Precautions.** Not recommended during first trimester of pregnancy.

IX. **Education.** Persistence of signs of vaginitis after 5 days of treatment indicate that another pathogen may be causing the condition; return to clinic.

MYCOLOG II CREAM AND OINTMENT (ANTIFUNGAL)

I. **Composition.** One gram of Mycolog contains nystatin 100,000 U and triamcinolone acetonide 1 mg.

II. **How supplied.** (Squibb) 15-gm, 30-gm, and 60-gm tubes or 120-gm jar.

III. **Route.** Topical.

IV. **Dosage and administration.** Age 2 months or older, rub sparingly into affected area bid.

V. **Action.** Triamcinolone has antiinflammatory, antipruritic, and vasoconstrictive actions; nystatin provides specific anticandidal activity.

VI. **Uses.**

A. Cutaneous candidiasis, superficial bacterial infections, infantile eczema, lichen simplex chronicus, pruritus ani, and pruritus vulvae.

B. Used in the following conditions when they are complicated by candidal and/or bacterial infection: atopic, eczematoid, stasis, nummular, contact, and seborrheic dermatitis; neurodermatitis, and dermatitis venenata.

VII. **Side effects.**

A. Burning local reactions, irritation, dryness, folliculitis, secondary infections, skin atrophy, striae, miliaria hypertrichosis, acneform eruptions, maceration of skin, and hypopigmentation.

B. Atotoxicity and nephrotoxicity.

VIII. **Contraindications.**

A. Viral diseases of the skin (vaccinia and varicella).

B. Fungal lesions (except candidiasis).

C. History of sensitivity to components of the drug.

D. Ophthalmic use or in external auditory canal with perforated tympanic membrane.

E. When circulation is impaired.

F. Pregnant patients or nursing mothers.

IX. **Precautions.**

A. Prolonged use may result in overgrowth of nonsusceptible organisms.

B. Stop use if irritation develops.

C. If external areas are treated, there may be systemic absorption.

X. **Education.**

A. Keep all medications out of children's reach.

B. Use sparingly, and only if necessary. Do not bandage or cover the area.

C. Do not use for a prolonged period of time.

D. Do not use tight-fitting diapers or plastic pants when treating diaper rash.

E. Not for ophthalmic use.

F. Store at room temperature.

MYCOSTATIN (ANTIFUNGAL)

I. **Generic name.** Nystatin.

II. Composition.

A. Ointment and cream. 100,000 U/gm.

B. Oral suspension. 100,000 U/ml in a vehicle containing 50% sucrose.

III. How supplied. (Squibb)

A. Cream and ointment—15-gm and 30-gm tubes.

B. Oral suspension—60-ml bottles with calibrated dropper.

IV. Route. Topical or PO.

V. Dosage.

A. Cream, ointment. Apply liberally to affected area bid until healed.

B. Oral suspension

1. Infants—2 ml qid (1 ml in each side of mouth).
2. Premature and low-birth-weight infants—1 ml qid.
3. Continue treatment 48 hours after perioral symptoms have disappeared.

VI. Action.

A. Nystatin probably acts by binding to sterols in the cell membrane of the fungus with a resultant change in membrane permeability, allowing leakage of intracellular components.

B. Exhibits no appreciable activity against bacteria or trichomonads.

VII. Uses.

A. Topical preparations. For treatment of cutaneous or mucocutaneous mycotic infections caused by *Candida albicans* and other candida species.

B. Oral suspension. For treatment of candidiasis in the oral cavity.

VIII. Side effects.

A. Topical preparations—Minor skin irritation.

B. Oral suspension—Diarrhea, GI distress, nausea, vomiting.

IX. Contraindications. Patients with hypersensitivity to the drug.

X. Precautions. Discontinue use immediately if hypersensitivity reaction occurs.

XI. Education.

A. Keep all medication out of children's reach.

B. Preparations do not stain skin or mucous membranes.

C. Store at room temperature; avoid freezing.

D. Apply oral suspension after feeding. Remember to keep bottle nipples and pacifiers clean, and use Mycostatin cream on breasts if nursing.

E. Return to office for follow-up after 1 weeks' treatment.

NIX (TOPICAL PEDICULICIDE)

I. Generic name. Permethrin 1% rinse.

II. Composition. Permethrin 10 mg/gm (1%); inactive ingredients are stearalkonium chloride, hydrolyzed animal protein, cetyl alcohol, polyoxyethylene 10 cetyl ether, hydroxyethylcellulose, balsam canada, fragrance, citric acid, and color.

III. How supplied. (Burroughs-Wellcome) 2-fl oz plastic squeeze bottles. Use enough to saturate hair and scalp; allow to remain on hair for at least 10 minutes before rinsing off with water. One single treatment is sufficient to eliminate head lice infestation. Combing of nits is not required but may be done for cosmetic reasons.

IV. Route. Topical.

V. Dosage. 1–2 oz as a cream rinse to be used after hair has been washed with shampoo and towel-dried (leave on 10 minutes only).

VI. Uses. For single-application treatment of head lice and nits. If live lice are observed at least 1 week following application, a second application may be given. Remove nits with the comb.

VII. Contraindications.

A. Patients with known sensitivity to any of the ingredients, to any synthetic pyrethroid or pyrethrin, or to chrysanthemums.

B. Pregnant or breast-feeding women.

C. Children under the age of 2 years.

VIII. Side effects. Head lice infestation is often accompanied by pruritus, erythema, and edema; treatment may temporarily exacerbate these conditions.

IX. Education.

A. Keep all medication out of children's reach.

B. Some itching, redness, or swelling of the scalp may occur after application of Nix.

C. Pruritus is the most common problem associated with Nix; the pruritus is actually caused by the lice itself.

D. If symptoms persist, do not use medication again; call your physician.

E. If sensitivity occurs, discontinue use.

F. If Nix is ingested, gastric lavage and general supportive measures are suggested.

G. Nix is not irritating to the eyes. However, contact with eyes during application should be avoided; flush eyes immediately with water if Nix gets in the eyes.

H. Discard remaining contents when treatment is finished.

I. Wash all linens, personal clothes in hot water and hot dryer, or dry clean if unable to wash.

J. Vacuum rooms used by patient and wash combs and brushes in hot soapy water.

K. Safety of use during pregnancy and for nursing mothers unknown.

L. All family members should be examined and treated.

NOVAHISTINE DMX (ANTITUSSIVE EXPECTORANT)

I. Composition. Each 5 ml contains dextromethorphan hydrobromide 10 mg, pseudoephedrine hydrochloride 30 mg, guaifenesin 100 mg, and alcohol 10% .

II. How supplied. (Dow Pharmaceuticals) 4-fl oz and 8-fl oz bottles.

III. Route. PO.

IV. Dosage. Not more than 4 doses qd. (No longer than 7 days.)

A. 2–5 years—1/2 tsp q4h.

B. 6–12 years—1 tsp q5h.

C. Over 12 years—2 tsp q4–6h.

V. Action. Cough suppressant—affects medulla of brain; nonanalgesic and nonaddictive.

VI. Uses. To control cough spasms or change a dry cough into a productive one. Helpful for cough—especially dry, nonproductive one—associated with mild upper respiratory infection, influenza, and bronchitis.

VII. Side effects. Nausea, dizziness, vomiting, mild stimulation.

VIII. Contraindications.

A. Patients with persistent or chronic cough (e.g., asthma) or with cough with excessive secretions.

B. Patients with heart problems, diabetes, high blood pressure, thyroid disease, or MAO inhibitor therapy.

C. Children under age 2.

D. Nursing mothers or during pregnancy.

IX. Precautions.

A. Refer to physician if cough persists longer than 1 week, recurs, or is associated with high fever, rash, or persistent headache.

B. Drugs containing dextromethorphan should not be given with monoamine oxidase inhibitors or antidepressants.

C. Dextromethorphan is incompatible with salicylates, tetracyclines, penicillin, and iodides.

X. Education.

A. Keep all medication out of children's reach.

B. If overdose occurs call Poison Control Center immediately.

C. Available over the counter.

D. Do not drive a car or operate machinery while on medication.

E. If cough persists longer than 1 week, call office.

PEDIACARE

I. Composition

A. PediaCare 1 (Children's Cough Relief Liquid). Dextromethorphan hydrobromide 5 mg/5 ml.

B. PediaCare 2 (Children's Cold Relief Liquid). Pseudoephedrine hydrochloride 15 mg and chlorpheniramine maleate 1 mg/5 ml.

C. PediaCare 3 (Children's Cold Relief).

1. Liquid—Pseudoephedrine hydrochloride 15 mg, chlorpheniramine maleate 1 mg, and dextromethorphan hydrobromide 5 mg.
2. Chewable tablets—Pseudoephedrine hydrochloride 7.5 mg, chlorpheniramine maleate 0.5 mg, and dextromethorphan hydrobromide 2.5 mg.

D. PediaCare Drops (Infants' Cold Relief Decongestant). Pseudoephedrine hydrochloride 7.5 mg/0.8 ml.

II. How supplied. (McNeil Consumer Products)

A. Liquid. 4-fl oz bottles (cherry-flavored).

B. Tablets. Bottles of 24 (fruit-flavored).

C. Drops. 1/2-fl oz bottles with calibrated dropper (cherry-flavored).

III. Route. PO.

IV. Dosage.

A. PediaCare Drops
   1. 0–3 months (6–11 lbs)—1/2 dropper (0.4 ml) q4–6h.
   2. 4–11 months (12–17 lbs)—1 dropper (0.8 ml) q4–6h.
   3. 12–23 months (18–23 lbs)—1 1/2 droppers (1.2 ml) q4–6h.

B. PediaCare 1-2-3
   1. 2–3 years (24–36 lbs)
      a. Liquid—1 tsp q4–6h.
      b. Tablets—2 q4–6h.
   2. 4–5 years (36–47 lbs)
      a. Liquid—1 1/2 tsp q4–6h.
      b. Tablets—3 q4-6h.
   3. 6–8 years (48–59 lbs)
      a. Liquid—2 tsp q4–6h.
      b. Tablets—4 q4–6h.
   4. 9–10 years (60–71 lb)
      a. Liquid—2 1/2 tsp q4–6h.
      b. Tablets—5 q4–6h.

C. PediaCare Night Rest Liquid
   1. 2–3 years—1 tsp
   2. 4–5 years—1 1/2 tsp
   3. 6–8 years—2 tsp
   4. 9–10 years—2 1/2 tsp
   5. 11 years—3 tsp

V. Uses

A. PediaCare 1: Cough due to minor irritation.

B. PediaCare 2: Nasal congestion or runny nose due to hayfever, or upper respiratory infection.

C. PediaCare 3: Nasal congestion, runny nose, hayfever, or cough.

VI. Contraindications. Children with heart disease, high blood pressure, thyroid disease, diabetes, glaucoma, asthma, or depression.

VII. Education.

A. Keep all medication of the children's reach.

B. Discontinue use after 7 days.

C. Call clinic if cough continues, high fever occurs, or headache or rash appears.

D. Medication may cause irritability and drowsiness.

E. Persistent cough is a sign of a serious illness; call physicain or nurse practitioner.

F. Do not exceed 6 doses in 24 hours.

G. Do not give to children on medication for high blood pressure.

H. Medication is not for nasal use; administer PO only.

I. If overdose occurs call Poison Control immediately.

J. Do not use medication if seal is broken, cap is open or carton is opened.

K. PediaCare Night Rest may be used every 6–8 hours.

PEDIALYTE (ORAL ELECTROLYTE SOLUTION)

I. **Composition.** Each liter contains:

Sodium	30 mEq
Potassium	20 mEq
Calcium	4 mEq
Magnesium	4 mEq
Chloride	30 mEq
Citrate	28 mEq
Dextrose	50 gm
Calories	200

II. **How supplied.** (Ross Laboratories) 8-fl oz bottles and 32-fl oz cans.

III. **Route.** PO.

IV. **Dosage.** Divide daily doses into frequent small feedings for rehydration.

A. 7–12 lbs—18–38 fl oz/day.

B. 13–19 lbs—47–53 fl oz/day.

C. 20–24 lbs—53–58 fl oz/day.

D. 24–30 lbs—58–69 fl oz/day.

E. 30–34 lbs—74–78 fl oz/day.

F. 34–40 lbs—83–85 fl oz/day.

V. **Action and uses.** To maintain and replace the normal electrolyte balance in infants and children who have moderate to severe diarrhea.

VI. **Precautions.** Do not recommend Pedialyte for very small infants (i.e., 1 month of age).

VII. **Education.**

A. Carefully calculate the amount needed according to the child's weight.

B. Discontinue all solid foods, and follow diarrhea protocol carefully.

C. Give frequent small feedings of Pedialyte.

D. Children age 4 years and older may have 2 qt a day.

PEDIAPROFEN

I. **Generic name.** Ibuprofen suspension.

II. **Composition.** 100 mg ibuprofen in 5 ml.

III. **How supplied.** Orange, berry, vanilla flavor in 4-fl oz. or 16-fl oz bottles.

IV. **Route.** PO.

V. **Dosage–temperature control.**

A. 6 months–12 years of age 5 mg/kl body weight for temperature <102.5°F

or

B. 10 mg/kg body weight for temperature >102.5°F.
Maximum daily dose 40 mg/kg.

C. For dysmenorrhea and mild to moderate pain in adults. Beginning with earliest onset of pain—400 mg PO.

D. Do not exceed 3,200 mg total daily dose.

VI. Action and uses. Recommended as a nonsteroidal, antiinflammatory agent. It possesses antipruritic and analgesic qualities. Especially successful in treating children's fevers, primary dysmenorrhea, rheumatoid arthritis, osteoarthritis and following dental extractions and procedures.

VIII. Side effects. Gastrointestinal symptoms, dizziness, headache, nervousness, tinnitus, rash, anorexia, abdominal pain, dry eyes and mouth and, in severe cases, hallucinations, bleeding episodes, gynecomastia, heart arrhythmias, serum sickness, lupus erythematosus syndrome, Schönlein-Henoch vasculitis or renal papillary necrosis.

IX. Contraindications.

A. In patients who have previously shown a reaction to ingredients in the medication or to aspirin or other antiinflammatory agents.

B. Not recommended for use during pregnancy or in nursing mothers.

C. Do not use in children under the age of 6 months.

D. Not recommended to be used with aspirin.

X. Precautions.

A. Blurred or diminished vision, scotomata or changes of color vision while taking medication indicate a need to discontinue the use of the medication and call the office immediately.

B. Use with caution in patients with previous history of hypertension or cardiac decompensation.

C. Medication can inhibit platelet aggregation. Use with caution in patients with coagulation defects or those on anticoagulant therapy.

XI. Education.

A. Keep all medication out of children's reach.

B. Medication is dispensed by prescription only.

C. Shake medication well before administration.

D. Store at room temperature.

E. Do not refrigerate medication.

F. Do not exceed recommended daily dose.

G. If gastrointestinal complaints occur, administer medication with food.

H. Patients need to discontinue use if the following symptoms occur: blurred vision, gastrointestinal bleeding, eye symptoms, skin rash, weight gain or edema, jaundice or severe hepatic reactions. Call office if these symptoms occur. If patient shows signs of aseptic meningitis consider the possibility of it being related to the medication.

PEDIAZOLE (ANTIBIOTIC)

I. Composition. Erythromycin ethylsuccinate 200 mg/5 ml and sulfisoxazole acetyl 600 mg/5 ml in oral suspension.

II. How supplied. (Ross) 100-ml, 150-ml, 200-ml, and 250-ml bottles; strawberry and banana flavors.

III. Route. PO.

IV. Actions and uses. Treatment of acute otitis media, particularly cases caused by susceptible strains of *Hemophilus influenzae,* including ampicillin-resistant strains.

V. **Side effects.** Rashes, erythema multiforme, periorbital edema, nausea, diarrhea, anorexia, headaches, tinnitus, vertigo, insomnia. Severe reactions, including Stevens-Johnson, toxic epidermal necrolysis, aplastic anemia and other blood disorders have occurred.

VI. **Contraindications.**

A. Children with allergies to erythromycin or sulfa drugs.

B. Infants less than 2 months of age.

C. Patients with impaired hepatic function.

D. Pregnant women and breast-feeding women.

VII. **Dosage.**

A. 18 lbs—1/2 tsp qid.

B. 35 lbs—1 tsp qid.

C. 53 lbs—1 1/2 tsp qid.

D. Over 100 lbs—2 tsp qid.

VIII. **Education.**

A. Pediazole in conjunction with high doses of theophylline may cause increased serum theophylline levels and even toxicity.

B. Increase fluid intake while on medication.

C. Discontinue medication if signs of rash or adverse reactions occur, i.e., fever, jaundice, purpura, sore throat or pallor.

D. Give full 10 days of medication even though symptoms of otitis media disappear.

E. May be given with meals.

F. Keep all medication out of children's reach.

G. Some reversible hearing loss has been noted in patients with renal insufficiency on high doses of erythromycin.

PENICILLIN V POTASSIUM (ANTIBIOTIC)

I. **Generic name.** Penicillin V potassium.

II. **Composition.**

A. Oral suspension—125 mg/5 ml and 250 mg/5 ml.

B. Tablets—250 mg and 500 mg.

III. **Route.** PO.

IV. **Dosage.**

A. Infants and small children—1–50 mg/kg/day in divided doses q6h.

B. Under 12–15 years— 50 mg/kg/day in divided doses q6h.

C. Over 12 years—125–300 mg q6h.

V. **Action and uses.**

A. Used for upper respiratory infections caused by streptococci, including pharyngitis and scarlet fever.

B. For pneumococcal infection of otitis media.

C. Used prophylactically in rheumatic fever and mild staphylococcal infection of soft tissue and skin.

VI. **Side effects.** Sore mouth and black tongue. Nausea, decreased appetite, vomiting, diarrhea, skin eruptions, urticaria.

VII. **Contraindications.** Patients with a known allergy to penicillin or ampicillin.

VIII. **Precautions.**

A. Use cautiously in patients with asthma or a history of allergies.

B. Order culture and test of sensitivity of skin infection before prescribing medication.

C. Order throat culture before treating in cases of strep pharyngitis.

IX. **Education.**

A. Keep all medications out of children's reach.

B. Advise patient to discontinue medication if there are any signs of rash, pruritus, or anaphylaxis.

C. May be administered with food, but blood levels are higher if given on an empty stomach.

D. Keep medication refrigerated and tightly capped.

E. Shake bottle well before pouring oral solutions.

F. Take medication for 10 full days even though symptoms disappear.

G. Order medication generically.

H. Discard any unused medication after 10 days.

PHENERGAN EXPECTORANT WITH CODEINE (COUGH FORMULA)

I. **Composition.** Syrup; promethazine hydrochloride 6.25 mg/5 ml and codeine phosphate 10 mg.

II. **Route.** PO.

III. **Dosage.**

A. Not to be used for children under 2 years of age.

B. Age 2–6 years—1/4–1/2 tsp, not to exceed 6.0 ml in 24 hours.

C. Age 6–12 years—1/2 tsp, q6h, not to exceed 8.0 ml in 24 hours.

IV. **Action and uses.** Antihistamine, antiemetic, and sedative qualities useful for persistent cough, perennial and seasonal allergic rhinitis, and allergic conjunctivitis.

V. **Precautions.** Doses of 75–125 mg of promethazine hydrochloride may cause paradoxical reaction, characterized by hyperexcitability and nightmares.

VI. **Education.**

A. Keep all medications out of children's reach.

B. Suggest using only at night to manage persistent cough in sleepless child. (No longer than 4 days.)

C. Order 4 oz—with no refills.

D. May be habit forming—carefully monitor medical plan.

E. Do not use during pregnancy or in nursing mothers.

F. Call office immediately if overdose.

G. Do not use with patients who have a history of drug dependency.

H. Medication may have a sedating effect—adults should not use medication when driving a vehicle or farm machinery; children should be discouraged from riding bikes when taking medication.

I. Do not use with tranquilizers, alcohol, or CNS depressants.

J. Overdose may result in respiratory depression, stupor or coma, cold clammy skin, bradycardia, Cheyne-Stokes respiration, pinpoint pupils, cardiac arrest, and death.

K. If cough continues, fever or course of illness worsens, discontinue medication and call for a medical appointment.

PONSTEL (ANALGESIC)

I. **Generic name.** Mefenamic acid.

II. **Composition.** 250 mg.

III. **How supplied.** (Parke-Davis) Bottles of 100 Kapseals.

IV. **Route.** PO.

V. **Dosage.** Children over 14 years. 500 mg initially, then 250 mg q6h as needed.

VI. **Action.** In clinical trials with animals, analgesic, antipyretic, and antiinflammatory activities were demonstrated.

VII. **Uses.** For relief of mild to moderate pain of primary dysmenorrhea when therapy does not exceed 1 week (usually only needed 2–3 days).

VIII. **Side effects.**

A. Nausea, GI discomfort, vomiting, gas, diarrhea.

B. Drowsiness, dizziness, nervousness, headaches, blurred vision, insomnia.

C. Urticaria, rash, facial edema, mild renal toxicity, dysuria, hematuria.

D. Severe autoimmune hemolytic anemia if used for prolonged periods of time.

E. Eye irritation, ear pain, perspiration, mild hepatic toxicity; an increased need for insulin in diabetics.

IX. **Contraindications.**

A. Children less than 14 years of age.

B. Patients hypersensitive to mefenamic acid.

C. Patients with ulcerations or chronic inflammation of either upper or lower GI tract.

D. During pregnancy or nursing mothers.

X. **Precautions.**

A. Administer with caution to patients with inflammatory disease of the GI tract or a history of kidney or liver disease.

B. Cases of autoimmune hemolytic anemia, may occur with continuous use 12 months or longer.

C. BUN values may rise during therapy.

D. If rash or diarrhea occurs, stop use of drug promptly.

E. May prolong prothrombin time.

F. May exacerbate asthma.

G. Produces false positive reaction for urinary bile in diazo tablet test.

XI. **Education**

A. Keep all medications out of children's reach.

B. Take medication with food.
C. Do not exceed 1 week of therapy.
D. If overdose occurs call Poison Control Center immediately.
E. If diarrhea occurs, reduce dose or discontinue use temporarily and call the office.

PROSTAPHLIN (ANTIBIOTIC)

I. **Generic name.** Oxacillin sodium.
II. **Composition.** Oral solution, 250 mg/5 ml.
III. **Route.** PO.
IV. **Dosage.** 50–100 mg/kg/day in 4 equal doses.
V. **Action and uses.**
A. Used for infections caused by penicillinase-producing staphylococci, beta-hemolytic streptococci, or pneumococci.
B. Very useful for therapy in suspected staphylococcal infection pending culture and sensitivity test.
VI. **Side effects.** Diarrhea, nausea, vomiting, pruritus, rash, hives, wheezing; elevated SGOT and SGPT; transient hematuria and superinfection.
VII. **Contraindications.**
A. Patients with sensitivity to penicillins or cephalosporins.
B. Premature infants and neonates.
C. Children with renal impairment.
VIII. **Precautions.** Use cautiously in children with a history of asthma.
IX. **Education.**
A. Keep all medications out of children's reach.
B. Give medication on an empty stomach 1 hour before or 2 hours after eating or drinking.
C. Keep medication tightly capped.
D. Keep medication in the refrigerator. (Solution remains stable for 14 days in the refrigerator.)
E. Take drug for required length of time as prescribed.
F. If rash or hives develop, discontinue medication and call the clinic.

PYRIDIUM (ANALGESIC)

I. **Generic name.** Phenazopyridine hydrochloride.
II. **Composition.** (Parke-Davis) Tablets—100 mg and 200 mg.
III. **Route.** PO.
IV. **Dosage.** Adults. 200 mg tid.
V. **Uses.** Helps relieve pain and symptoms of urinary dysuria in adolescents; especially helpful during time interval between diagnosis and treatment.
VI. **Side effects.** Mild GI symptoms.

VII. Precautions. Yellowish tinge of skin or sclera may indicate decline in renal function. Not recommended during pregnancy or in nursing mothers. Discontinue use if headache, rash, pruritis or GI disturbance. If overdose call the office immediately.

VIII. Contraindications. Patients with renal insufficiency or sensitivity to ingredients in medication.

IX. Education.

A. Keep all medication out of children's reach.

B. Take medication tid after meals.

C. The medication will give urine a reddish-orange tint and may stain fabric.

D. Use only as long as symptoms persist.

E. Do not exceed 2 days on medication.

RONDEC-DM (ANTIHISTAMINE/DECONGESTANT/ANTITUSSIVE)

I. Composition.

A. Drops. Each 1-ml dropperful contains carbinoxamine maleate 2 mg/pseudoephedrine hydrochloride 25 mg, dextromethorphan hydrobromide 4 mg, and less than 0.6% alcohol.

B. Syrup. Each 5 ml (1 tsp) contains carbinoxamine maleate 4 mg, pseudoephedrine hydrochloride 60 mg, dextromethorphan hydrobromide 15 mg, and less than 0.6% alcohol.

II. How supplied. (Ross Laboratories)

A. Drops—30-ml bottles with dropper (grape-flavored).

B. Syrup—4-fl oz and 16-fl oz bottles (grape-flavored).

III. Route. PO.

IV. Dosage.

A. Drops

1. 1–3 months—1/4 dropperful qid.
2. 3–6 months—1/2 dropperful qid.
3. 6–9 months—3/4 dropperful qid.
4. 9–18 months—1 dropperful qid.

B. Syrup

1. 18 months–5 years—1/2 tsp (2.5 ml) qid.
2. 6 years and over—1 tsp (5 ml) qid.

V. Action and uses. Relief of symptoms of nasopharyngitis, common cold, bronchitis, bronchial cough, and recurrent cough; nonnarcotic, antitussive, decongestive and antihistaminic.

VI. Side effects. Sedation, moderate drowsiness, dizziness, vomiting, headache, nausea, dysuria, polyuria, cardiac arrhythmias, respiratory difficulty, tremors, hallucinations, weakness, pallor.

VII. Contraindications. Children with glaucoma, urinary retention, ulcer, or coronary disease. Hypertension or ischemic heart disease. Patient's taking MAO inhibitors or during asthmatic attacks.

VIII. **Precautions.** Use with caution in patients with a history of asthma, diabetes, or hyperthyroidism. Not recommended during pregnancy, use with caution in nursing mothers.

IX. **Education.**

A. Keep all medicine out of childrens reach.

B. If overdose occurs, call Poison Control immediately.

C. May be given with analgesics and antibiotics.

D. Suggest giving tid if side effects occur.

E. Avoid exposure of medication to excessive heat.

F. Keep liquid cool and dark.

G. Keep tightly capped.

H. Antihistamine may enhance the effects of barbiturates, alcohol, antidepressants or other CNS depressants.

I. If cough worsens or fever ensues, call the office immediately.

SEBULEX (MEDICATED SHAMPOO)

I. **Composition.** 2% sulfur and 2% salicylic acid in surface-active cleansers and wetting agents.

II. **How supplied.** (Westwood) 4-oz and 8-oz bottles.

III. **Route.** Topical.

IV. **Dosage and administration.**

A. Shake shampoo well.

B. Apply moderate amount to wet scalp.

C. Allow lather to remain on scalp for 5 minutes.

D. Rinse carefully.

V. **Action and uses.** For itchy scalp, seborrhea, cradle cap, and dandruff.

VI. **Contraindications.** Patients who develop skin irritation.

VII. **Education.**

A. Keep all medications out of children's reach.

B. Avoid contact with eyes; rinse carefully away from face.

C. May be repeated every 3 days for 1 week.

D. May be purchased over the counter.

SODIUM SULAMYD (10% OPHTHALMIC SOLUTION AND OPHTHALMIC OINTMENT)

I. **Generic name.** Sulfacetamide sodium 10%.

II. **Composition.**

A. Solution. Each milliliter of 10% solution (sterileaqueous) contains 100 mg sulfacetamide solution, 3.1 mg sodium thiosulfate and 5 mg methylcellulose, with 0.5 mg methylparaben and 0.1 mg prophylparaben added as preservatives and monobasic sodium phosphate added as buffer.

B. Ointment. Same ingredients as in solution in a bland, unctuous petrolatum base.

III. **How supplied.** (Schering)

A. Solution—5-ml bottles with dropper.

B. Ointment—3.5-gm tubes.

IV. **Route.** Apply topically to eye.

V. **Dosage.**

A. Solution—1–2 gtt into lower conjunctival sac 3–4 times a day for 5 days.

B. Ointment—Apply small amount to lower conjunctiva 4 times a day for 5 days.

VI. **Actions and uses.** Used for both gram-positive and gram-negative microorganisms causing conjunctivitis, corneal ulcer, and other occular infections.

VII. **Precautions.**

A. Sodium Sulamyd is incompatible with silver preparations.

B. Ophthalmic ointments may retard corneal healing.

C. If signs of sensitivity or other untoward reactions occur, stop use of preparation.

VIII. **Education.**

A. Keep medications out of children's reach.

B. Store in refrigerator.

C. Solution will discolor with age; if it is discolored, it should be discarded.

D. Do not touch conjunctiva with dropper or tube during application.

E. The ointment may be used adjunctly with solution.

F. Be aware of expiration date on container, discard after date is reached.

SUDAFED (ADRENERGIC)

I. **Generic name.** Pseudoephedrine hydrochloride.

II. **Composition**

A. Syrup—30 mg/5 ml.

B. Tablets—30 mg and 60 mg.

III. **How supplied** (Burroughs-Wellcome)

A. Syrup. 4-oz and 1-pt bottles.

B. Tablets. Boxes of 24.

IV. **Route.** PO.

V. **Dosage.** Do not exceed daily dosage. Do not exceed 4 doses in 24 hours.

A. Age 2–6 years—1/2 tsp of syrup q4–6 hours.

B. 6–12 years—1 tsp of syrup q4–6 hours.

C. Over 12 years—two 30-mg tablets qid.

VI. **Action and uses.**

A. Used for nasal congestion, bronchial congestion, acute coryza, rhinitis, and serous otitis media with eustachian tube congestion.

B. May be used in combination with antibiotics, analgesics, antihistamines, or expectorants in cases of allergic rhinitis, sinusitis, acute otitis media, and tracheobronchitis.

VII. **Side effects.** Mild stimulation and nausea.

VIII. **Contraindications.** Patients with hypertension, diabetes, or hyperthyroidism.

IX. **Precautions.** Sudafed interacts with monoamine oxidase inhibitors and guanethidine.

X. **Education.**

A. Keep all medications out of children's reach.

B. Sudafed is an over-the-counter drug; no prescription is needed.

C. Do not take any nonprescription drug with Sudafed without approval of provider.

D. Avoid giving medication at bedtime; it may cause restlessness and sleeplessness.

E. Discontinue medication if extreme restlessness, agitation, tachycardia, or anorexia occurs.

F. Do not give product more then 7 days.

G. Call immediately, if accidental overdose.

H. If symptoms do not improve, cough is worse, or fever ensues call medical provider.

I. Store medication 59°–77°F and protect from light.

SUPRAX

I. **Generic name.** Cefixime. A semisynthetic cephalosporin antibiotic.

II. **Composition.**

A. Oral suspension 100 mg/5 cc

B. Scored 200-mg and 400-mg film-coated tablets

III. **Route.** PO.

IV. **Dosage.** Children dose 8/mg/kg q day.

A. A normal guide for treating otitis media:

	Weight	Daily Dose
50-ml bottle	7 lbs	1/4 tsp
	14 lbs	1/2 tsp
	21 lbs	3/4 tsp
	28 lbs	1 tsp
100-ml bottle	35 lbs	1 1/4 tsp
	42 lbs	1 1/2 tsp
	49 lbs	1 3/4 tsp
	56 lbs	2 tsp

B. Children age 12 and over should be treated with adult dose.

C. Children with otitis media should be treated with suspension rather than tablets (peak flow is higher on suspension rather than tablets).

D. Not recommended in children less than 6 months of age.

E. Adult dose 400 mg daily (1 tab q day or 2 200 mg bid)

V. **Action and uses.** Used for the treatment of:

A. Uncomplicated urinary tract infections caused by *Escherichia coli* and *Proteus mirabilis.*

B. Otitis media caused by *Haemophilus influenzae, Moraxella catarrhalis,* and *Streptococcus pyogenes.*

C. Pharyngitis and tonsillitis caused by *Streptococcus pyogenes.*

D. Active bronchitis and acute exacerbations of chronic bronchitis caused by *Streptococcus pneumoniae* and *Haemophilus influenzae.*

VI. **Side effects.**

A. Gastrointestinal—adverse reactions such as diarrhea, abdominal pain, nausea and vomiting.

B. CNS—headaches and dizziness.

C. Hypersensitivity reactions—skin rashes, urticaria, or pruritus.

D. Hepatic—may have elevated SGPT, SGOT, and alkaline phosphatase, BUN or creatinine.

E. *In severe cases cephalosporins may trigger seizures.*

VII. **Contraindications.** In persons with known allergy to the cephalosporin group of antibiotics, penicillin allergy. (A cross hypersensitivity in up to 10% of people with penicillin allergy may occur.)

VIII. **Precautions.** Safety of use in pregnancy has not been established. It is not known if Suprax is excreted in human milk. Safety and effectiveness in children under the age of six months of age has not been established.

IX. **Education**

A. Take medication for the allotted time of 10 days even though symptoms disappear.

B. Shake the suspension well before using.

C. The suspension may be kept for 14 days at room temperature or may be refrigerated.

D. Keep bottle tightly capped.

E. Discard unused portion of medication after 14 days.

F. Medication may be taken with or without food.

TAVIST SYRUP

I. **Generic name.** Clemastine fumarate.

II. **Composition.** Each tsp (5 ml) contains 0.67 mg of clemastine fumarate.

III. **Route.** PO.

IV. **Dosage.** (Sandoz) Supplied in citrus flavor, 4-fl oz bottle.

A. Children age 6–12 years of age—1 tsp bid for symptoms of allergic rhinitis, 2 tsp bid starting dose for urticaria and angioedema. Do not exceed 6 teaspoons in 24-hour period.

B. Children age 12 and over—2 tsp bid for symptoms of allergic rhinitis, 4 tsp bid for symptoms of urticaria and angioedema. Do not exceed 12 teaspoonsful over 24-hour period.

V. **Action and uses.** Recommend for the relief of allergic rhinitis and allergic pruritus, urticaria, and angioedema.

VI. **Side effects.** Dryness of mouth, nose and throat; drug rash, headache, sleepiness, anorexia.

VII. **Contraindicated.**

A. In patients hypersensitive to the drug or other antihistamines.

B. Do not use in newborns or premature infants.

C. Use with caution in patients with narrow angle glaucoma, stenosing peptic ulcer, pyloroduodenal obstruction or bladder neck obstruction.

D. Not recommended for use with hypnotics, sedatives, tranquilizers or with alcohol.

E. Not recommended for use when operating machinery or driving a car.

F. Use with caution in patients with hypertension, bronchial asthma, increased intraocular pressure, hyperthyroidism or cardiovascular disease.

VIII. **Education.**

A. Do not exceed recommended dose.

B. Signs of antihistamine toxicity in children include fixed, dilated pupils, dry mouth, flushed face, fever, excitation/agitation, hallucinations, ataxia, incoordination, tonic/clonic convulsions and post ictal depression.

C. In overdose antihistamines can cause hallucinations, convulsions and death.

D. Safety of medication during pregnancy is unknown.

E. Medication is excreted in breast milk. Not recommended for use in nursing mothers.

F. Keep medications out of the reach of children.

G. Store medication in tightly closed container in dry, cool place, away from sunlight and heat.

H. MAO inhibitors prolong and increase intensity of anticholinergic effects of antihistamines.

I. Patients should be questioned regarding a history of glaucoma, urinary retention, peptic ulcer, or pregnancy, before suggesting antihistamine use.

J. Patients may not take alcohol, sleeping pills, sedatives or tranquilizers while taking antihistamines.

K. Medication can cause dizziness, headache, drowsiness, dry mouth, blurred vision, nausea or nervousness in some people.

TETRACYCLINE CAPSULES (ANTIBIOTIC)

I. **Generic name.** Tetracycline hydrochloride.

II. **Composition.**

A. Capsules—250 mg or 500 mg.

B. Suspension—125 mg/5 ml.

III. **Route.** PO.

IV. **Dosage.**

A. Children 9 years and over—15–25 mg/lb/day in 4 divided doses.

B. Adults—1 or 2 capsules in 4 divided doses.

V. **Action and uses.**

A. Inhibits protein synthesis.

B. Active against a broad range of gram-positive and gram-negative organisms, especially *Mycoplasma pneumoniae, Escherichia coli, Shigella, Hemophilus influenzae, Klebsiella.*

C. Also used for intestinal amebiasis and in severe acne.

VI. **Side effects.** Nausea, vomiting, diarrhea, glossitis, enteritis, monilial overgrowth, loss of appetite.

VII. **Contraindications.**

A. Patients with hypersensitivity to any tetracyclines or with renal impairment.

B. Children under 9 years of age, in whom it may cause permanent discoloration of teeth.

C. Women in the first trimester of pregnancy.

VIII. **Education.**

A. Keep all medications out of children's reach.

B. Take medication on an empty stomach 1 hour before or 2 hours after eating.

C. Do not take tetracycline with any milk products or iron preparations.

D. Avoid prolonged exposure to sunshine.

E. Tetracycline is present in the breast milk of lactating women taking the medication, and is not recommended during breast feeding.

F. Avoid oral antacids and diuretics when taking tetracycline.

G. Take medication for the prescribed period of time.

H. Order generically to save cost.

I. Limit refills of tetracycline when treating for acne to ensure follow-up visits.

J. Do not take during pregnancy.

K. Do not take medication during the summer—over exposure to sun can have adverse effects.

L. Acne may take at least 1 month treatment before noticeable affect, if it seems worse discontinue use and call the office.

THEO-DUR SPRINKLE

I. **Generic name.** Anhydrous theophylline.

II. **Composition.** Sustained-action capsule contains 50-mg, 75-mg, 125-mg, or 200-mg anhydrous theophylline in the form of long-acting, microencapsulated beads within a hard gelatin capsule.

III. **How supplied.** (Key Pharmaceutical) 50-mg, 75-mg, 125-mg, and 200-mg sustained-action capsules in bottles of 100.

IV. **Route.** PO.

V. **Dosage and administration.**

A. Carefully open capsule and sprinkle a spoonful of contents on soft food (applesauce or pudding). Swallow the food immediately without chewing and then drink a glass of cool water or juice. The small amount of food used will not affect bioavailability.

B. Dividing the daily dose into 3 every hours may be indicated if symptoms occur repeatedly.

C. Initial dosage. 16 mg/kg/24 h or 400 mg/24 h (whichever is less) in 2 divided doses at 12-hour intervals.

D. Dosage should not exceed the following.

Age	Daily Dose	Dose/12 h
6–9	24 mg/kg/day	12.0 mg/kg
9–12	20 mg/kg/day	10.0 mg/kg
12–16	18 mg/kg/day	9.0 mg/kg
16+	13 mg/kg/day or 900 mg (whichever is less)	6.5 mg/kg

Note: Dosage should be calculated on the basis of lean ideal body weight; Theo-Dur does not distribute to fatty tissue.

E. Medication should not be given with food; administer 1 hour before or 2 hours after meals.

F. Dosing requires two stages:

1. Initiation of therapy.
2. Titration, adjustment, and chronic maintenance of medication.

VI. Use. For the relief or prevention of mild to moderate symptoms of asthma or bronchitis. Theo-Dur sprinkles are not intended for the treatment of acute respiratory symptoms of asthma, chronic bronchitis, or emphysema, which require rapid relief.

VII. Side effects. Nausea, vomiting, epigastric pain, hematemesis, diarrhea; headache, irritability, restlessness, insomnia, convulsions, palpitations, tachycardia, hypotension, circulatory failure, ventricular arrhythmias; albuminuria, increased RBC, ADH syndrome, rash.

VIII. Contraindications.

A. Persons who have shown hypersensitivity to theophylline or any capsule components.

B. Pregnant patients.

C. Nursing mothers.

D. Use in children under age 6.

IX. Precautions.

A. Most patients are able to obtain a safe therapeutic result with Theo-Dur when serum levels are maintained between 10 and 20 g/ml, particularly during initiation of therapy. It is important that each dosage be individually planned and that serum levels be titrated and monitored. *Serum sample should be measured at the time of peak absorption and repeated often (5–10 hours after dosing).*

B. When it is not possible to obtain serum levels, very low doses of Theo-Dur should be given.

C. Any medication-food mixture should be used immediately and not saved or stored for further use.

D. Subdividing the contents of a capsule is not recommended.

E. Capsule contents should not be crushed or chewed.

F. Children weighing less than 25 kg should be maintained on a liquid preparation to allow for small dosage increments.

G. Safety and effectiveness in children under the age of 6 years have not been established.

H. Do not try to maintain any dose of Theo-Dur that is not tolerated.

I. Theo-Dur must be used cautiously in patients with cardiac disease, hypertension, congestive heart disease, alcoholism, and liver disease, and in the elderly.

X. **Education.** Keep all medications out of children's reach.

A. Drug interactions

1. Lithium carbonate; increased excretion of lithium carbonate.
2. Propranolol: increased theophylline serum level is associated with antagonism of propranolol.
3. Troleandomycin or erythromycin: increased theophylline level.

B. Overdose

1. Immediately call physician.
2. If no seizure occurs
   a. Induce vomiting.
   b. Administer a cathartic.
   c. Activated charcoal may be suggested.
   d. Monitor vital signs, maintain blood pressure, and provide adequate hydration.
3. If seizure occurs
   a. Establish an airway.
   b. Administer oxygen.
   c. Monitor vital signs.
   d. Await instruction remedications to be administered.

TINACTIN (ANTIFUNGAL)

I. **Generic name.** Tolnaftate.

II. **Composition**

A. Cream 1%—10 mg/gm.

B. Solution 1%—Each 1 ml contains tolnaftate 10 mg and butylated hydroxytoluene 1 mg.

C. Powder 1%—10 mg/gm.

III. **How supplied.** (Schering)

A. Cream—15-gm tubes.

B. Solution—10-ml bottles.

C. Powder—45-gm containers.

IV. **Route.** Topical.

V. **Dosage and administration.** Wash and dry infected area bid, then apply.

A. Cream—Rub 1/2-inch ribbon of cream gently on infected area.

B. Solution—Massage 2–3 drops gently to cover infected area.

C. Powder—Sprinkle powder liberally on all infected areas and in shoes and socks.

VI. **Action.** The active ingredient in Tinactin is a highly active synthetic fungicidal agent that is effective in the treatment of superficial fungus infections of the skin. It is inactive systemically, is virtually nonsensitizing, and does not ordinarily sting or irritate intact or broken skin, even in the presence of acute inflammatory reactions.

VII. **Uses.** Effective in treating superficial fungus infections of the skin that cause tinea pedis (athlete's foot), tinea cruris (jock itch), and tinea corporis (body ringworm).

VIII. **Side effects.** None.

IX. **Precautions.**

A. If burning or itching does not improve within 10 days or becomes worse or if irritation occurs, discontinue use and consult physician.

B. Tinactin products are for external use only. Keep out of eyes.

C. Cream and solution are not recommended for nail or scalp infections.

D. Powder is not recommended for use on scalp.

X. **Education.**

A. Keep all medications out of children's reach.

B. These products are odorless and greaseless and do not stain or discolor the skin, hair, or nails.

C. All forms begin to relieve burning, itching, and soreness within 24 hours. Symptoms are usually cleared in 2–3 weeks.

D. Where skin is thickened, treatment may take 4–6 weeks.

E. To help prevent recurrence, continue treatment for 2 weeks after disappearance of all symptoms.

F. Do not use in children under age 2.

G. If overdose call physician immediately.

H. Children under age l2 should be supervised in the use of Tinactin.

I. Store product between 36° and 86°F.

TOFRANIL (ANTIDEPRESSANT)

I. **Generic name.** Imipramine hydrochloride.

II. **Composition.** 10-mg, 25-mg, and 50-mg tablets.

III. **How supplied.** (Geigy Pharmaceuticals) Bottles of 100, 1,000, and 5,000.

IV. **Route.** PO.

V. **Dosage.** 25–50 mg given 1 hour before bedtime. Dose should not exceed 2.5 mg/kg/day.

A. Children age 6 and over. Start medication at 25 mg for 1 week. If no response, increase dosage to 50 mg nightly.

B. Children over 12 years. Up to 75 mg.

C. After 3 months decrease medication, slowly withdrawing over a 3-month period.

D. If child has a breakthrough, maintain 50-mg level for a full 6 months.

VI. **Action.** Unknown.

VII. **Uses.** Used for nocturnal enuresis in children age 6 years and over; given only after appropriate tests have ruled out any possible organic disease.

VIII. **Side effects.** Nervousness, sleep disorders, mild GI symptoms, constipation, anxiety, emotional outbursts, skin rash, petechiae, urticaria, itching, dry mouth, black tongue, jaundice.

IX. **Contraindications.** Hyperthyroid patients and patients with a history of urinary retention, seizure disorder, glaucoma, or cardiovascular disease.

X. **Education.**

A. Imipramine requires some time before it has full therapeutic effect.

B. Lower doses recommended in adolescents.

C. Store tablets in a tightly closed container.

D. Return to office for follow-up at 1-month intervals.

E. Blood and urine levels of imipramine may not correlate with the degree of intoxication and are not dependable indicators in clinical management.

F. Do not use with alcohol.

G. Medication may impair mental or physical abilities required to operate a car, farm machinery.

H. Safety for use in children other than nocturnal enuresis is not established.

I. Write prescription for lowest amount possible.

J. Prior to elective surgery, discontinue medication for as long as possible.

K. Do not use with decongestants or local anesthetics.

L. High exposure to sunlight may cause photosensitization on Tofranil.

M. Both elevation and lowering of blood sugar can happen on Tofranil. Call office immediately if overdose occurs and call Poison Control regarding treatment.

TUSSI-ORGANIDIN DM

I. **Composition.** Each 5 ml contains Organidin (iodinated glycerol) 30 mg (15 mg organically bound iodine) and dextromethorphan hydrobromide.

II. **How supplied.** Liquid in 1-pt bottle or 1-gallon bottle.

III. **Route.** PO.

IV. **Dosage.**

A. Children—1/2 to 1 tsp q4h

B. Adults—1–2 tsp q4h

V. **Action.** Antitussive and expectorant formula for the common cold and upper respiratory conditions.

VI. **Contraindications.**

A. An individual with a marked sensitivity to iodides or other ingredients.

B. Not recommended for newborns, during pregnancy, or for nursing mothers.

C. If pregnant, discontinue medication and inform regarding risk to the fetus.

D. Any person with a history of thyroid disease.

VII. **Precautions.**

A. Children with cystic fibrosis appear to experience exaggerated susceptibility to the goitrogenic effect of iodides.

B. Iodides may cause flare up of adolescent acne.

C. Iodide may increase the hypothyroid effect of lithium and other antithyroid drugs.

VIII. **Side effects.** Little or none.

IX. **Education.**

A. Keep all medications out of the reach of children.
B. Store at controlled room temperature (do not freeze or expose to heat).
C. Keep bottle tightly closed.
D. Discontinue use if rash appears and call the office immediately.
E. Do not use over prolonged period of time.
F. Do not exceed recommended dose.
G. If cough worsens, fever ensues or cold symptoms do not improve in a few days, discontinue use and call the office.

TYLENOL–CHILDREN'S (ANALGESIC)

I. **Generic name.** Acetaminophen.

II. **Composition.**

A. Tablets—80 mg.
B. Elixir—160 mg/5 ml and 7% alcohol.
C. Drops— 80 mg/0.8 ml and 7% alcohol.
D. Junior strength chewable tablets—160 mg acetaminophen.

III. **How supplied.** (McNeil)

A. Tablets—Bottles of 30 (fruit flavored).
B. Elixir—2-fl oz and 4-fl oz bottles (cherry flavored).
C. Drops— 1/2-oz (15-ml) bottles (fruit flavored).
D. Junior strength chewable tablets. Package of 24 in blister packaging.

IV. **Route.** PO.

V. **Contraindications.** Anyone with sensitivity to acetaminophen.

VI. **Uses.** Anagelsic-antipuretic, for reduction of fever and discomfort of colds and teething.

VII. **Dosage.** Administer the following tid–qid, but not more than 5 doses in 24 hours.

Age	Weight	Drops (Dropperful)	Elixir	Tablets	Jr. Tab
0–3 mos	6–11 lbs	0.4 ml	—	—	—
4–11 mos	12–17 lbs	0.8 ml	1/2 tsp	—	—
12–23 mos	18–23 lbs	1.2 ml	3/4 tsp	1 1/2	—
2–3 yrs	24–35 lbs	1.6 ml	1 tsp	2	—
4–5 yrs	36–47 lbs	2.4 ml	1 1/2 tsp	3	—
6–8 yrs	48–59 lbs	4	2 tsp	4	2 tabs
9–10 yrs	60–71 lbs	5	2 1/2 tsp	5	2 1/2 tabs
11–12 yrs	72–75 lbs	—	3 tsp	6	3 tabs

VIII. **Education.**

A. Keep all medications out of children's reach.
B. Consult provider if administered to child under 2 years of age.
C. Do not use longer than 10 days.

D. Do not exceed recommended daily dosage.

E. Call office immediately if overdose occurs.

F. Call medical provider if fever persists more than 3 days or pain persists.

G. Do not use if carton, cap, overwrap or if printed bottle wrap is broken or missing.

H. All packages have child resistant safety caps.

VENTOLIN INHALER (AEROSOL BRONCHODILATOR)

I. **Generic name.** Albuterol (international generic name is salbutamol).

II. **Composition.** a[1][(tert-butylamino) methyl]-4-hydroxy-m-a, a[1]-diol); 90 µg/actuation.

III. **How supplied.** (Glaxo) Metered dose aerosol unit; 17-gm canister.

IV. **Route.** PO inhalation aerosol.

V. **Dosage and administration.** Two inhalations of albuterol taken approximately 15–20 minutes before exercise; may be repeated once every 4–6 hours. More frequent doses or larger number of inhalants are not recommended. Some patients find one inhalation sufficient to control bronchospasm.

VI. **Uses.** For relief of bronchospasm in teenagers or adults who have reversible obstructive airway disease and for prevention of exercise-induced bronchospasm.

VII. **Side effects.** Heart palpitations, tachycardia, increased blood pressure, tremor, nausea, vomiting, vertigo, insomnia, unusual drying of the mouth; occasionally rash, urticaria, bronchospasm, or oropharyngeal edema may occur.

VIII. **Contraindications.**

A. Patients who show a hypersensitivity to the ingredients.

B. Children under the age of 12.

C. Nursing mothers.

D. During pregnancy, labor, or delivery.

IX. **Precautions.**

A. Use of albuterol inhaler in pregnancy may affect development of the fetus.

B. Inhalant should be used with caution in patients with a history of diabetes mellitus, hyperthyroidism, cardiovascular disorder, and hypertension.

C. Safe and effective use in children under the age of 12 is not established.

D. Albuterol should be administered with caution to patients being treated with monoamine oxidase inhibitors or tricyclic antidepressants.

X. **Education**

A. Use of adrenergic aerosols is sometimes associated with paradoxical bronchospasm; if this should occur, discontinue the medication immediately.

B. Death may result from overuse of the inhalant; strict adherence to dosage and frequency must be followed to ensure its safety.

C. Do not use other aerosol bronchodilators or epinephrine with this inhalant.

D. The Ventolin Inhaler can be useful for the treatment of recurrent bouts of bronchospasm; when it is used judiciously, it is safe over a period of years.

E. If the recommended dosage of the albuterol inhalant does not work effectively, discontinue use and call or see physician or nurse practitioner immediately.

F. Overdose is indicated by intense anginal pain and hypertension.

G. Store at 59°–86°F.

H. Therapeutic effect of medication may increase when canister is cold *Shake well* before using.

VENTOLIN SYRUP (BRONCHODILATOR)

I. **Composition.** Albuterol sulfate 2 mg/5 ml; other ingredients include citric acid monohydrate, FD&C yellow No. 6, saccharin sodium, sodium benzoate, and sodium citrate.

II. **How supplied.** (Glaxo) 16-fl oz bottles (strawberry flavored).

III. **Route.** PO.

IV. **Dosage.**

A. 2–6 years—0.1 mg/kg of body weight tid (not to exceed 1 tsp tid).

B. 6–14 years—1 tsp tid–qid.

C. Over 14 years—1–2 tsp tid–qid (not to exceed 8 mg qid).

V. **Uses.** For relief of bronchospasm in children 2 years of age or more with reversible obstructive airway disease.

VI. **Contraindications.**

A. Patients with a history of sensitivity to any components.

B. Patients who have cardiovascular disease, hypertension, hyperthyroidism, or diabetes mellitus.

VII. **Precautions.**

A. Use with extreme caution in patients being treated with monoamine oxidase inhibitors.

B. This agent has an inhibited effect when used with beta-receptors and blocking agents.

VIII. **Education.**

A. Keep medication out of children's reach.

B. Albuterol is longer acting than isoproterenol; it may last up to 6 hours.

C. Do not increase dose or frequency of medication without medical consultation.

D. The most common adverse reaction to the medication is tremor; other side effects include headache, dizziness, sleeplessness, epistaxis, tachycardia, dilated pupils, irritable behavior, sweating, chest pain, and weakness. If any of these symptoms occur, discontinue the medication and call the nurse practitioner or physician; it may be necessary to decrease the dosage.

E. Increased fluid intake will diminish dry mouth effect.

F. Keep medication in cool environment.

VERMOX CHEWABLE TABLETS (ANTHELMINTIC)

I. **Generic name.** Mebendazole.

II. **Composition.** 100 mg.

III. **How supplied.** (Janssen) Boxes of 12 tablets.

IV. **Route.** PO.

V. **Dosage.** Adults and children over 2 years of age:

- **A.** Pinworm. 1 tablet once.
- **B.** Roundworm, whipworm, hookworm. 1 tablet bid for 3 consecutive days.

VI. **Action.** Vermox blocks glucose uptake by the susceptible helminths, thereby depleting the energy level until it is inadequate for survival.

VII. **Uses.**

- **A.** For the treatment of:
  1. *Trichuris trichiura* (whipworm).
  2. *Enterobius vermicularis* (pinworm).
  3. *Ascaris lumbricoides* (roundworm).
  4. *Necator americanus* (American hookworm).
  5. *Ancylostoma duodenale* (common hookworm).
- **B.** In single or mixed infections, efficacy varies.

VIII. **Side effects.** Transient symptoms of abdominal pain and diarrhea in cases of massive infection.

IX. **Contraindications.**

- **A.** Pregnant patients; may produce fetal damage.
- **B.** Patients with hypersensitivity to the drug.

X. **Precautions.** Consider the benefits and risks if administering to a child less than 2 years of age. (Do not treat children under age 2 without physician's consent.)

XI. **Education.**

- **A.** Keep all medication out of children's reach.
- **B.** Tablets may be chewed, swallowed, or crushed.
- **C.** If patient is not cured 3 weeks after treatment, a second course of treatment is advised.
- **D.** Discuss contagiousness/hygiene and how disease is transmitted or reinfected.
- **E.** In case of overdose call Poison Control Center immediately.
- **F.** Same dosage for adults and children.
- **G.** Often all family members are treated at the same time.

VI-DAYLIN/F (MULTIVITAMINS/FLUORIDE)

I. **Composition.** 1 dropperful (1 ml) contains:

Fluoride	0.25 mg
Vitamin A	1500 IU
Vitamin D	400 IU
Vitamin E	5 IU
Vitamin C	35 mg
Thiamine (vitamin B_1)	0.5 mg
Riboflavin (vitamin B_2)	0.6 mg
Niacin	8 mg
Vitamin B_6	0.4 mg
Alcohol	< 0.1%

II. How supplied. (Ross Laboratories)

A. Liquid route—50-ml bottles.

B. Tablets—bottle of 100.

III. Route. PO.

IV. Dosage. One dropperful qd or chewable tablet.

A. 0–1 year—Vitamin with fluoride, 0.25 mg, 1 dropperful.

B. 1–3 years—Fluoride, 0.25 mg, 1 dropperful.

C. 3–5 years—Fluoride, 0.50 mg, 1/2 chewable tablet.

D. 5–12 years—Fluoride, 1 mg, 1 chewable tablet.

E. Iron added as necessary at 4 months.

V. Action and uses. As aid in the prophylaxis of appropriate vitamin deficiencies as well as in the prevention of dental caries.

VI. Contraindications. When fluoride contact in drinking water is known to be 0.7 parts per million or less.

VI. Precautions

A. Do not exceed daily recommended dose, since excessive amounts of fluoride cause mottling of tooth enamel and osseous changes.

B. Acute ingestion of 10–20 mg of sodium fluoride may cause excessive salivation and GI disturbances; 500 mg may be fatal.

VII. Education

A. Keep all medicine out of children's reach.

B. Overdose—call Poison Control Center. In children acute ingestion of 10–20 mg of sodium fluoride may cause excessive salivation and GI disturbances; 500 mg may be fatal.

REFERENCES

Govaini, L.E. and Hayes, D.E. *Drugs and Nursing Implications.* Appleton-Century-Crafts.

Mandell-Douglas-Bennett. *Handbook of Antimicrobial Therapy 1992.* McNeil Pharmacology.

Nelson, John D. *1991–1992 Pocketbook of Pediatric Antimicrobial Therapy* (9th ed.). Williams & Wilkins Pub.

Physicians Desk Reference 1993 (46th ed.) Oradell, NJ: Medical Economics.

Appendices

APPENDIX A: CONVERSION TABLES

TEMPERATURE

°Fahrenheit	°Centigrade
0	-17.8
32.0	0
97.0	36.1
98.0	36.7
98.6	37. 0
99.0	37.2
99.5	37.5
100.0	37.7
100.4	38.0
101.0	38.3
102.0	38.8
103.0	39. 4
104.0	40. 0
105.0	40.5

Conversion for above 0°C
°F to °C: subtract 32, multiply by 5, divide by 9 or 5/9 (°F - 32).
°C to °F: multiply by 9, divide by 5, add 32 or (% x °C) + 32.

LENGTH

Inches	Centimeters	Centimeters	Inches
1	2.5	1	0.4
2	5.1	2	0.8
4	10.2	3	1.2
6	15.2	4	1.6
8	20.3	5	2.0
10	25.0	6	2.4
12	30.5	8	3.1
18	46.0	10	3.9
24	61.0	15	5.9
30	76.0	20	7.9
36	91.0	30	11.8
42	107.0	40	15.7
48	122.0	50	19.7
54	137.0	60	23.6
60	152.0	70	27.6
66	168.0	80	31.5
72	183.0	90	35. 4
78	198.0	100	39.4

1 inch = 2.54 cm
1 cm = 0.3937 inch

WEIGHT

Pounds	*Kilograms*	*Kilograms*	*Pounds*
4	1.8	1	2.2
6	2.7	2	4.4
8	3.6	3	6.6
10	4.5	4	8.8
15	6.8	5	11.0
20	9.1	6	13.2
25	11.4	8	17.6
30	13.6	10	22
35	15.9	15	33
40	18.2	20	44
45	20.4	25	55
50	22.7	30	66
55	25.0	35	77
60	27.3	40	88
65	29.5	45	99
70	31.8	50	110
80	36.3	55	121
90	40.9	60	132
100	45.4	65	143
125	56.7	70	154
150	68.2	80	176
175	79.4	90	198
200	90.8	100	220

1 lb = 0.454 kg.
1 kg = 2.204 lb.

APPENDIX B: GROWTH CHARTS

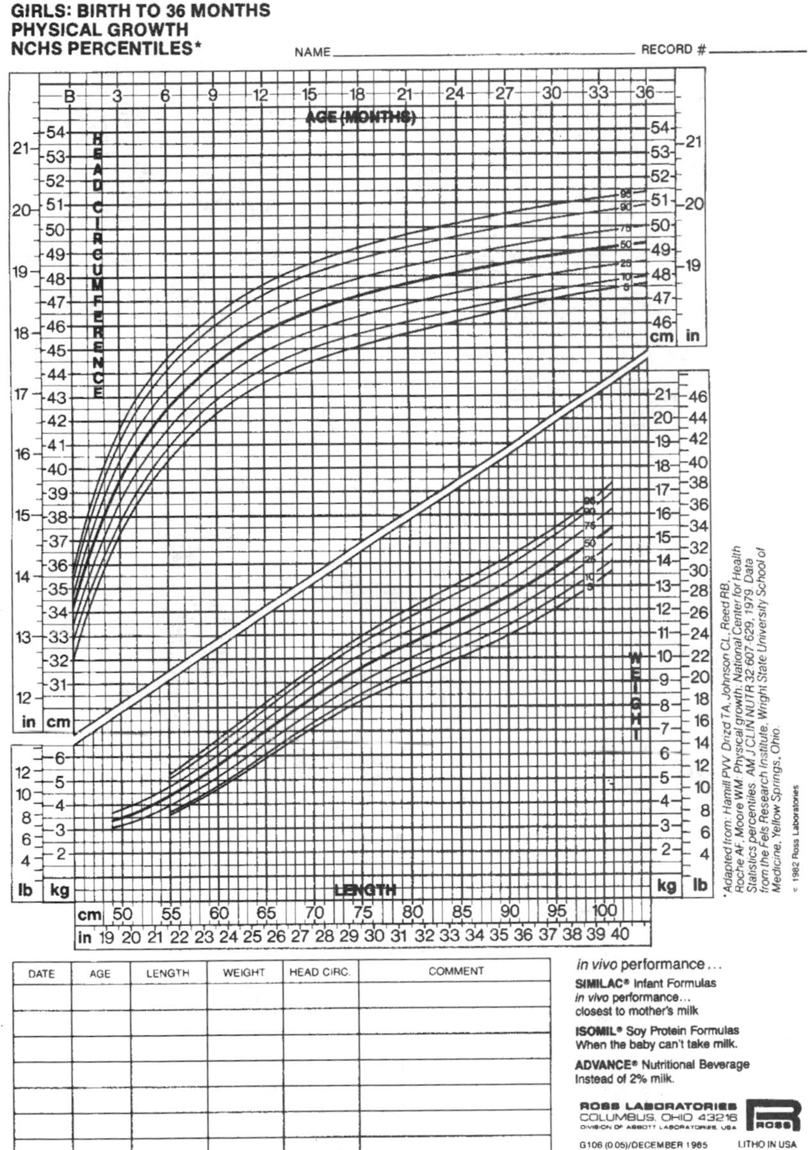

Source: Ross Laboratories, Columbus, Ohio, 43216. Adapted from Hamill PVV, Drizd TA, Johnson CL, Reed RB, Roche AF, Moore WM: Physical growth: National Center for Health Statistics percentiles. *AM. J. CLIN. NUTR.* 32:607–629, 1979. Data from the Fels Longitudinal Study, Wright State University School of Medicine, Yellow Springs, Ohio. © 1982 Ross Laboratories. Reprinted with permission.

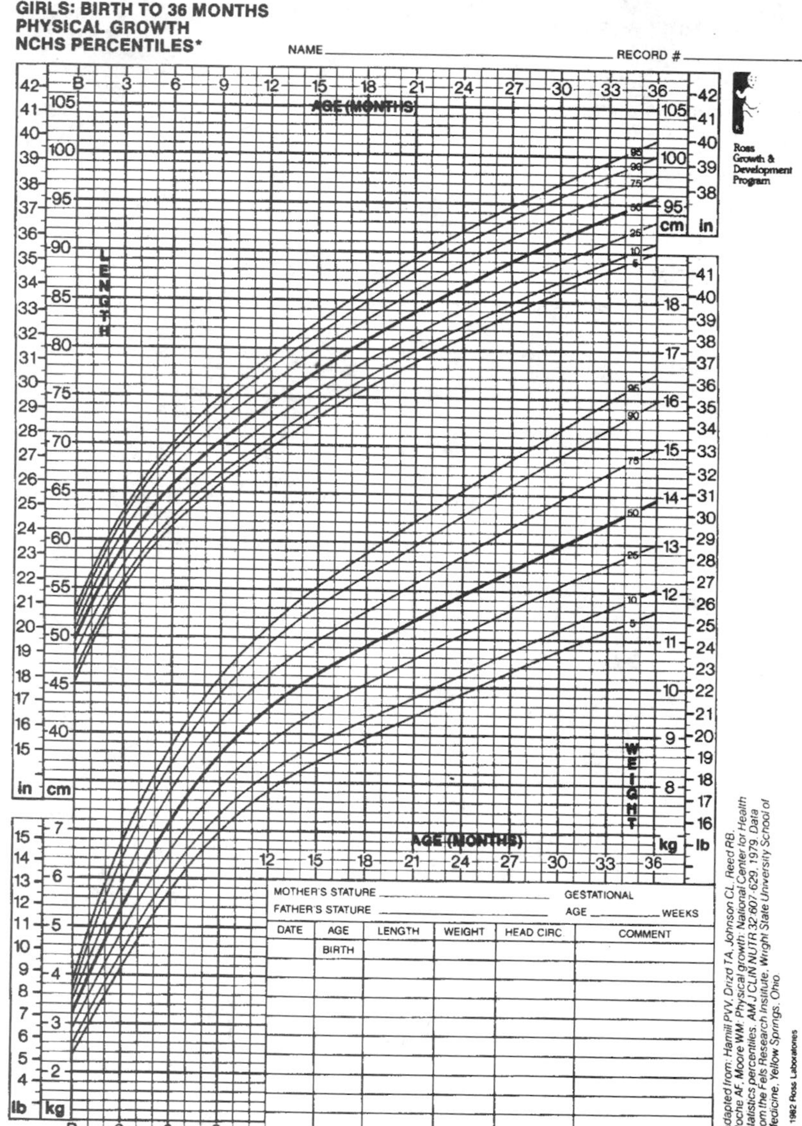

Source: Ross Laboratories, Columbus, Ohio, 43216. Adapted from Hamill PVV, Drizd TA, Johnson CL, Reed RB, Roche AF, Moore WM: Physical growth: National Center for Health Statistics percentiles. *AM. J. CLIN. NUTR.* 32:607–629, 1979. Data from the Fels Longitudinal Study, Wright State University School of Medicine, Yellow Springs, Ohio. © 1982 Ross Laboratories. Reprinted with permission.

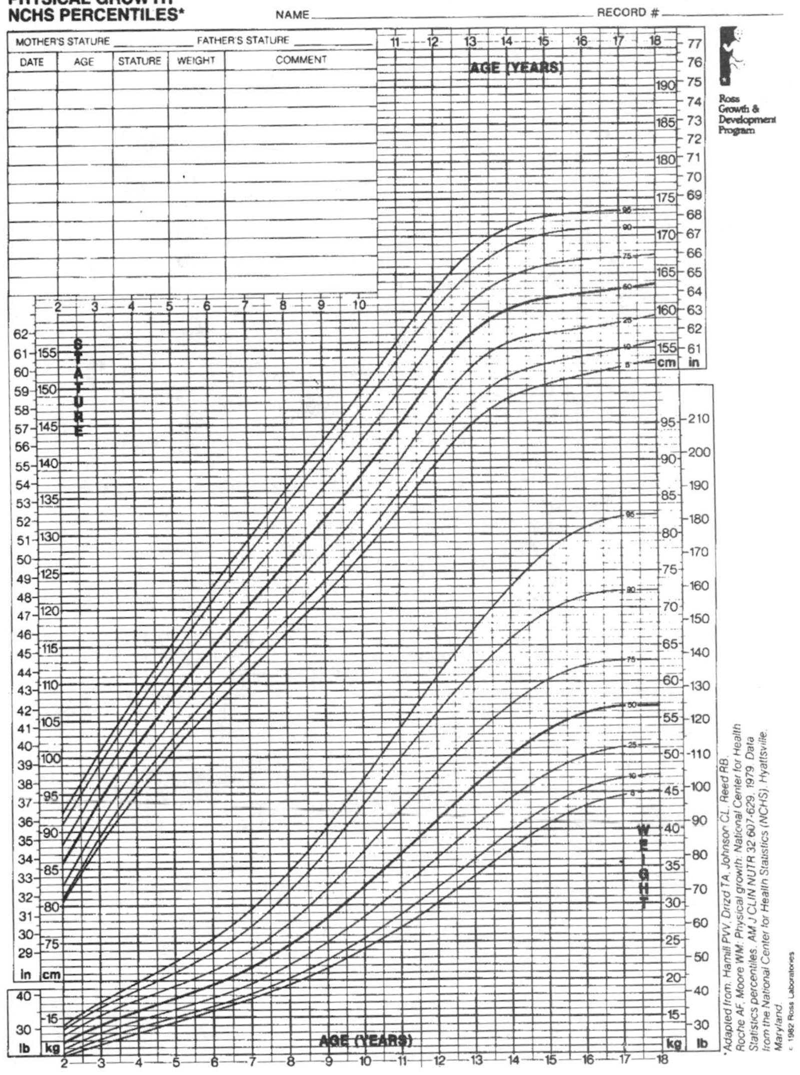

Source: Ross Laboratories, Columbus, Ohio, 43216. Adapted from Hamill PVV, Drizd TA, Johnson CL, Reed RB, Roche AF, Moore WM: Physical growth: National Center for Health Statistics percentiles. *AM. J. CLIN. NUTR.* 32:607–629, 1979. Data from the National Center for Health Statistics (NCHS), Hyattsville, Maryland. © 1982 Ross Laboratories. Reprinted with permission.

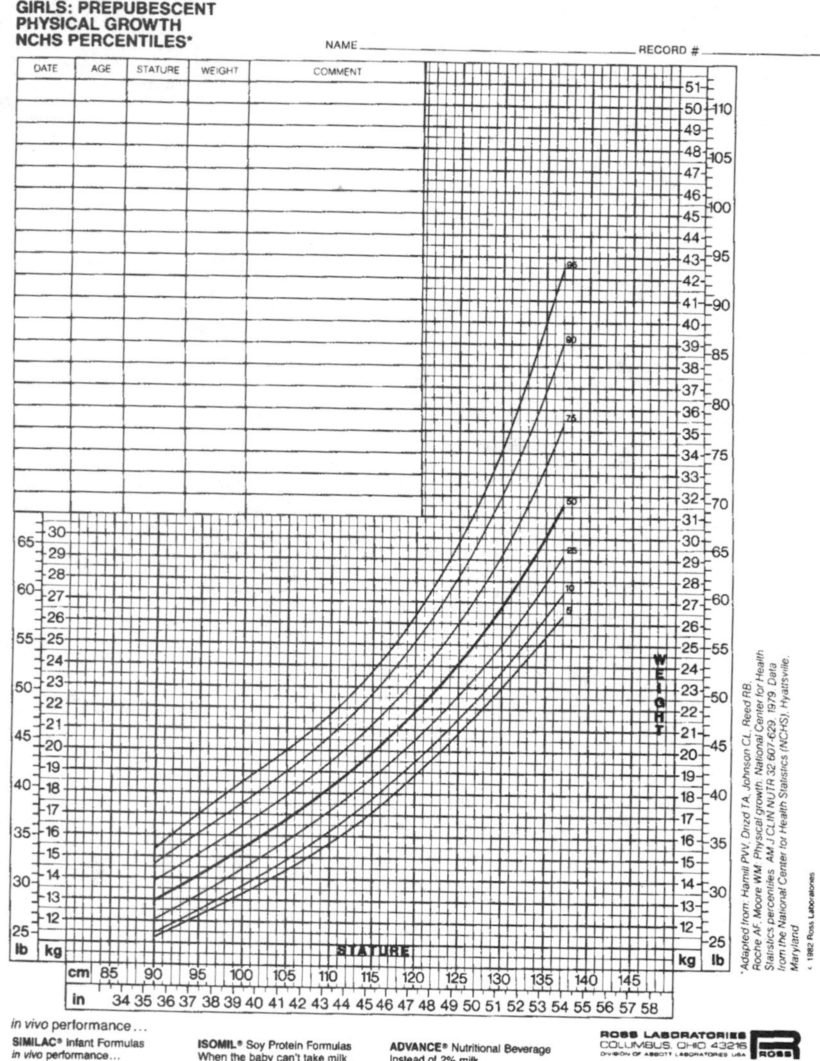

Source: Ross Laboratories, Columbus, Ohio, 43216. Adapted from Hamill PVV, Drizd TA, Johnson CL, Reed RB, Roche AF, Moore WM: Physical growth: National Center for Health Statistics percentiles. *AM. J. CLIN. NUTR.* 32:607–629, 1979. Data from the National Center for Health Statistics (NCHS), Hyattsville, Maryland. © 1982 Ross Laboratories. Reprinted with permission.

BOYS: BIRTH TO 36 MONTHS PHYSICAL GROWTH NCHS PERCENTILES*

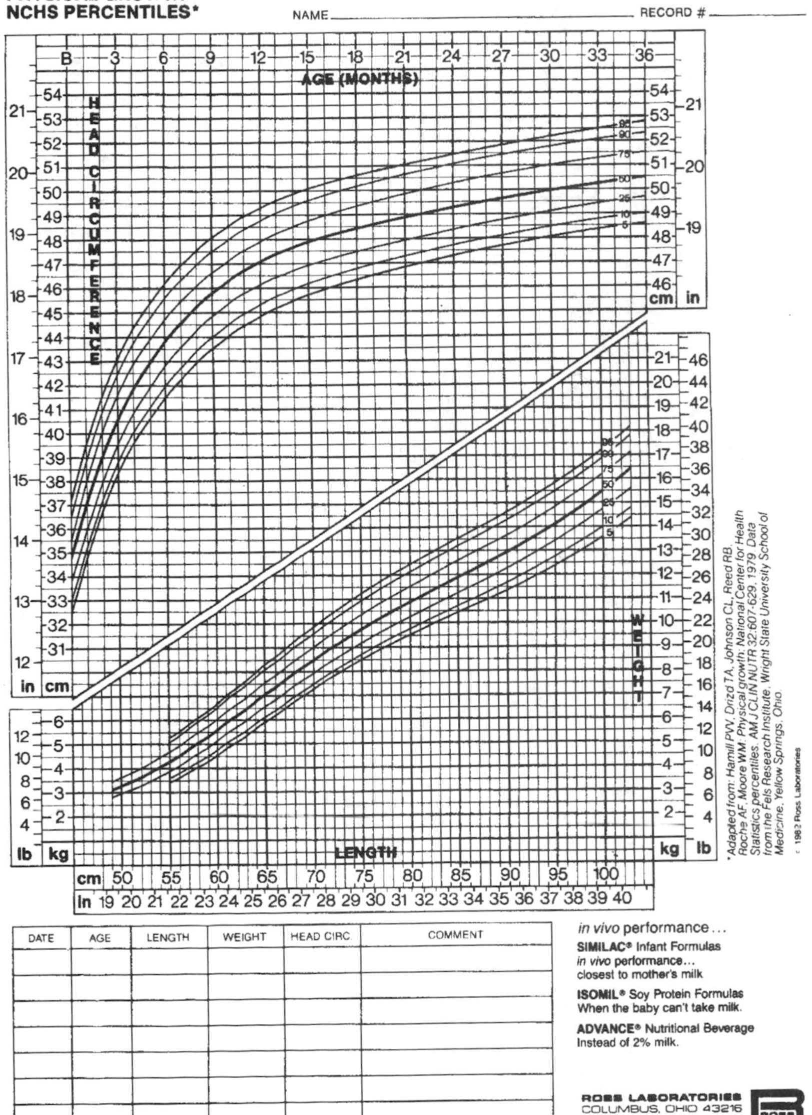

DATE	AGE	LENGTH	WEIGHT	HEAD CIRC.	COMMENT

Source: Ross Laboratories, Columbus, Ohio, 43216. Adapted from Hamill PVV, Drizd TA, Johnson CL, Reed RB, Roche AF, Moore WM: Physical growth: National Center for Health Statistics percentiles. *AM. J. CLIN. NUTR.* 32:607–629, 1979. Data from the Fels Longitudinal Study, Wright State University School of Medicine, Yellow Springs, Ohio.

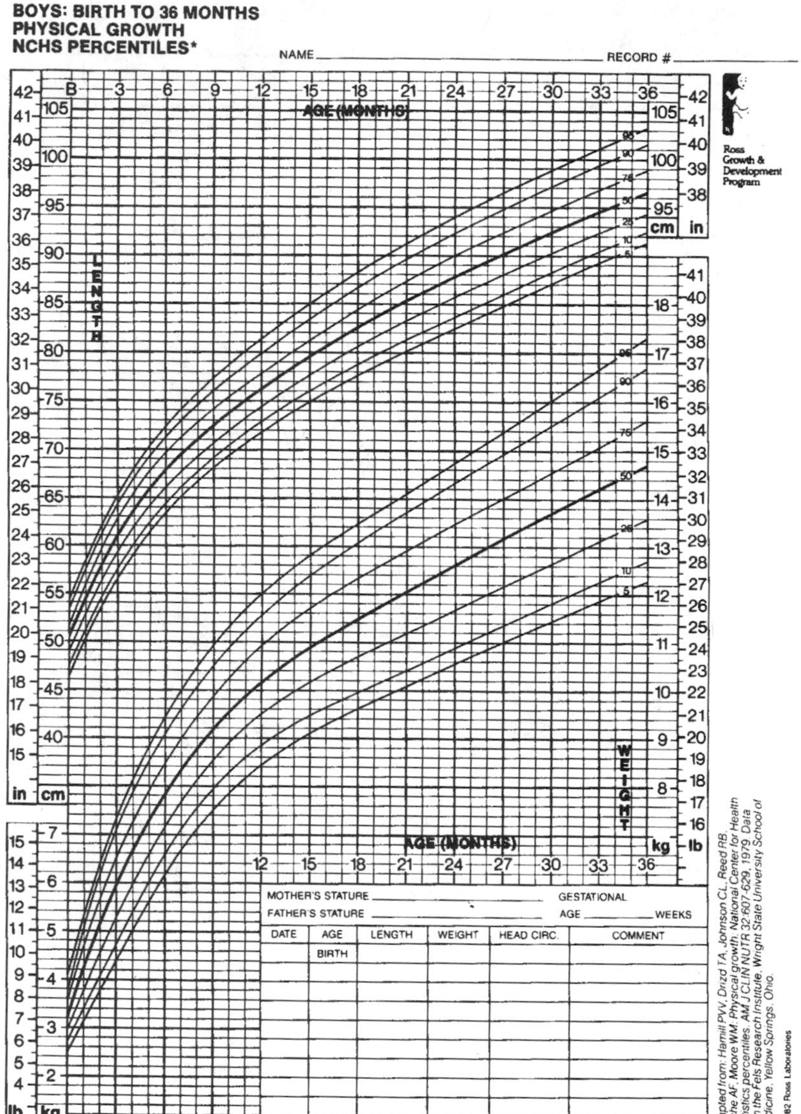

Source: Ross Laboratories, Columbus, Ohio, 43216. Adapted from Hamill PVV, Drizd TA, Johnson CL, Reed RB, Roche AF, Moore WM: Physical growth: National Center for Health Statistics percentiles. *AM. J. CLIN. NUTR.* 32:607–629, 1979. Data from the Fels Longitudinal Study, Wright State University School of Medicine, Yellow Springs, Ohio. © 1982 Ross Laboratories. Reprinted with permission.

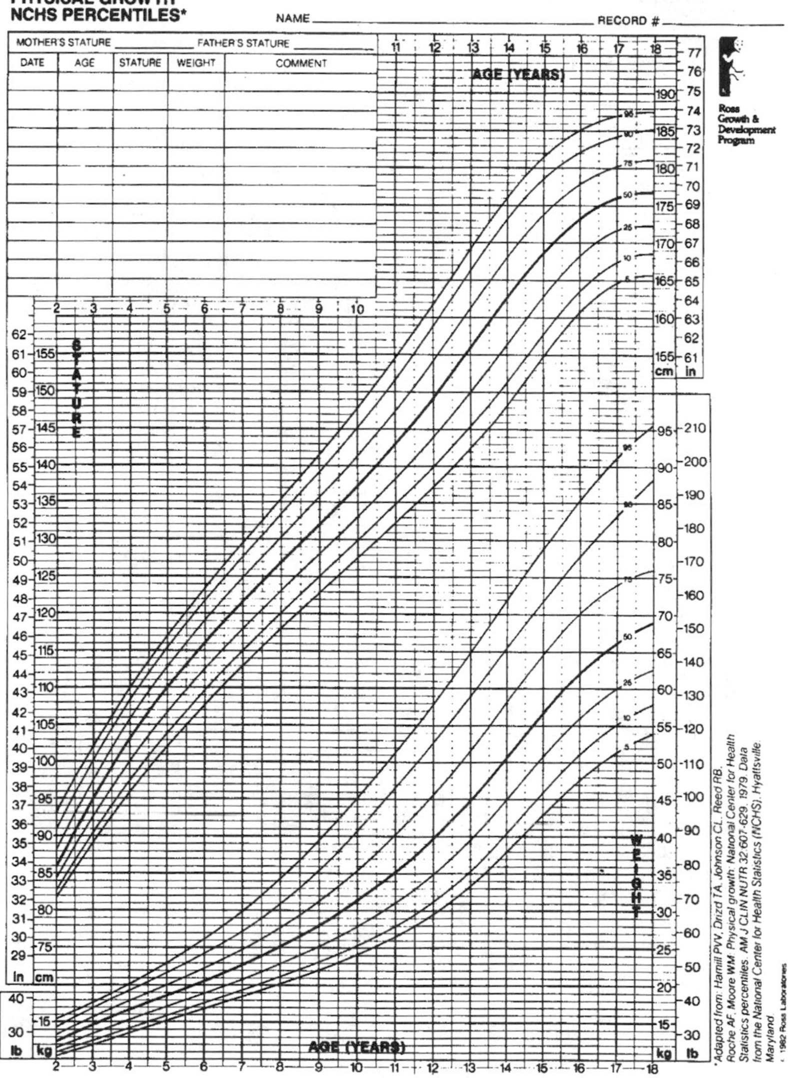

Source: Ross Laboratories, Columbus, Ohio, 43216. Adapted from Hamill PVV, Drizd TA, Johnson CL, Reed RB, Roche AF, Moore WM: Physical growth: National Center for Health Statistics percentiles. *AM. J. CLIN. NUTR.* 32:607–629, 1979. Data from the National Center for Health Statistics (NCHS), Hyattsville, Maryland. © 1982 Ross Laboratories. Reprinted with permission.

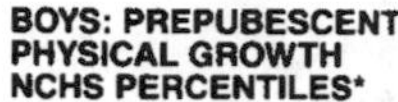

BOYS: PREPUBESCENT PHYSICAL GROWTH NCHS PERCENTILES*

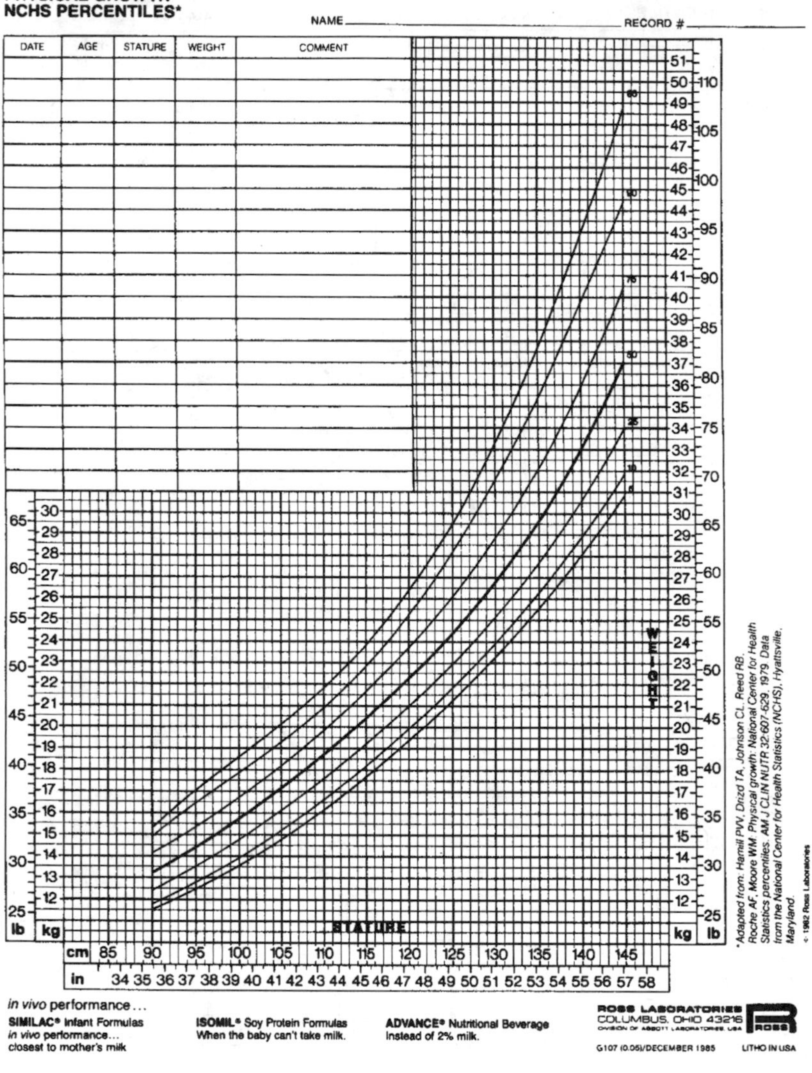

NAME ______________________ RECORD # __________

DATE	AGE	STATURE	WEIGHT	COMMENT

WEIGHT

STATURE

cm 85 90 95 100 105 110 115 120 125 130 135 140 145

in 34 35 36 37 38 39 40 41 42 43 44 45 46 47 48 49 50 51 52 53 54 55 56 57 58

kg 12 13 14 15 16 17 18 19 20 21 22 23 24 25 26 27 28 29 30 31 32 33 34 35 36 37 38 39 40 41 42 43 44 45 46 47 48 49 50 51

lb 25 30 35 40 45 50 55 60 65 70 75 80 85 90 95 100 105 110

*Adapted from: Hamill PVV, Drizd TA, Johnson CL, Reed RB, Roche AF, Moore WM: Physical growth: National Center for Health Statistics percentiles. AM J CLIN NUTR 32:607-629, 1979. Data from the National Center for Health Statistics (NCHS), Hyattsville, Maryland.

Source: Ross Laboratories, Columbus, Ohio, 43216. Adapted from Hamill PVV, Drizd TA, Johnson CL, Reed RB, Roche AF, Moore WM: Physical growth: National Center for Health Statistics percentiles. *AM. J. CLIN. NUTR.* 32:607–629, 1979. Data from the National Center for Health Statistics (NCHS), Hyattsville, Maryland. © 1982 Ross Laboratories. Reprinted with permission.

APPENDIX C: RECOMMENDED SCHEDULE FOR IMMUNIZATION OF NORMAL INFANTS AND CHILDREN

	Birth	*1–2 mos*	*2 mos*	*4 mos*	*6 mos*	*6–18 mos*	*15 mos*	*4–6 yrs*	*14–16 yrs*
Hep. B[1]	1st dose	2nd dose				3rd dose			
DTP[2]			1st dose	2nd dose	3rd dose		4th dose	5th dose	
Polio[3]			1st dose	2nd dose			3rd dose	4th dose	
Hib[4]			1st dose	2nd dose	3rd dose		4th dose		
MMR[5]							1st dose	2nd dose at 7th grade	
Td[2]									1st dose

Vaccine Administration Notes

[1] **Hepatitis B:** Recommended for all children born after January 1, 1992 and required for day care attendence for children in this age group. Schedule may vary depending on hepatitis B status of mother.

[2] **DTP-DT-Td:** Fourth dose of DTP can be given at 18 months. Half doses are not acceptable. DT is only acceptable when accompanied by a letter stating there is a medical contraindication to DTP. First Td needed 10 years after last DTP and every 10 years thereafter.

[3] **Polio:** Third dose of polio can be given at 18 months. Fourth dose should be administered by entry into kindergarten (4–6 years).

[4] **Hib:** Number of doses required varies depending on age child starts immunization. Doses 3 and 4 should be given according to manufacturer's guidelines.

[5] **MMR:** Although first dose is recommended at 15 months, requirement will be met if given on or after first birthday. Second dose is required at entry to 7th grade only and must be given at least 30 days after the first dose.

(CHILDREN WHO ARE BEHIND SCHEDULE OR MISSED VACCINE, SEE NEXT PAGE)

Massachusetts Department ol Public Health—Revised July 1992

For all products used, consult manufacturer's package insert for instructions for storage, handling, and administration.

(Cont'd)

RECOMMENDED IMMUNIZATION SCHEDULE FOR CHILDREN STARTING LATE (< 7 YEARS OLD)

Age at start of vaccination	*Vaccine given at 1st visit*	*Timing and Vaccines for Later Visits*				
		1 mo after 1st visit	*2 mos after 1st visit*	*4 mos after 1st visit*	*6–12 mos after previous dose*	*Preschool (4–6 yrs)*
2–6 mos	DTP		DTP	DTP	DTP	DTP
	Polio		Polio		Polio	Polio
	Hib[2]		Hib[2]	Hib[2]	Hib booster at ≥15 mos[2]	
	Hep B[1]	Hep B[1]		Hep B[1]		
					MMR at age 15 mos[4]	
7–11 mos	DTP		DTP	DTP	DTP	DTP
	Polio		Polio		Polio	Polio
	Hib[2]		Hib[2]	Hib booster at age ≥ 15 mos[2]		
	Hep B[1]	Hep B[1]		Hep B[1]		
				MMR at age 15 mos[4]		
12–14 mos	DTP		DTP	DTP	DTP	DTP
	Polio		Polio		Polio	Polio
	Hib[2]		Hib[2]			
	Hep B[1]	Hep B[1]		Hep B[1]		
		MMR at age 15 mos[4]				
15–59 mos	DTP		DTP	DTP	DTP	DTP[3]
	Polio		Polio		Polio	Polio[3]
	Hib[2]					
	Hep B[1]	Hep B[1]		Hep B[1]		
	MMR[4]					
5–6 yrs	DTP		DTP	DTP	DTP	
	Polio		Polio		Polio	
	MMR	Second dose of MMR due at entry to 7th grade[4]				
	(Hib vaccine is not routinely recommended for children 5 years [60 ms or older])					

RECOMMENDED SCHEDULE FOR CHILDREN STARTING AT AGE 7 OR OLDER

Vaccine	*First visit*	*2 months after 1st visit*	*8–14 months after 1st vislt*	*At entry to 7th grade*	*High school and every 10 ysr thereafter*
Td	First dose	Second dose	Third dose		Additional doses
Polio	F'irst dose	Second dose	Third dose		
MMR[4]	First dose			Second dose	

Vaccine Administration Notes

[1]Hepatitis B vaccine recommended for children born on or after January 1, 1992.

[2]Hib schedule varies depending on when child starts vaccination.

[3]Fifth dose of DTP and fourth dose of polio are not needed if previous doses were given after fourth birthday.

[4]Second dose of MMR must be given at least 30 days after first dose and is required for entry to 7th grade.

APPENDIX D: CLINICAL SIGNS OF DEHYDRATION

Sign	*Mild*	*Moderate*	*Severe*
Weight loss (% of body weight)	3–5%	6–9%	10–15%
Fontanelle	Flat		Sunken
Fever (in absence of infection)	Variable	Present	Present
Skin			
Turgor	Normal	↓	Tenting
Color	Normal	Pallor	Pallor
Mucous membranes	Slightly moist	Dry	Parched
Tears	Present	Variable	Absent
Thirst	Slight	Moderate to marked	Marked
Pulse	May be normal	↑	↑
Intake	↓ – < output	↓ – < output	↓ – < output
Urinaryoutput	↓	↓	↓ to oliguria
Urine specific gravity	Slightly changed	Increased	Markedly increased up to 1.03
Neurologic status	Normal	Irritable	Hyperirritable or lethargic

APPENDIX E: NORMAL RED BLOOD CELL VALUES

Age	*Hgb (gm/100 ml)*	*Hemato-crit (%)*	*Reticulo-cytes (%)*	*Mean Corpuscular Volume (μ^3)*	*Mean Corpuscular Hgb ($\mu\mu g$)*	*Mean Corpuscular Hgb Conc. (%)*
Newborn	16–24	47–60	4.1–6.3	106	38	36
3 mos	10–15	31–41	0.5–1.0	82	27	34
6 mos–6 yrs	11–14	33–42	0.5-1.0	82	27	34
7–12 yrs	11–16	34–40	0.5–1.0	82	27	34
Adolescent						
Female	14	37–47	0.5–1.8	80–94	27–32	33–38
Male	16	42–52	0.5–1.8	80–94	27–32	33–38

APPENDIX F: SAMPLE PEAK EXPIRATORY FLOW RATE NOMOGRAM

MEN
75
72
69
66
63
Ht. (ins.)
STANDARD DEVIATION MEN = 48 litres/min.
STANDARD DEVIATION WOMEN = 42 litres/min.
WOMEN
69
66
63
60
57
Ht. (ins.)
IN MEN, VALUES OF PEF UP TO 100 LITRES/MIN. LESS THAN PREDICTED, AND IN WOMEN LESS THAN 85 LITRES/MIN. LESS THAN PREDICTED, ARE WITHIN NORMAL LIMITS
PEF L/min.
660
650
640
630
620
610
600
590
580
570
560
550
540
530
520
510
500
490
480
470
460
450
440
430
420
410
400
390
380
15
20
25
30
35
40
45
50
55
60
65
70
Age in Years

Data from: Nunn, AJ, Gregg, I, *Brit. Med. J.* 1989; 298:1068-70

+95%
MEAN
−95%
Peak Flow Rate (l/min.)
700
650
600
550
500
450
400
350
300
250
200
150
100
100
110
120
130
140
150
160
170
180
190
Height (cm)

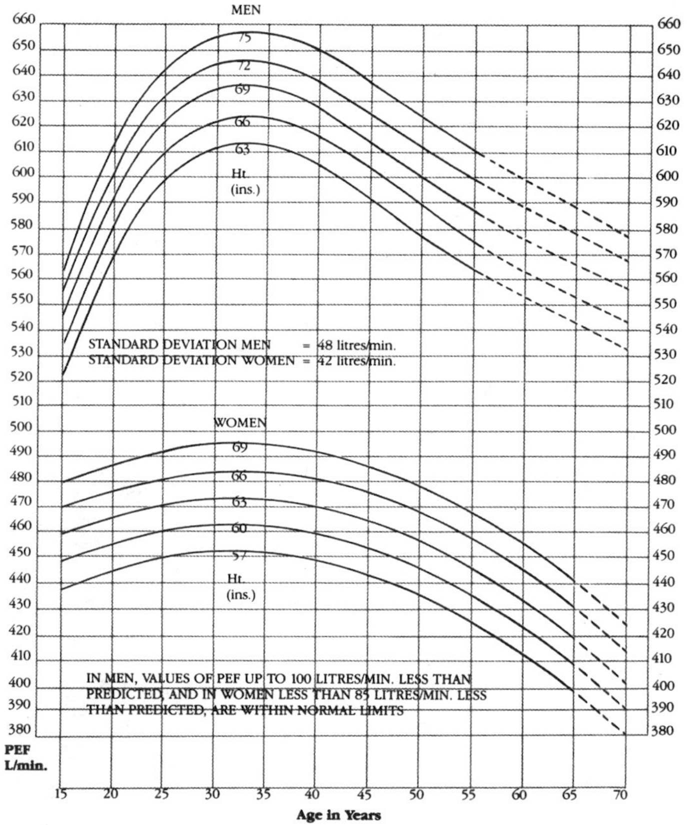

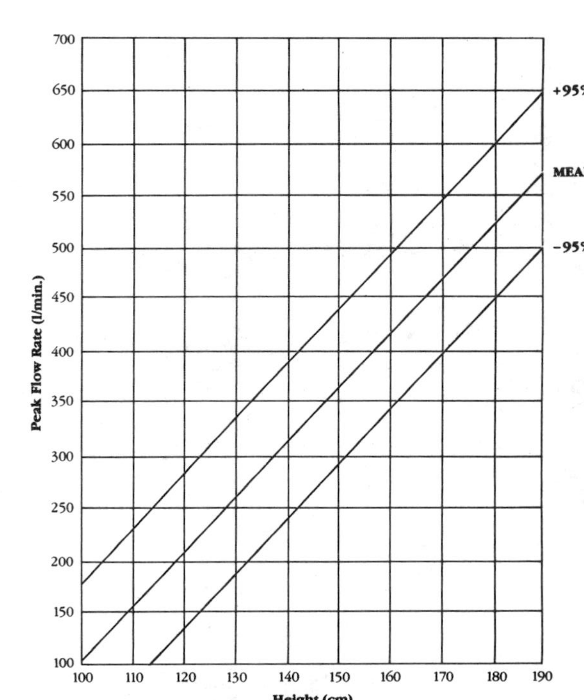

Data from: Godfrey S. et al., *Brit. J. Dis. Chest,* 1970; 64:15-24.

Table 1
Predicted Average Peak Expiratory Flow for Normal Males

(liters per minute)

Age	Height				
	60''	65''	70''	75''	80''
20	554	602	649	693	740
25	543	590	636	679	725
30	532	577	622	664	710
35	521	565	609	651	695
40	509	552	596	636	680
45	498	540	583	622	665
50	486	527	569	607	649
55	475	515	556	593	634
60	463	502	542	578	618
65	452	490	529	564	603
70	440	477	515	550	587

Data from: Leiner GC, et al.: Expiratory peak flow rate. Standard values for normal subjects. Use as a clinical test of ventilatory function. *Am Rev Resp Dis* 88:644, 1963.

Table 2
Predicted Average Peak Expiratory Flow for Normal Females

(liters per minute)

Age	Height				
	55''	60''	65''	70''	75''
20	390	423	460	496	529
25	385	418	454	490	523
30	380	413	448	483	516
35	375	408	442	476	509
40	370	402	436	470	502
45	365	397	430	464	495
50	360	391	424	457	488
55	355	386	418	451	482
60	350	380	412	445	475
65	345	375	406	439	468
70	340	369	400	432	461

Data from: Leiner GC, et al.: Expiratory peak flow rate. Standard values for normal subjects. Use as a clinical test of ventilatory function. *Am Rev Resp Dis* 88:644, 1963.

Table 3
Predicted Average Peak Expiratory Flow for Normal Children and Adolescents

(liters per minute)

Height (inches)	Males & Females	Height (inches)	Males & Females
43	147	56	320
44	160	57	334
45	173	58	347
46	187	59	360
47	200	60	373
48	214	61	387
49	227	62	400
50	240	63	413
51	254	64	427
52	267	65	440
53	280	66	454
54	293	67	467
55	307		

Data from: Polger, G, Promedhat V: *Pulmonary function testing in children: Techniques and standards.* Philadelphia, W.B. Saunders, 1971.

Note: These tables are averages and are based on tests with a large number of people. An individual's PEFR may vary widely. Further, many individuals' PEFR values are consistently higher or lower than the average values. It is recommended that PEFR objectives for therapy be based upon each individual's "personal best," which is established after a period of PEFR monitoring while the individual is under effective treatment.

Reproduced with permission from Guidelines and Management of Asthma—Publication # 91-3042, Objective measures of lung function, p. 23. Bethesda: U.S. Department of Health and Human Services, 1991.

APPENDIX G

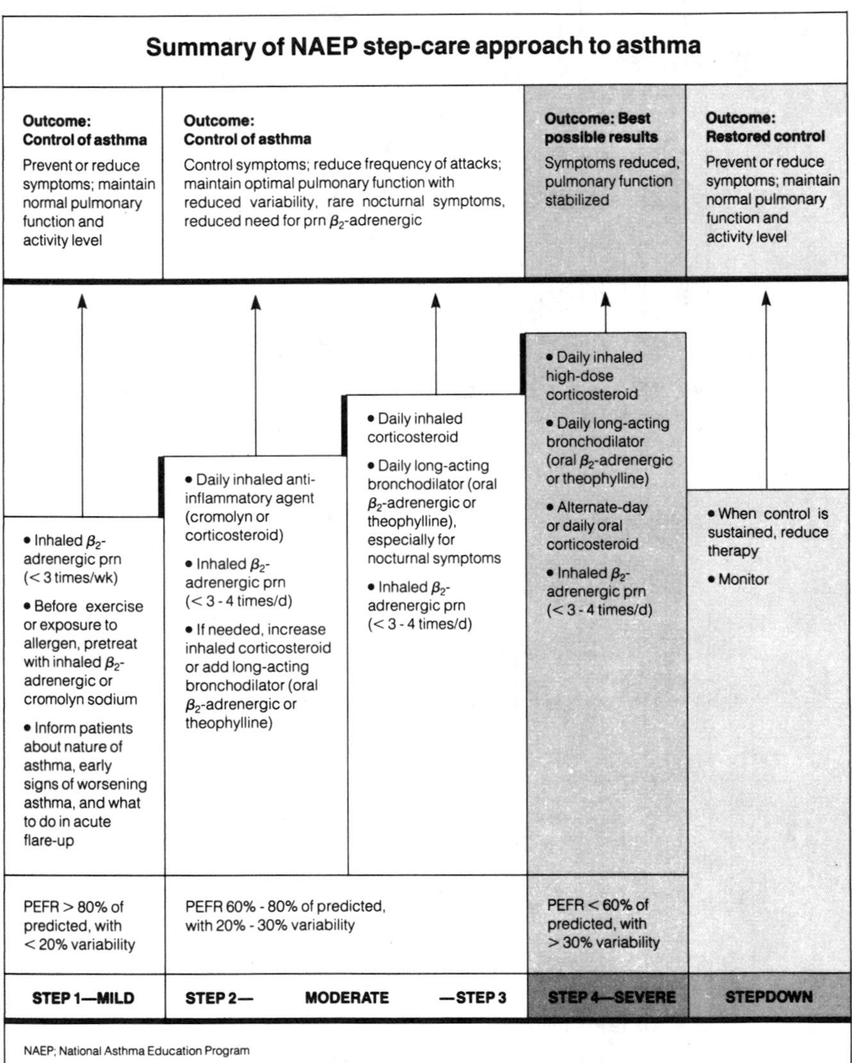

Reproduced with permission from Sheffer, A. L. (1992). Where β_2-adrenergics fit into step-care for asthma. *J Respir Dis* 13:10 (Suppl); S51.

APPENDIX H: ABSTRACT OF NEW HAMPSHIRE REPORTING LAW

I. Reporting is mandatory. New Hampshire Law (RSA 169-C-29:30) requires that any person who has reason to suspect that a child under the age of 18 has been abused or neglected must report the case to the Local District Office New Hampshire Division of Welfare.

II. An abused child is one who has

A. Been sexually molested.

or

B. Been sexually exploited.

or

C. Been intentionally physically injured.

or

D. Been psychologically injured such that he exhibits symptoms of emotional problems generally recognized to result from consistent mistreatment or neglect.

III. A neglected child is one

A. Who has been abandoned by his parents, guardian, or custodian.

or

B. Who is without proper parental care or control, subsistence, education as required by law, or other care or control necessary for his physical, mental, or emotional health, when it is established that his health has suffered or is very likely to suffer serious impairment; and the deprivation is not due primarily to the lack of financial means of the parents, guardian, or custodian.

or

C. Whose parents, guardian, or custodian is unable to discharge his responsibilities to and for the child because of incarceration, hospitalization, or other physical or mental incapacity.

NOTE: A child who is under treatment solely by spiritual means through prayer, in accordance with the tenets of a recognized religion by a duly accredited practitioner thereof, shall not for that reason alone be considered to be neglected.

IY. Nature and content of report

A. Oral. Immediately by telephone or otherwise.

B. Written. Within 48 hours if requested.

C. Content (if known):

1. Name and address of the child suspected of being neglected or abused.
2. Names of parents or person caring for child.
3. Specific information indicating neglect or nature of abuse (including any evidence of previous injuries).
4. Identity of parents or persons suspected in being responsible for neglect or abuse.
5. Any other information that might be helpful or is required by the bureau.

V. Immunity from liability. Anyone who makes a report in good faith is immune from any liability, civil or criminal. The same immunity applies to participation in any investigation by the bureau or judicial proceedings resulting from such a report.

APPENDIX I: YOUR CHILD AND ORGANIZED SPORTS

A. Be sure your child is ready for an organized sports program.
B. Weigh the time spent on sports against that for other important activities.
C. Consider what your child's participation will mean for your family's mealtime, vacation time, weekends.
D. Know how many hours and months your child will be involved in practices, games, tournaments.
E. Find out about the goals and qualifications of adults in the program.
F. Know the health and safety policies of the program.
G. Know that children are appropriately matched for maturity, size, and skill.
H. Know that each player on the team gets to play.
I. Plan on how you will behave when your child is a loser, a "bench warmer," or wants to quit.
J. Ask if parents are expected at practices or games.
K. Be ready for the expenses of uniforms, fees, transportation.
L. Observe how parents, coaches, spectators behave in front of children.

Source: From "Your Child and Organized Sports." © 1981 Ross Laboratories. Reprinted with permission of Ross Laboratories, Columbus, OH 43216.

APPENDIX J: ARE YOU DYING TO BE THIN?

The following questionnaire will give you an indication of whether or not you are living a lifestyle that indicates anorexic and/or bulimic tendencies. Anorexia nervosa (key symptom: extreme weight loss due to self-starvation) and bulimia (key symptom: binging followed by purging) are becoming more and more openly acknowledged as publicity increases public awareness and understanding.

Answer the following questions honestly. Write the number of your answer in the space at the left.

____ 1. I have eating habits that are different from those of my family and friends.
1. Often 2. Sometimes 3. Rarely 4. Never

____ 2. I find myself panicking if I cannot exercise as I planned for fear of gaining weight.
1. Almost always 2. Sometimes 3. Rarely 4. Never

____ 3. My friends tell me I am thin but I don't believe them because I feel fat.
1. Often 2. Sometimes 3. Rarely 4. Never

____ 4. (Females only) My menstrual period has ceased or become irregular due to no known medical reasons.
1. True 2. False

____ 5. I have become obsessed with food to the point that I cannot go through a day without worrying about what I will or will not eat.
1. Almost always 2. Sometimes 3. Rarely 4. Never

____ 6. I have lost more than 25% of the normal weight for my height (e.g., 30 lbs from 120 lbs).
1. True 2. False

____ 7. I would panic if I got on the scale tomorrow and found out I had gained two pounds.
1. Almost always 2. Sometimes 3. Rarely 4. Never

____ 8. I find that I prefer to eat alone or when I am sure no one will see me thus am making excuses so I can eat less and less with friends and family.
1. Often 2. Sometimes 3. Rarely 4. Never

____ 9. I find myself going on uncontrollable eating binges during which I consume large amounts of food to the point that I feel sick and make myself vomit.
1. 20 or more times/day 2. 1–2 times/week 3. Rarely 4. Never

____ 10. I use laxatives as a means of weight control.
1. On a regular basis 2. Sometimes 3. Rarely 4. Never

____ 11. I find myself playing games with food (e.g., cutting it up into tiny pieces; hiding food so people will think I ate it; chewing it and spitting it out without swallowing), telling myself certain foods are bad.
1. Often 2. Sometimes 3. Rarely 4. Never

____ 12. People around me have become very interested in what I eat and I find myself getting angry at them for pushing food on me.
1. Often 2. Sometimes 3. Rarely 4. Never

____ 13. I have felt more depressed and irritable recently than I used to and/or have been spending an increasing amount of time alone.
1. True 2. False

____ 14. I keep a lot of my fears about food and eating to myself because I am afraid no one would understand.

1. Often 2. Sometimes 3. Rarely 4. Never

____ 15. I enjoy making gourmet, high-calorie meals or treats for others as long as I don't have to eat any myself.

1. Often 2. Sometimes 3. Rarely 4. Never

____ 16. The most powerful fear in my life is the fear of gaining weight or becoming fat.

1. Often 2. Sometime 3. Rarely 4. Never

____ 17. I find myself totally absorbed when reading books about dieting, exercising and calorie counting to the point that I spend hours studying them.

1. Often 2. Sometimes 3. Rarely 4. Never

____ 18. I tend to be a perfectionist and am not satisfied with myself unless I do things perfectly.

1. Often 2. Sometimes 3. Rarely 4. Never

____ 19. I go through long periods of time without eating anything (fasting) as a means of weight control.

1. Often 2. Sometimes 3. Rarely 4. Never

____ 20. It is important to me to try to be thinner than all of my friends.

1. Often 2. Sometimes 3. Rarely 4. Never

Scoring

Add scores together and compare with the table below: Also, if #6 is True (1), subtract 8 points from total. Or if #6 is False (2), use total as it is.

Under 30—Strong tendencies toward anorexia nervosa

30–45—Strong tendencies toward bulimia

45–55—Weight conscious, not necessarily with anorexia and bulimic tendencies

Over 55—No need for concern

If you scored below 45, it would be wise for you to (1) seek more information about anorexia nervosa and bulimia and (2) contact a counselor, pastor, or physician, to determine what kind of assistance would be most helpful for you. Anorexia nervosa and bulimia are potentially life-threatening disorders which can be overcome with the proper support and counsel. The earlier you seek help the better, although it is never too late to start on the road to recovery.

For more information contact:

K. Kim Lampson Reiff, Ph.D.,
Sherwood Forest Office Park #104
2661 Bel-Red Road
Bellevue, WA 98008.

INDEX